Food is MEDICINE
Food is INFORMATION
Food is LIFE TO OUR BODIES

It's that simple
WE ARE WHAT WE EAT

come to the table

MEGAN B. KALKSTEIN

photography • design
TARA HOPE THOMPSON

Copyright © 2020
Megan B. Kalkstein
www.megankalkstein.com
Baltimore, Maryland

All rights reserved. No part of this book may be reproduced or transmitted in any form or by any means, electronic or mechanical, including photocopying, recording, or any information storage and retrieval system, without permission in writing from the author.

ISBN: 978-0-578-78239-3

Cover Art • Photography • Design
Tara Hope Thompson
www.tarahopephotography.com

Printed in the United States of America
Ironmark- Pre-Press & Printing
www.Ironmarkusa.com

dedication

To Keller, Ryder, Major, Walker, Charlotte, and those yet to come...

May the bounty that will succeed, grace your family's tables, to nourish and enlighten for many generations to come.
~MaeMae

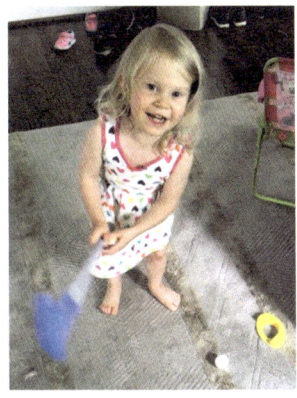 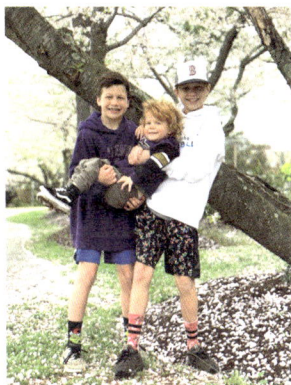 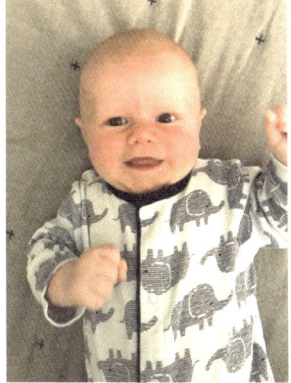

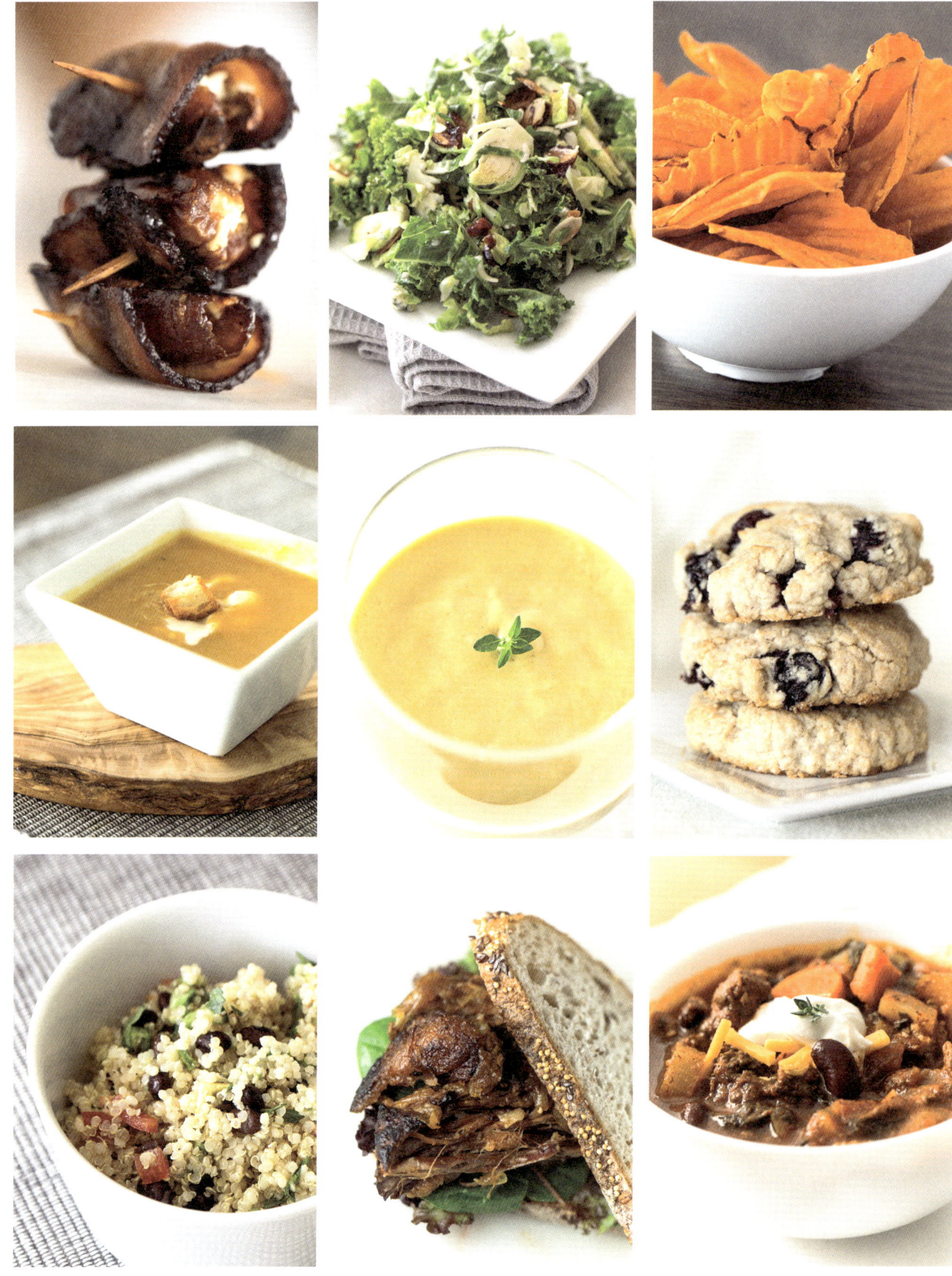

contents

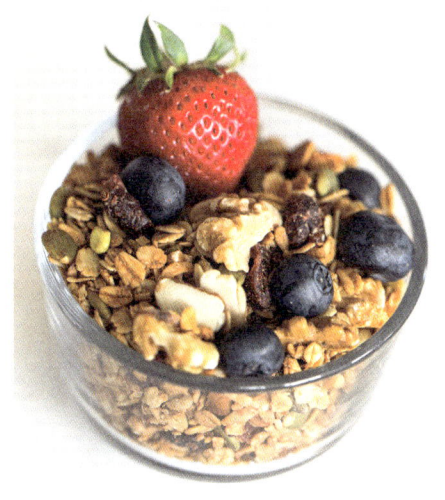

introduction 9
my pantry 14

CHAPTER 1 breakfast & smoothies 16

CHAPTER 2 appetizers 34

CHAPTER 3 soups 56

CHAPTER 4 salads & dressings 84

CHAPTER 5 main courses 112

CHAPTER 6 sides 164

CHAPTER 7 muffins & biscuits 192

CHAPTER 8 desserts 206

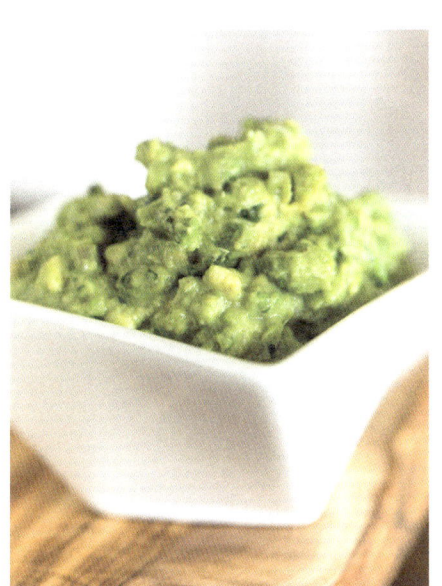

giving thanks 238
children's letters 240
index 244

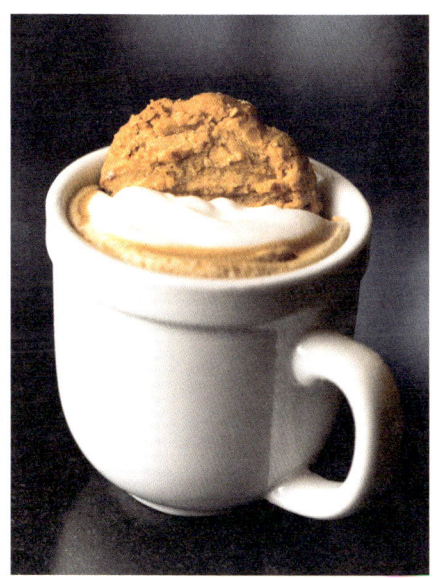

GF = Gluten-Free
DF = Dairy-Free
V = Vegan
LS = Low Sugar

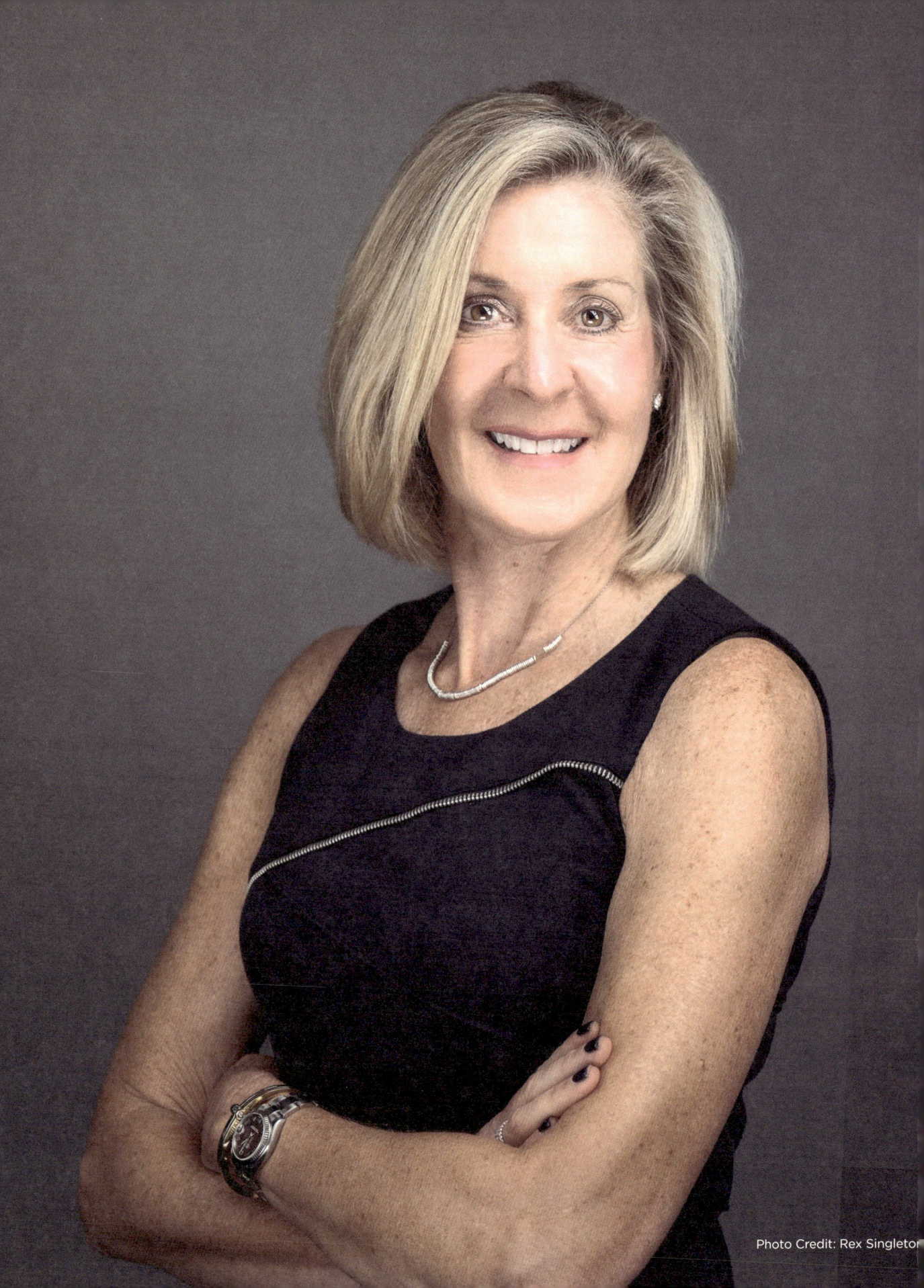

Photo Credit: Rex Singleton

introduction

Growing up in a big family set the stage for eating a whole-foods, nutritious diet throughout my life. My grandfather was a livestock farmer and weekly trips to his farm brought home fresh chicken and eggs, along with a side of beef by the whole or half cow. Two large freezers in our basement were always packed with farm-fresh, grass-fed meat, that had recently been processed, dressed and packaged. We were the Blakeslee family and ours was just one of many homes in a beautiful neighborhood filled with children.

My Mom and Dad loved to eat well. We always sat down for dinner as a family, Sunday through Thursday at 6:00 o'clock. And there were 12 of us - four brothers and six sisters, so organization was key. Mom always had all of the food bases covered, which included a healthy protein, a salad, a vegetable, bread and a starch. We operated like clockwork and on a rotation, so everyone had a job and knew his or hers without question: set, clear, load or wash, then rotate. When I tell people that my mother could have run a big business really well, she did - that was our family. These dinners set the foundation for enjoying the ritual and pleasure of a meal. Cooking is a passion and a treasured hobby for most of my siblings. And even to this day, whether at home or traveling, reconnecting always includes planning the dinner meal.

The table where you eat is truly the core of family time. It's where you connect and nourish your mind and body. It's where you laugh and enlighten. The kitchen or dining table is the one place in a home where you can have the most significant impact on the relationships and the health of those you love the most. It's where you share stories, influence behavior and feed your offspring. Over the years, while raising my four children, I saw this tradition in other families erode to busy lives filled with over-scheduled children and parents who lost interest in cooking. Fast or fastcasual food became the norm for family dinner. Thanks to the foundation my parents laid, I carried on the tradition and love for cooking, feeding and providing nutrition for my family. With four active children, three of whom continued their athletic pursuits in college, they needed big, nourishing meals to fuel their bodies and brains. Dinner was always organized and prepared long before the last hungry one came through the door.

The years to influence our children's lives go quickly, but teaching them about health and wellness through food choices sets a foundation for lifetimes of good health. I am grateful my children continue the tradition of quality dining, cooking with their families and appreciate the importance of a healthy lifestyle.

It is no surprise I was interested in becoming a nutritionist at an early age. I was always observing the power of healthy foods and the effects of eating the unhealthy foods. When a doctor said foods don't make your skin break out, I disagreed and eliminated the ones I knew to cause problems. When I developed headaches in my early teens, I eliminated meats with nitrates from my diet and the headaches related to those toxins ceased. I always had an innate awareness of the power of food and how important what we chose to eat really is.

It wasn't until many years later, that I finally set out to learn the science behind what I believed to be true. When I was 50, I completed my masters in nutrition, but my love for learning has never stopped and my education is ongoing. I see clients on a regular basis and their diet-related issues run the gamut - weight, inflammation, depression, autoimmune diseases, familial cholesterol, etc. A lot of these issues potentially stem from lifestyle, dietary habits, and choices. *Food is medicine, food is information, food is life to our bodies.* It can be that simple: *We are what we eat.*

In addition to the scientific research I am immersed in as a nutritionist, I am always improving my skills in the kitchen. Cooking is a joy and eating is a greater joy, but sharing a meal is the greatest joy of all. Becoming a good cook is a lifetime journey. Times change. Where once I used low-fat products, I now only use full-fat ones. And now my kitchen is almost completely organic, because of increasing access to healthy foods. I have improved techniques by learning from other cooks, chefs and educators. My grains are from artisanal sources, my meat is pasture-raised and my fish is wild-caught. There is a food revolution occurring and access to healthy food is becoming more readily available to a larger percentage of the population. There is no longer an excuse to ignore the impact of food on the health of our community. I focus on anti-inflammatory foods. I take traditional dishes and add extra vegetables to make them more nutritious. I also use organic products in 90 percent of the ingredients.

This collection of recipes does not follow any particular diet that is currently trending. It follows my whole-foods principles, where the quality of ingredients trump everything else. It does not address people who cannot eat dairy or gluten, are diabetic, eat a very low-carb diet, have nut allergies, sugar addiction and so on. If a specific recipe is gluten-free, dairy-free, vegan, or low in sugar, it is labeled as such. These are nutrient-rich recipes that have fed my family for 35 years. They have entertained countless friends and large family gatherings.

My family, friends and clients have asked for this book for a long time and I am thrilled to have finally pulled this collection of recipes together. Now is the time to cook healthy meals with quality ingredients and entice families to get into their kitchens and cook together, to come to the table.

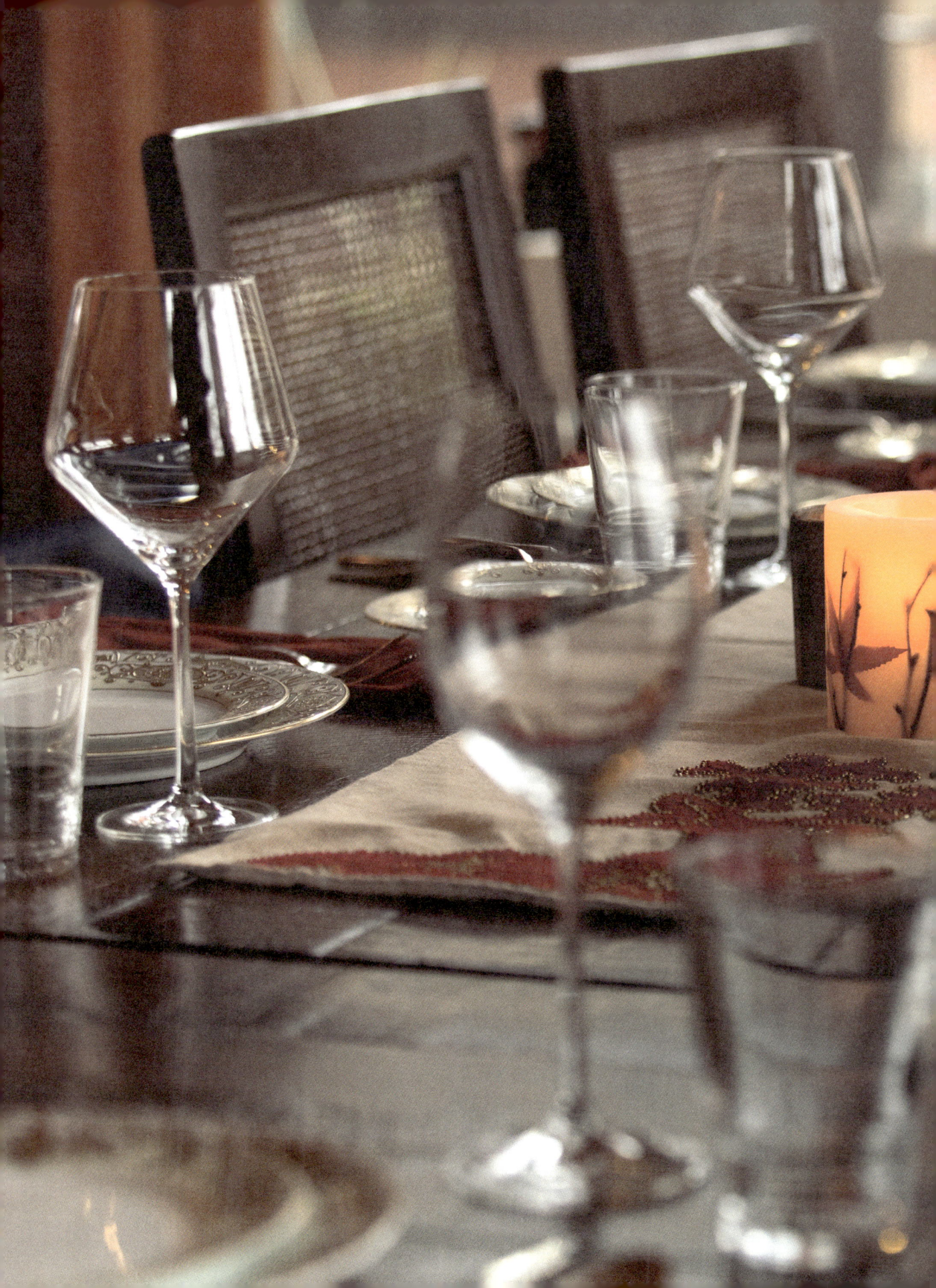

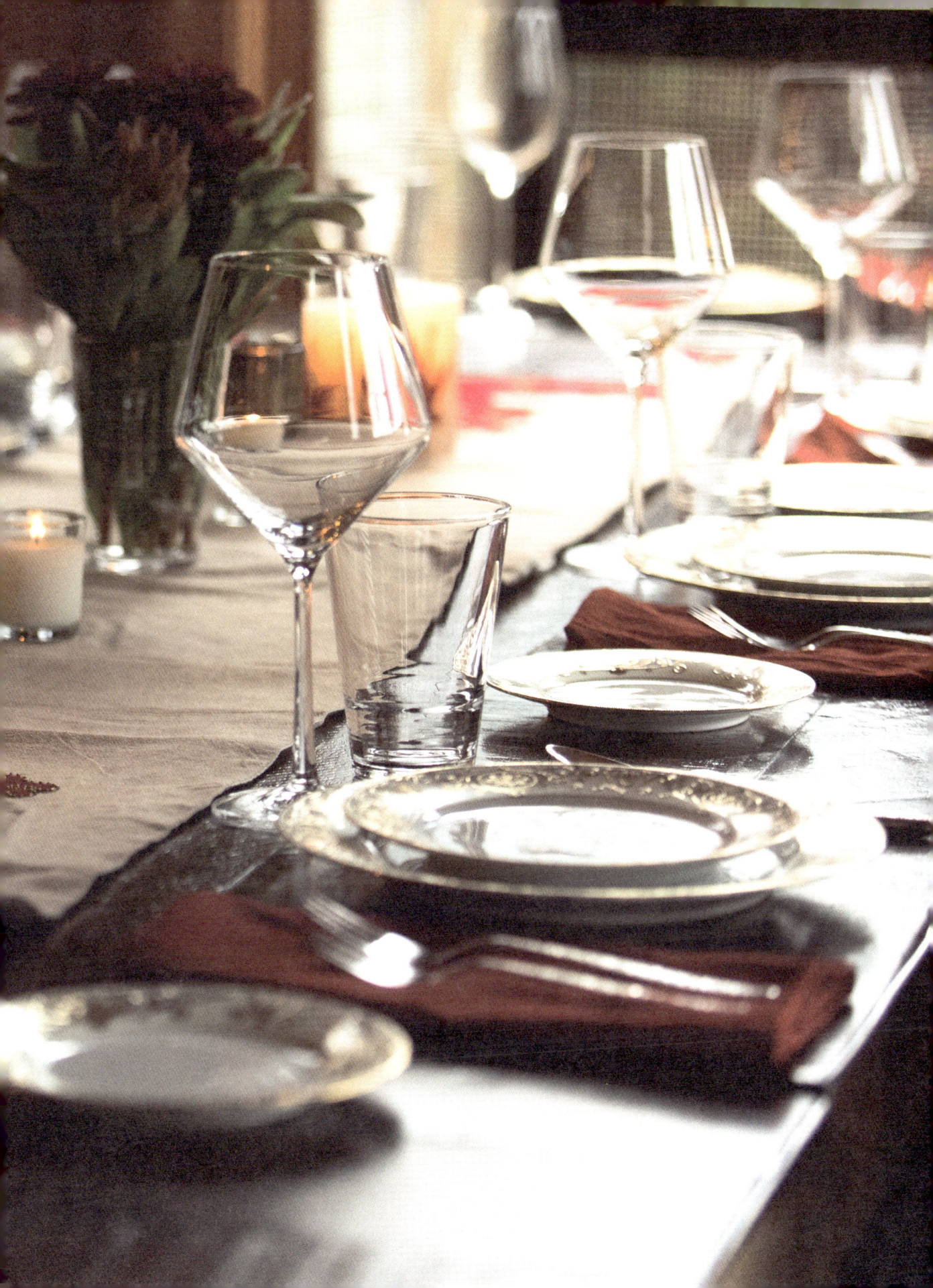

the big pantry shop

- ☐ organic extra virgin olive oil *(several varieties)*
- ☐ organic coconut oil
- ☐ organic avocado oil
- ☐ spray for cooking and baking: olive oil • coconut oil
- ☐ vinegars: balsamic • champagne • cider • red wine
- ☐ a large variety of organic dried spices
- ☐ sea salt • fine salt
- ☐ whole peppercorn black pepper
- ☐ chicken stock: low sodium • regular *(organic varieties sold in boxes)*
- ☐ vegetable stock
- ☐ beef stock
- ☐ organic canned beans: black • kidney • northern • garbanzo
- ☐ low sodium organic non-GMO soy sauce
- ☐ organic mayonnaise *(I prefer avocado mayonnaise)*
- ☐ tomato paste
- ☐ diced tomatoes
- ☐ tomato sauce *(organic preferred)*
- ☐ canned tomatoes: San Marzano is my #1 choice
- ☐ sustainable canned tuna in water, lightly salted
- ☐ almonds • walnuts • cashews • pecans
- ☐ pistachios: whole • shelled
- ☐ pumpkin seeds
- ☐ sesame seeds
- ☐ flax seeds: whole • ground
- ☐ hemp seeds
- ☐ Matcha tea powder
- ☐ cocoa powder
- ☐ lentils
- ☐ raisins and other dried fruits *(blueberries, cranberries, and cherries)*
- ☐ organic rice: wild rice • basmati • brown rice • jasmine

- ☐ organic pasta *(several sizes and shapes including orzo)*
- ☐ good quality bread crumbs, gluten-free if preferred
- ☐ organic, gluten-free oatmeal
- ☐ organic blue corn chips, lightly salted
- ☐ whole-grain crackers
- ☐ gluten-free crackers
- ☐ flour: whole wheat • unbleached white *(organic preferred)*
- ☐ almond flour
- ☐ cornmeal
- ☐ organic non-GMO cane sugar: brown • fine white
- ☐ coconut sugar
- ☐ non-sweetened organic coconut flakes
- ☐ garlic
- ☐ onions
- ☐ shallots
- ☐ potatoes: sweet and regular
- ☐ organic whole milk
- ☐ almond milk
- ☐ coconut milk
- ☐ organic cream
- ☐ coconut water
- ☐ organic butter: salted • unsalted
- ☐ frozen organic spinach, corn, peas, and shelled edamame
- ☐ frozen organic blueberries and raspberries

CHAPTER 1

breakfast & smoothies

sesame-nut bars   19

Christmas pecan sour cream coffee cake   20

asparagus frittata   23

homemade granola   24

oatmeal muffins   26

all-day energy smoothie   29

morning power smoothie   29

blueberry kale smoothie   30

berry chocolate protein powerhouse smoothie   30

BREAKFAST HAS BECOME SOMEWHAT CONTROVERSIAL in my business, with many nutritionists talking about intermittent fasting and delaying your first meal until the lunch hour. That's all fine if it works for you, but I still like breakfast to start my day. I need some healthy protein before I go workout and I have never been one to exercise or drink my morning coffee without something in my stomach. I also never eat or snack after dinner, so I tend to wake up hungry!

These are a few of my go-to breakfast recipes and I can always find the ingredients for them in my refrigerator, freezer or pantry.

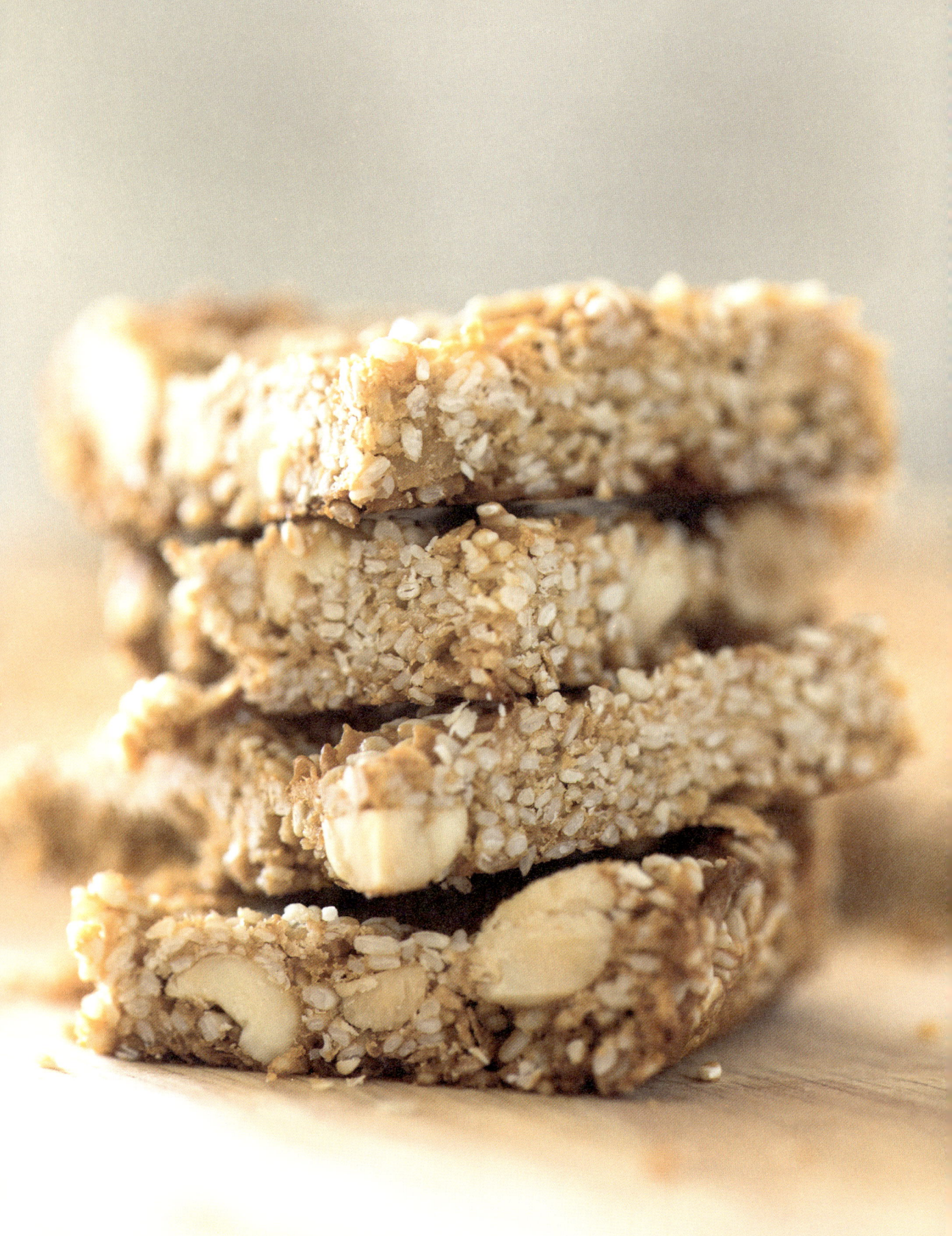

sesame-nut bars

16 bars

THESE BARS ARE A GREAT ALTERNATIVE for a hurried breakfast or a quick bite before rushing to the gym. They are packed with protein, not too sweet, and taste great with your morning beverage. Keep them in an airtight container for up to 6 weeks in your pantry.

1¼ cups white and/or black sesame seeds

¾ cup unsweetened shredded coconut

¼ cup peanuts (*or cashews*)

¼ tsp. salt

¼ cup honey

2 Tbsp. creamy peanut butter

¼ tsp. vanilla

MBK'S TIPS

Be certain to purchase organic creamy peanut butter with no added sugar. Make sure your sesame seeds are fresh, as they go rancid very quickly.

1. Preheat oven to 350°.

2. Spray an 8x8 glass baking dish with cooking oil. Line with parchment paper, leaving a generous overhang on all sides.

3. Mix the first 4 ingredients together in a medium-size mixing bowl.

4. Mix honey, peanut butter, and vanilla together in a small bowl, then add to dry ingredients and mix well.

5. Spread mixture evenly into prepared pan, pressing firmly into an even layer. Bake for 20-25 minutes until golden around the edges.

6. Transfer to a wire rack and let cool until firm, 30-40 minutes. Lift out of baking dish and cut into 16 bars. Store tightly wrapped at room temperature.

Enjoy!

NUTRITION EXTRAS

Low in sugar and high in plant protein.

GF
DF
V
LS

christmas pecan sour cream coffee cake

THIS CAKE HARDLY QUALIFIES AS BREAKFAST. But on Christmas morning, it is our traditional coffee cake that we indulge in, while opening our gifts. Kind of the breakfast before the real breakfast. I make this only on Christmas and the family looks forward to the treat every year. I can't imagine not nibbling on this delight, while playing Santa and passing out the gifts.

CAKE

- 2 cups all-purpose flour
- 1¼ teaspoon baking soda
- ½ teaspoon cinnamon
- ½ teaspoon ground nutmeg
- ½ teaspoon salt
- ½ cup unsalted room temperature butter
- 1⅓ cup packed golden brown sugar
- 1 teaspoon vanilla
- 2 large eggs
- 1 cup sour cream

MBK'S TIPS

It can be made the day before and warmed in the oven the next day on a low temperature of 300° for 15 minutes.

Cover with foil before putting in oven.

1. Preheat oven to 350° and position rack in center of oven.
2. Butter or spray a 9x13x2 inch or 12-inch round baking pan.
3. Combine flour, baking soda, cinnamon, nutmeg, and salt. Set aside.
4. Beat butter, sugar, and vanilla in large bowl until well blended, approximately 2 minutes.
5. Add eggs one at a time, mixing after each. Slowly add flour and mix just until incorporated.
6. Fold in sour cream, carefully, as not to overmix.
7. Spoon half the mixture into the bottom of the prepared pan. Top with half of the pecan mixture. Add the second half of cake batter and top with remaining pecan mix.
8. Bake until topping is brown and tester inserted into the center of cake comes out clean, 45-55 minutes. Cool before serving.

Enjoy!

PECAN MIX TOPPING

⅔ cup packed dark brown sugar

⅔ cup all purpose flour

¾ teaspoon cinnamon

8 tablespoons unsalted butter, melted and cooled

⅔ cup chopped pecans, toasted

1. Combine sugar, flour, and cinnamon with melted butter.
2. Mix with fork until well blended.
3. Add pecans and set aside.

Photo Credit: MBK

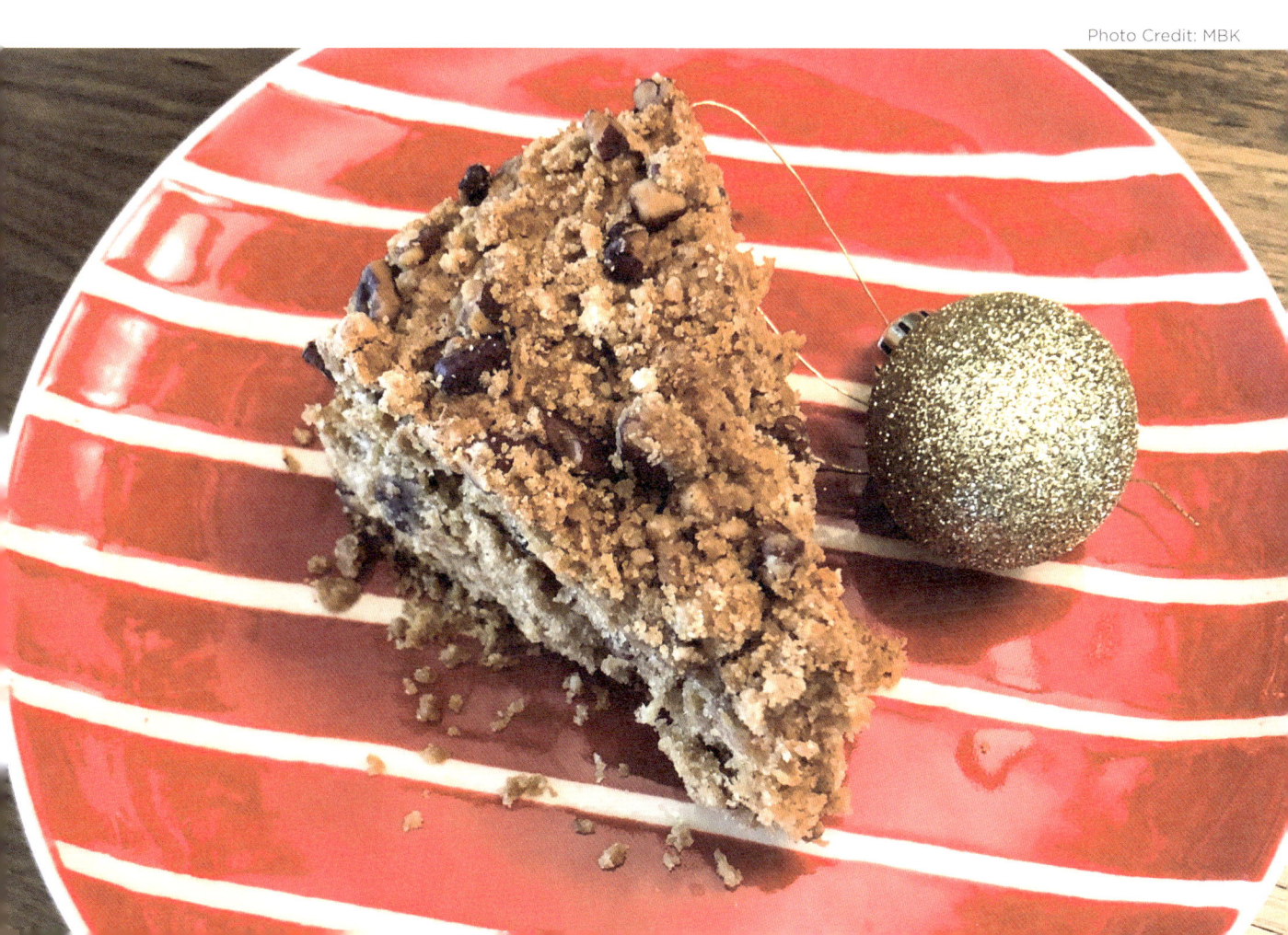

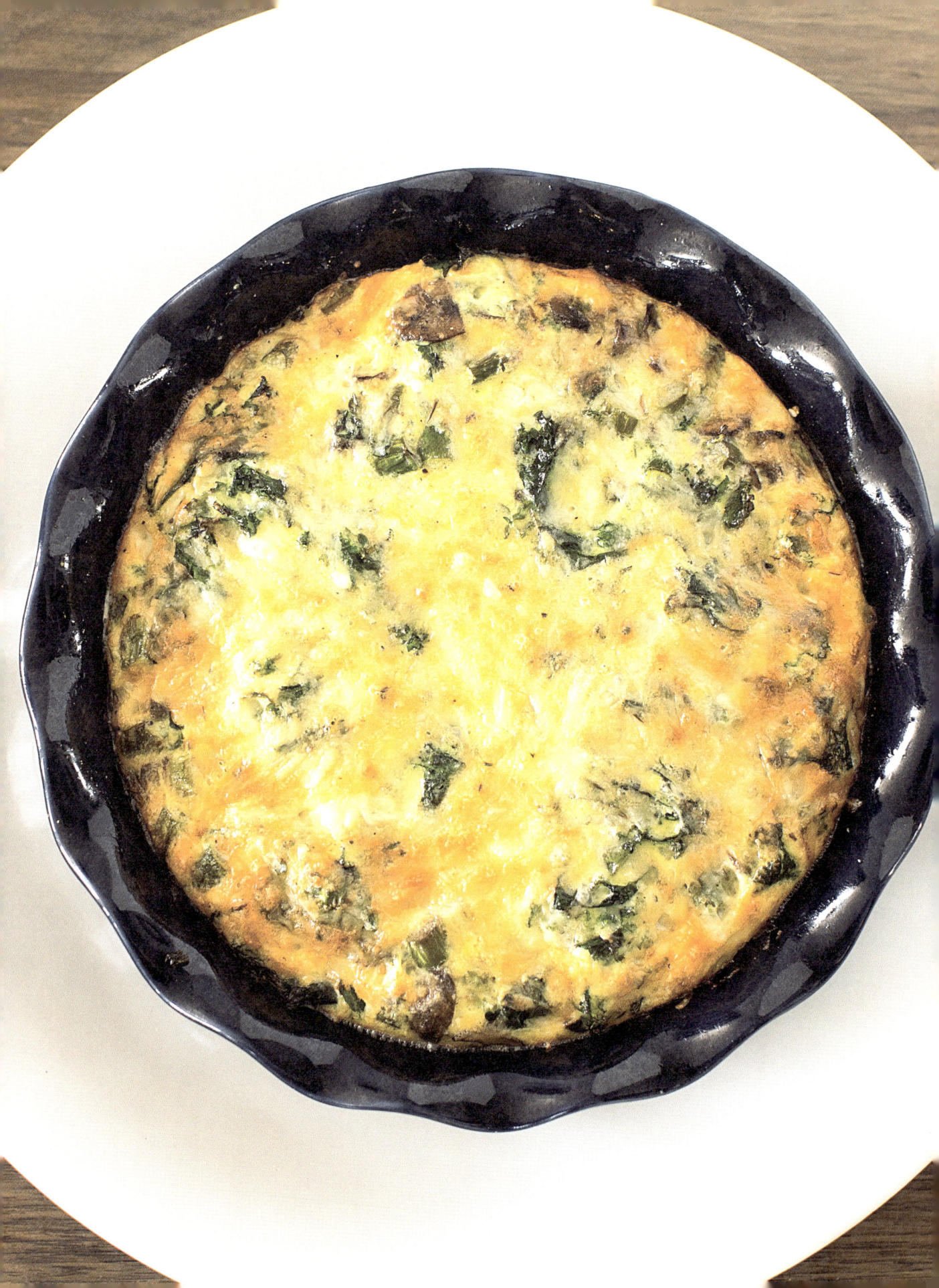

asparagus frittata

Makes 6 servings

I MAKE A FRITTATA ALMOST WEEKLY and my recipe changes weekly. The basics are outlined below, but you can add any number of vegetables and proteins of your choice. I typically get sausage from my summer farmers market and tend to use ground pork or turkey, instead of bacon, during that season. Vegetable choices vary on what sounds good and are fresh at the time. Peppers, onions, mushrooms, asparagus, spinach, kale, or broccoli. Any combination of these is always delicious with eggs.

4 pieces nitrate-free bacon

olive oil for sautéing vegetables

⅔ pound asparagus, cleaned, trimmed, and diced

1 cup baby bella mushrooms, sliced

2 cups spinach or kale, cleaned, trimmed, and chopped

7 eggs

1 cup whole milk

¼ cup cream

salt and pepper to taste

¾ cup shredded gruyere cheese

2 tablespoons fresh herbs, thyme or chives *(optional)*

1. Preheat oven to 375°.
2. Spray deep dish quiche pan with olive oil and set aside.
3. Cook the bacon, chop and set aside.
4. Heat 1 tablespoon olive oil in a non-stick pan and saute vegetables on medium heat until tender and starting to brown, approximately 6 minutes.
5. In a separate bowl beat eggs, milk, cream, and seasoning until well blended.
6. Lay an even layer of chopped bacon in the bottom of the dish. Spread cooked vegetables on top of the bacon. Pour the egg mixture to cover completely. Top with grated cheese and fresh herbs.
7. Cook for 25- 30 minutes or until middle is firm. Do not over bake.

Enjoy!

MBK'S TIPS

I always have two clean deep dish quiche pans available, in case I am feeding a crowd and need to double the recipe.

NUTRITION EXTRAS

Eggs are my number one choice of protein for breakfast, with each egg containing 7 grams.

The egg is a powerhouse of disease-fighting nutrients, including lutein, zeaxanthin, and cartenoids, which are known to protect the eyes. They are also loaded with choline, a brain nutrient that about 90% of people aren't getting enough of.

GF
LS

homemade granola

I RARELY EAT GRANOLA AS A STAND ALONE for breakfast. I might snack on some with my coffee if I'm not particularly hungry, but never do I sit down to a large bowl of granola covered in milk. It's generally an added topping that I keep in the pantry to top a serving of cottage cheese or yogurt. I always keep a fresh batch for times when I'm looking for a little something sweet or an in-between meal snack. It's easy to make and stays fresh for long periods of time when sealed in an airtight container.

MBK'S TIPS

Be sure to rotate pan to ensure even cooking. Watch carefully as it cooks quickly at the end of the estimated time.

The granola will become crunchy once it has cooled.

1 large egg white, beaten

3 cups old-fashioned rolled oats

1½ cups raw unsalted nuts, chopped *(almonds, pistachios, pecans or walnuts)*

1½ cups unsweetened coconut flakes

½ cup raw seeds *(sesame, pumpkin or flax)*

½ cup agave or maple syrup

¼ cup coconut oil, warmed to liquid

2 tablespoons coconut sugar

¾ teaspoon salt

1 teaspoon cinnamon

1 cup of dried fruit *(raisins, blueberries or cranberries)*

NUTRITION EXTRAS

High in fiber and a moderate amount of plant-based protein.

GF

1. Preheat oven to 300°.

2. In a large bowl, toss all ingredients, except fruit, until well combined.

3. Spread granola evenly on a rimmed baking sheet and bake for 40-50 minutes, stirring every 10 minutes, until granola is golden brown.

4. Remove from oven and let cool completely before adding fruit.

Enjoy!

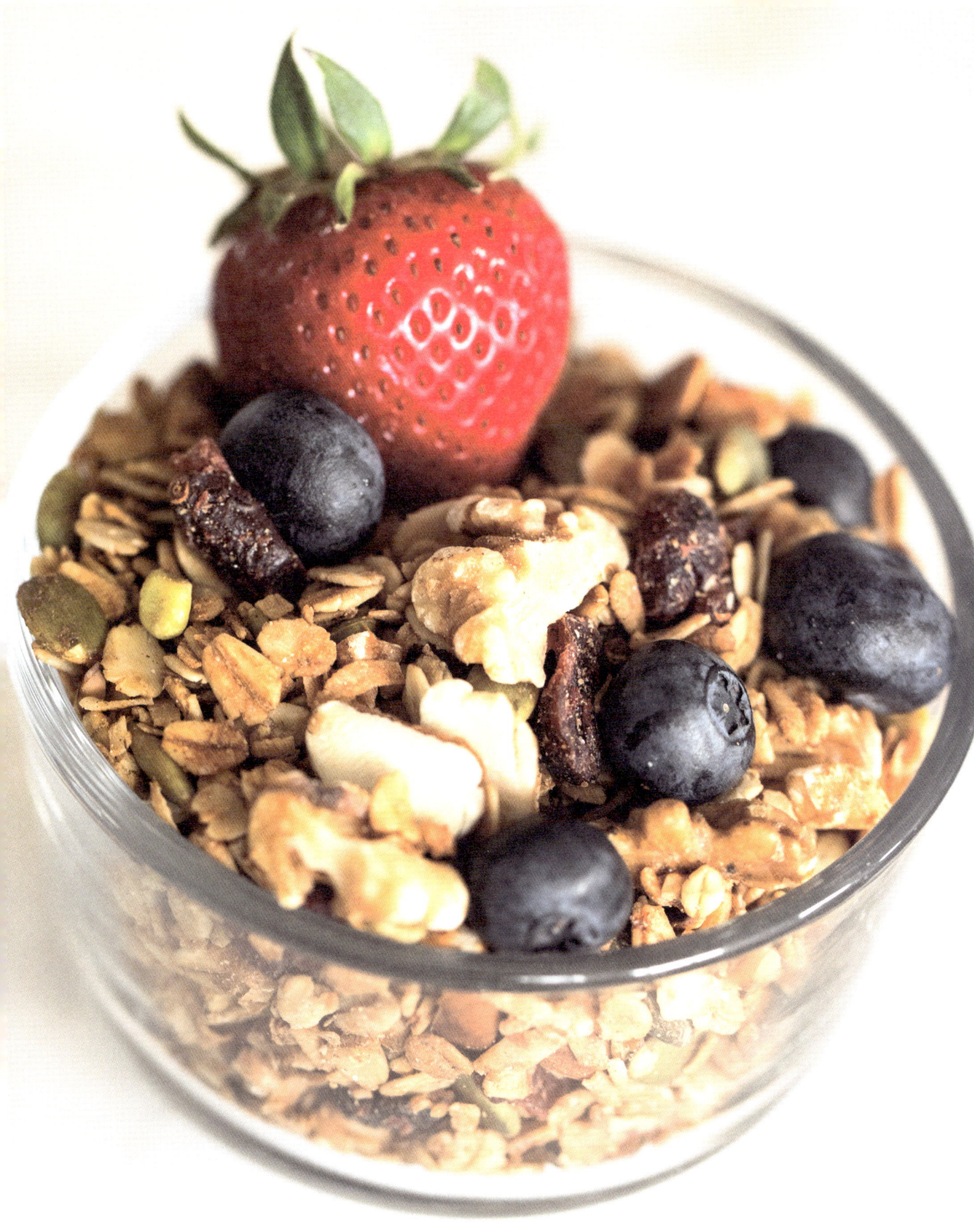

oatmeal muffins

12-15 muffins

I HAVE BEEN MAKING THESE MUFFINS FOR YEARS, for countless guests at our lake house, and they are always a hit. Many have requested the recipe and now also make these muffins as part of their morning repertoire. The recipe calls for multiple grains, but once you purchase the ingredients, it's easy to assemble. You may find that you will want to keep these in your freezer at all times for a quick and easy breakfast.

MBK'S TIPS

If you are not using your flours for long periods of time, store in the freezer, to maintain freshness. Just pull out an hour before intended use.

- 2⅓ cups old-fashioned oats
- 1 cup whole wheat flour
- 1 cup nuts, chopped *(pecans or walnuts preferred)*
- 1 cup coconut sugar
- 2 tablespoons oat bran
- 2 tablespoons wheat bran
- 2 teaspoons cinnamon
- 1½ teaspoons baking soda
- ¾ teaspoon salt

- 1 cup buttermilk
- ½ cup coconut oil, warmed to liquid
- 1 large egg
- 1 teaspoon vanilla extract
- ⅓ cup boiling water
- 1 cup of dried fruit *(blueberries or cherries preferred)*

NUTRITION EXTRAS

These are packed with plant-based protein and healthy fats and can stand alone for a quick and delicious breakfast.

1. Preheat oven to 375°.
2. Line a 12-cup muffin pan with paper muffin cups.
3. Whisk oats and next 8 ingredients in a large mixing bowl.
4. Add buttermilk, coconut oil, egg, and vanilla and whisk to blend.
5. Stir in boiling water and let stand for 5 minutes.
6. Fold in fruit and divide batter among prepared muffin cups.
7. Bake until a tester comes out clean, approximately 18-20 minutes for standard muffins. Let cool before eating.

Enjoy!

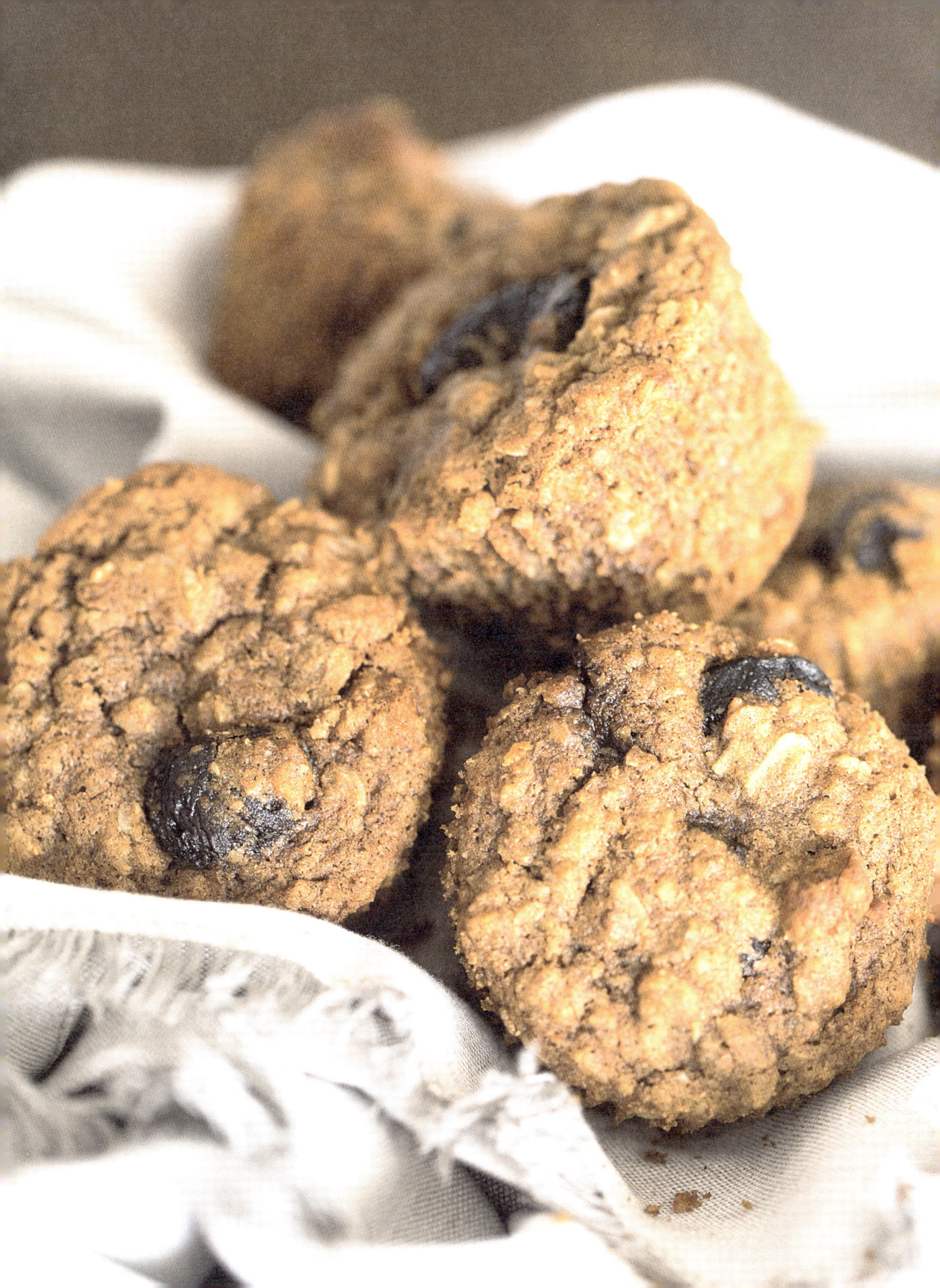

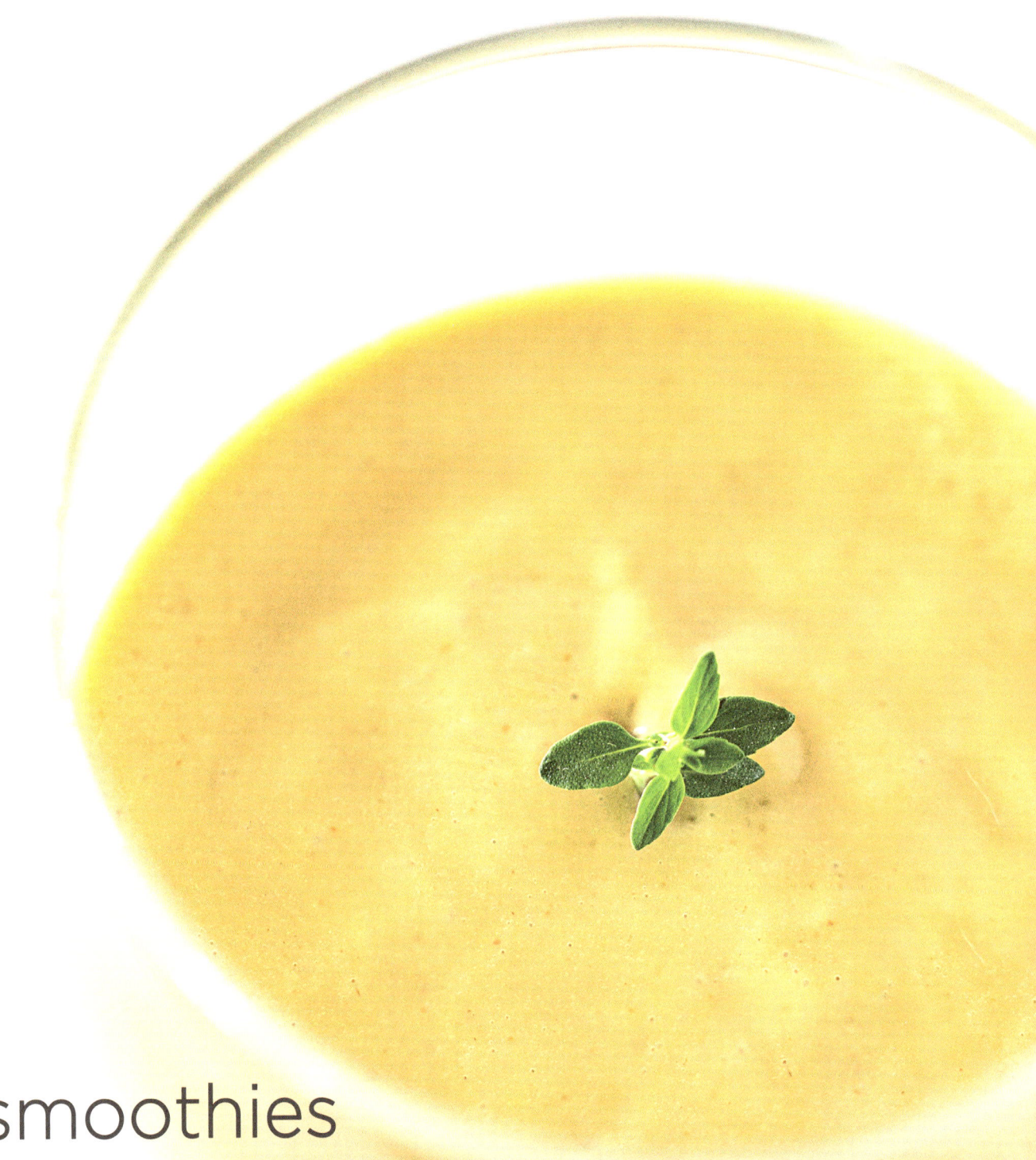

smoothies

SOMETIMES A SMOOTHIE JUST SOUNDS GOOD AND REFRESHING for breakfast. Not in the mood for eggs and need a lift before a workout? A quick smoothie for the drive to the gym can be just what you need. These are not too sweet and have lots of protein to get you through a busy AM. You can always add more liquid if it gets too thick, but add slowly in 1/4 cup increments. Smoothies can quickly go from thick to watery and lose their taste if measurements are off.

all-day energy

1 teaspoon Matcha green tea powder

¼ ripe avocado

1 frozen banana

1½ cup almond or cashew hemp milk

1 Medjool date, pitted

½ teaspoon vanilla

1. Wash and prep all ingredients.
2. Blend until smooth.

Enjoy!

MBK'S TIPS

A vitamix is a wonderful addition to any kitchen, but it is quite costly. A simple mixer or non-commercial bullet works just fine.

moring power

1 cup coconut water

1 scoop pea protein powder

1 tablespoon flax or chia seed

½ cup frozen spinach

½ cup frozen mixed berries (*blueberry, strawberry, raspberry*)

1 small or ½ large frozen banana

1. Mix all the ingredients in a blender until smooth.

Enjoy!

NUTRITION EXTRAS

High in protein and loaded with phytochemicals, providing multiple vitamins.

These smoothies cover multiple micro-nutrients in one serving, including vitamins A and C.

GF
DF
V

blueberry kale

MBK'S TIPS

A vitamix is a wonderful addition to any kitchen, but it is quite costly. A simple mixer or non-commercial bullet works just fine.

1 cup almond milk or coconut water

¾ cup frozen blueberries

1 banana *(can be frozen)*

1 tablespoon ground flax seeds

1 tablespoon of preferred protein powder

2 cups loosely packed kale or other dark leafy greens

1. Blend all ingredients until desired consistency.
2. Add water or ice if smoothie is too thick.

Enjoy!

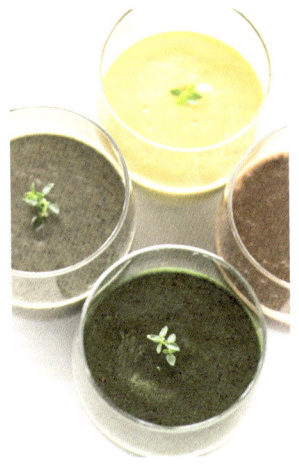

berry chocolate protein powerhouse

NUTRITION EXTRAS

High in protein and loaded with phytochemicals, providing multiple vitamins.

These smoothies cover multiple micro-nutrients in one serving, including vitamins A and C.

GF
DF
V

1 large frozen banana

1 cup frozen blueberries

1 cup almond milk or coconut water

2 tablespoons hemp seeds

1 scoop pea protein powder

2 tablespoons cocoa powder

1 cup kale, leaves only, tightly packed

1. Wash and prep all ingredients.
2. Blend and serve.

Enjoy!

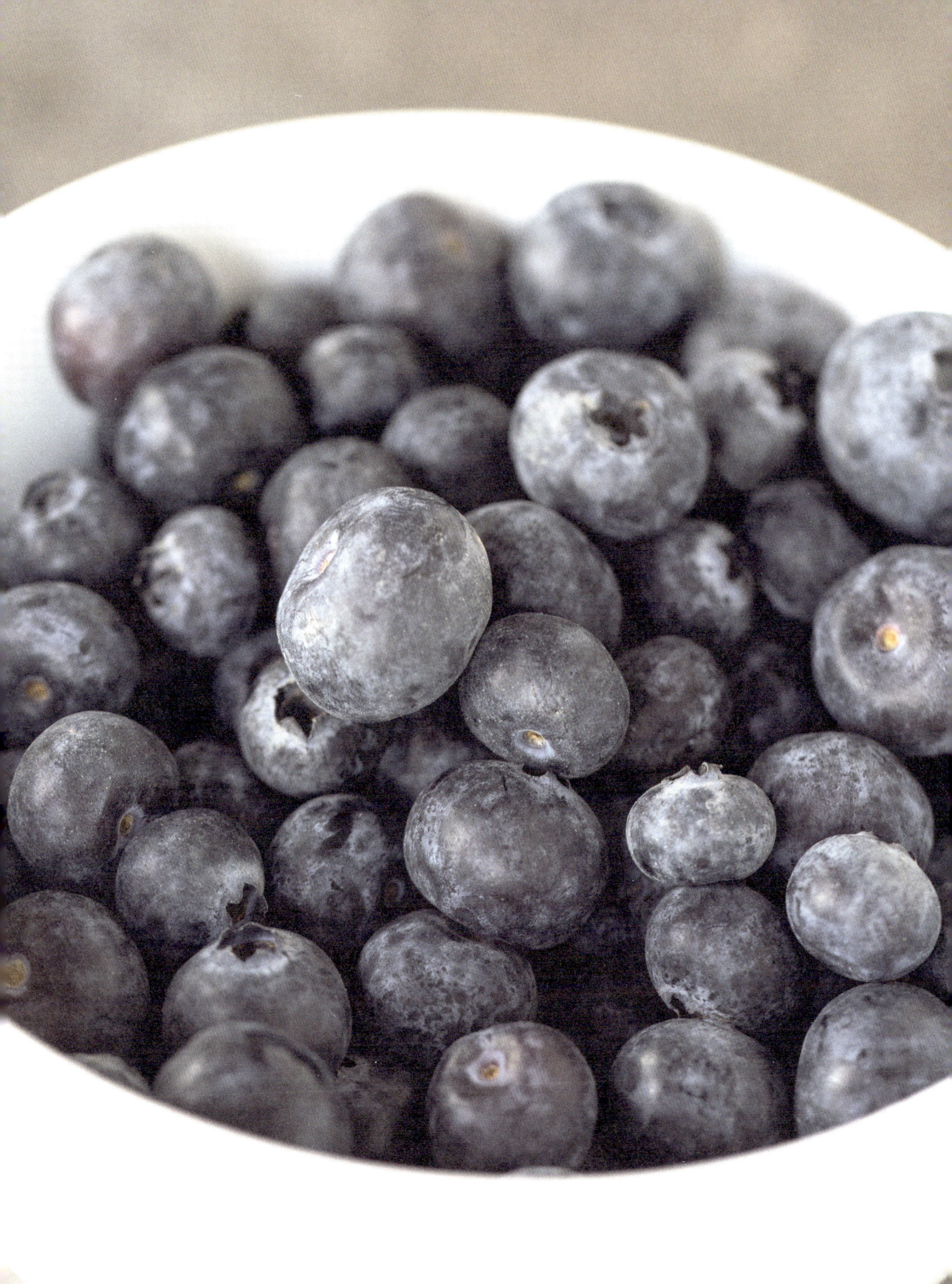

herbs & spices

Turmeric, oregano, basil, garlic, ginger..... and more!

Herbs and spices make foods tastier, while boosting your health. They have long been touted for their medicinal qualities. They are rich in phytochemicals, which are healthful plant chemicals, that fight inflammation and reduce damage to the body's cells. Because they are so flavorful, they make it easy to cut back on the use of too much salt, sugar and fat. The use of fresh herbs for flavor helps in maintaining a nutritious diet.

Your pantry should be full of organic dried spices to experiment with and have available for a variety of recipes. Your garden or weekly trip to the farmers market should bring home an array of fresh organic herbs to flavor and enhance your cooking. Dried spices and fresh herbs both season your recipes and change the flavor with very different methods. I tend to use spices when slow cooking a dish and fresh-cut herbs for finishing a plate. Fresh herbs are a game-changer when it comes to intensifying the outcome of your dish.

The simple act of throwing fresh cut basil on a finished plate of pasta or adding mint to a green salad is sometimes exactly what you need.

Good food tastes good and it's good for you! Winner winner!

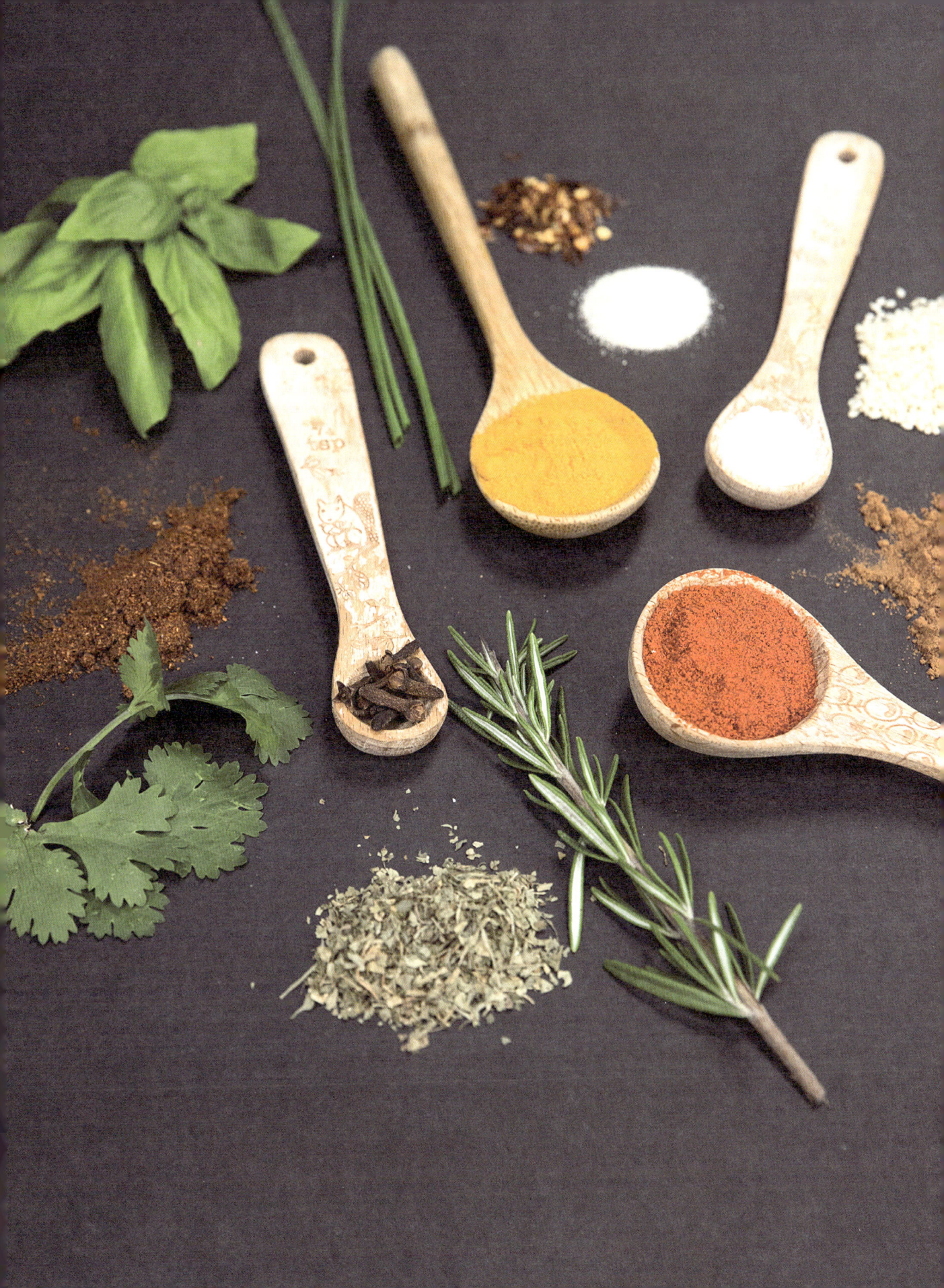

CHAPTER 2
appetizers

bacon-wrapped dates with goat cheese 36

guacamole 39

hot and spicy Mexican dip appetizer 40

summer salsa 43

roasted carrot hummus 44

lime and avocado sea scallops 47

spicy shrimp 48

sweet potato chips 51

baked tequila lime chicken drumsticks 52

I ALWAYS LIKE AN APPETIZER IF HAVING A GLASS OF wine and feel that wine is meant to be enjoyed in the company of good food and never alone. Most times, I am good to go with artisanal cheeses, local or homemade hummus, cut vegetables and crudités. But truthfully, there are many delicious appetizers that make for wonderful noshing with friends and family.

I can't say appetizers are my strong suit, but I have my regulars that have been standards in my kitchen for many years. I have picked a few that are easy to assemble with common ingredients. Make a couple of these ahead of time for guests, and you are ready for an appetizer only gathering. One of my favorite ways to entertain!

bacon-wrapped dates
with goat cheese

THIS APPETIZER HAS THREE INGREDIENTS and a flavor punch that will wow a crowd. The sweet and salty taste of the bacon and date, along with the creaminess of goat cheese, is the perfect combination. It is a crowd stunner! Rich and satisfying and easy to make. This will quickly become a favorite, as it has for my dearest friend Michele, who continues to share with friends and family.

MBK'S TIPS

Make ahead of time and cook before guests arrive. Perfectly delicious served at room temperature.

NUTRITION EXTRAS

Make sure to get a good quality thick-cut nitrate-free bacon. I love a peppered, applewood-smoked variety.

GF

18 large Medjool pitted dates

4 ounces goat cheese

6 strips thick cut, nitrate free bacon

1. Preheat oven to 400°.
2. Cut bacon into thirds.
3. Slice dates lengthwise and add a small piece of goat cheese.
4. Close tightly and wrap with bacon, securing with a wooden toothpick.
5. Bake in the oven for 14-17 minutes on a wire rack, turning halfway through the cooking process.

Enjoy!

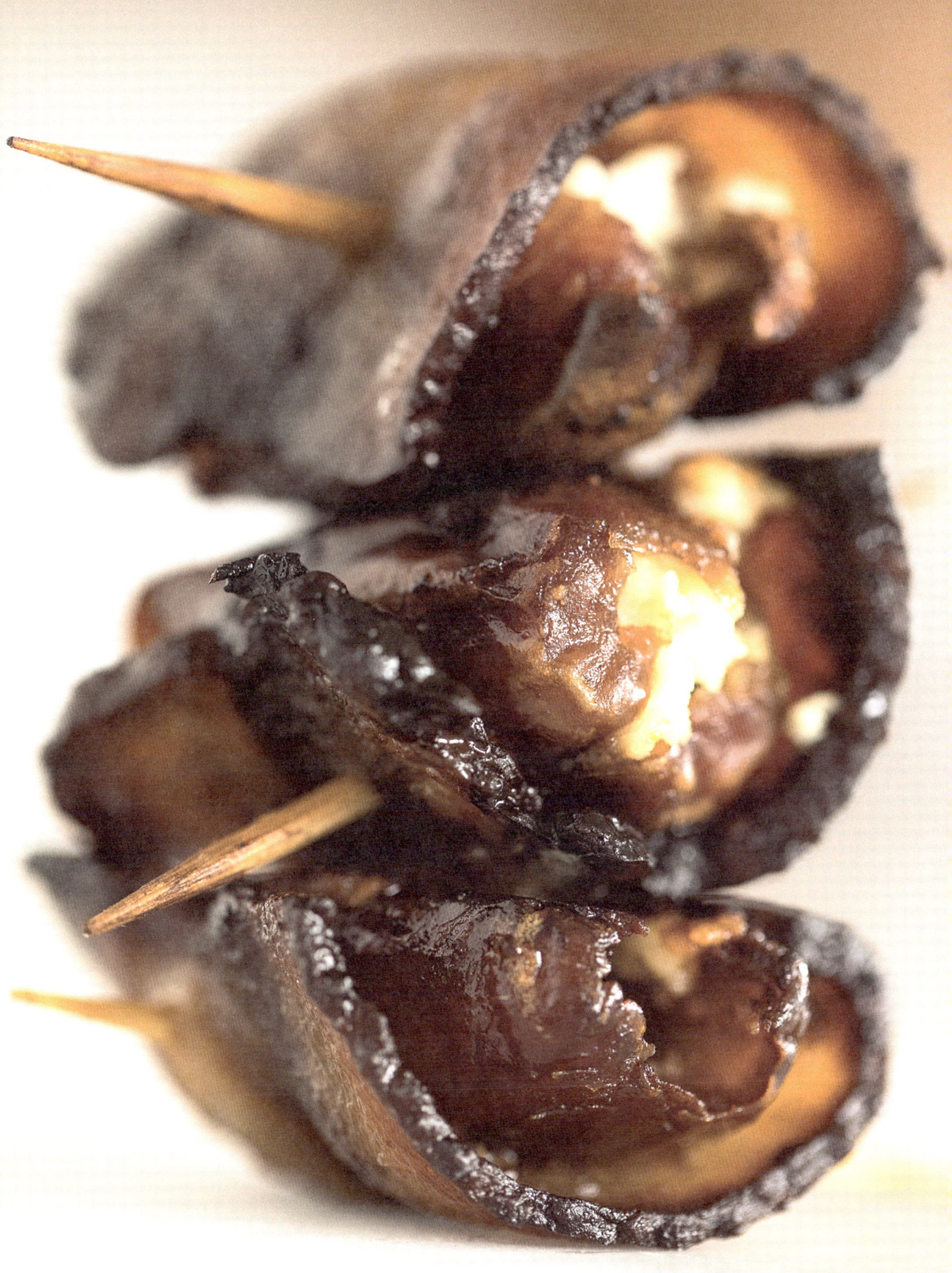

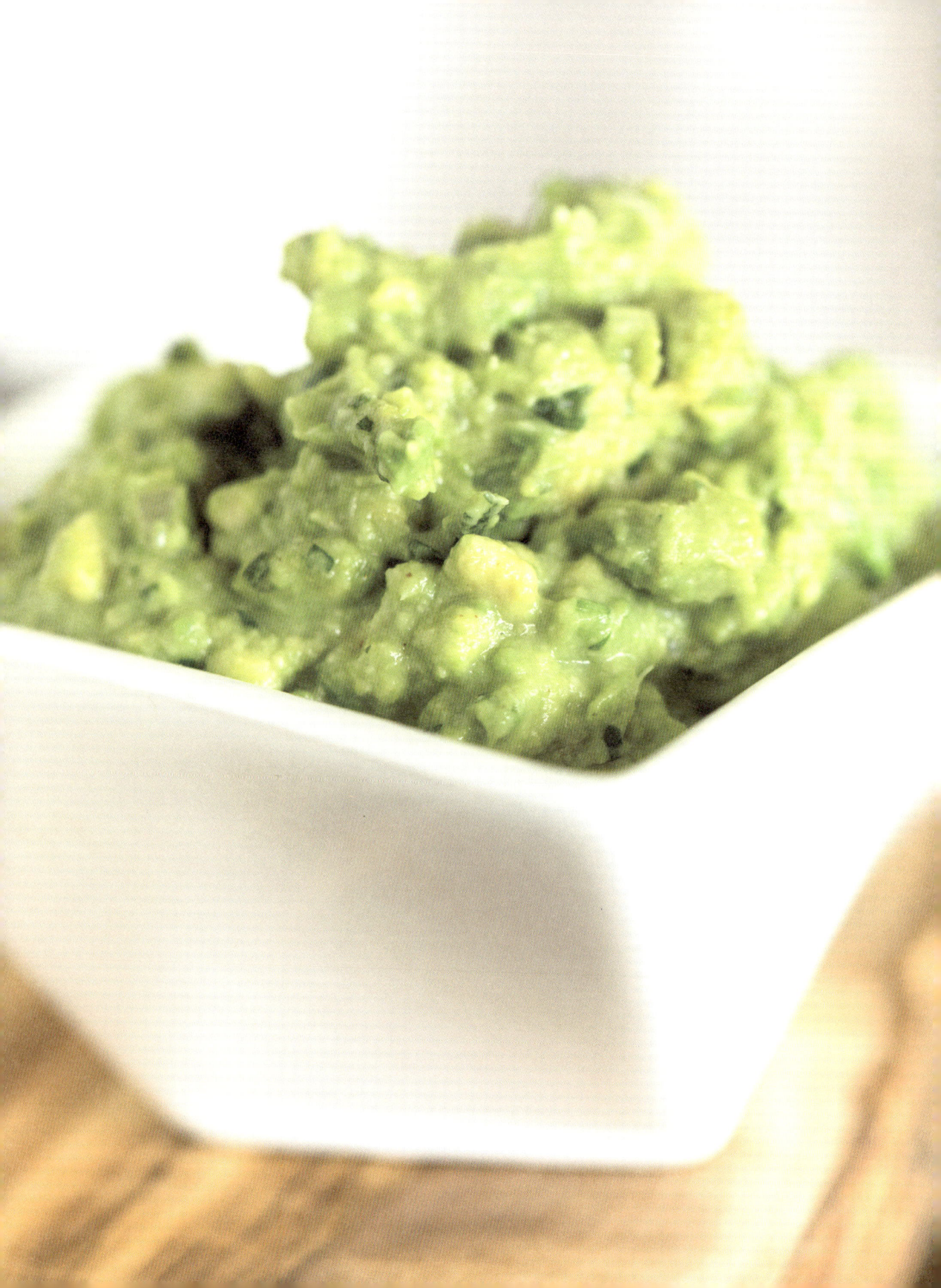

guacamole

THIS IS MY SISTER SARAH'S VERSION OF GUACAMOLE. She is the person who introduced the family to the taste of this little unknown fruit in the 1990's. Believe it or not, most people were not eating avocados 20 years ago. We all make a different spin on this recipe depending on how much heat, raw garlic or spice one prefers. If you are new to making this dish, follow these measurements to a tee, and you will be sold. This is how I always make my version - crowd-pleasing and always on hand.

4 avocados

3 limes, juiced

⅓ cup fresh picked cilantro, chopped

¼ cup shallots, finely chopped

1 garlic clove, minced

1 teaspoon cumin

½ teaspoon sea salt

1 serrano pepper, diced

1. Cut ripe avocados in half, seed, and scoop into medium-size serving dish.

2. Squeeze juice of limes over avocados.

3. Add cilantro, shallots, garlic, spices, and serrano pepper.

4. Using a pastry whisk smash all ingredients together to desired consistency. Do not over mix *(some chunky pieces will remain)*.

5. Serve with fresh tortilla chips.

Enjoy!

MBK'S TIPS

Make it fresh, as guacamole turns brown rather quickly, once exposed to the elements *(keeping the nut in the bowl until used, is said to delay oxidation)*.

Be sure to pick avocados that are fresh and slightly soft.

Roast the pepper for a more intense flavor.

NUTRITION EXTRAS

The healthiest fat you can eat.

Plant-based and rich in Vitamins A, C, and E. Also rich in fiber.

GF
DF
V
LS

hot and spicy mexican dip

THIS DIP IS ADDICTIVELY DELICIOUS, however it can be messy to prepare and present. Be sure to let this sit for a good hour after it has cooked to absorb all the moisture. It will be plenty warm enough served at room temperature. I love having this left over in the refrigerator, as it just gets better with age, and can be perfect to add to a quesadilla.

1 can vegetarian refried beans

1 large sweet onion, diced

2 large or 3 medium tomatoes, chopped and drained of excess water *(you can use canned tomatoes, but be sure to drain in a colander so extra moisture is released)*

3 jalapeño peppers, seeded and diced *(can be roasted first)*

1 poblano pepper, roasted and diced

1 serrano pepper for extra heat, diced

1 tablespoon chili powder

1 tablespoon cumin

1 teaspoon cayenne pepper *(optional)*

½ teaspoon salt

1 cup sour cream

2-3 cups sharp cheddar cheese, shredded

NUTRITION EXTRAS

A plant-based appetizer that pleases a vegetarian crowd.

GF

1. Preheat oven to 325°.
2. In large 9x12 ovenproof dish spread refried beans to cover the bottom completely.
3. Layer vegetables starting with onions, then tomatoes, jalapeños, poblano, and serrano. Sprinkle spices evenly over the layered dish.
4. Spread sour cream to cover, then top with grated cheese.
5. Bake in preheated oven for 45 minutes, until vegetables are completely cooked through and boiling. Remove from oven and let cool for approximately 45 minutes, until liquid is absorbed and the mixture is completely cool.
6. Serve at room temperature with fresh tortilla chips.

Enjoy!

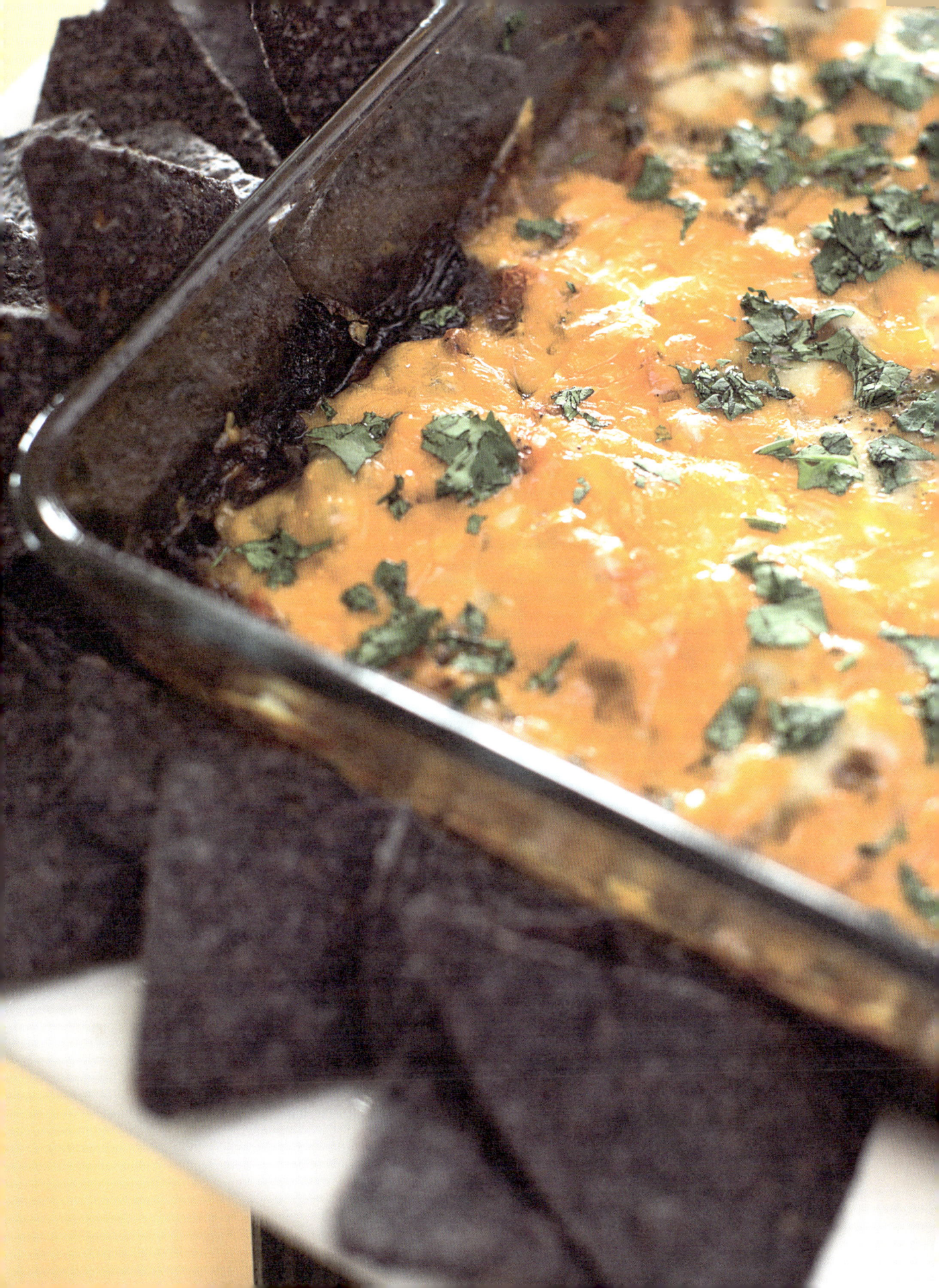

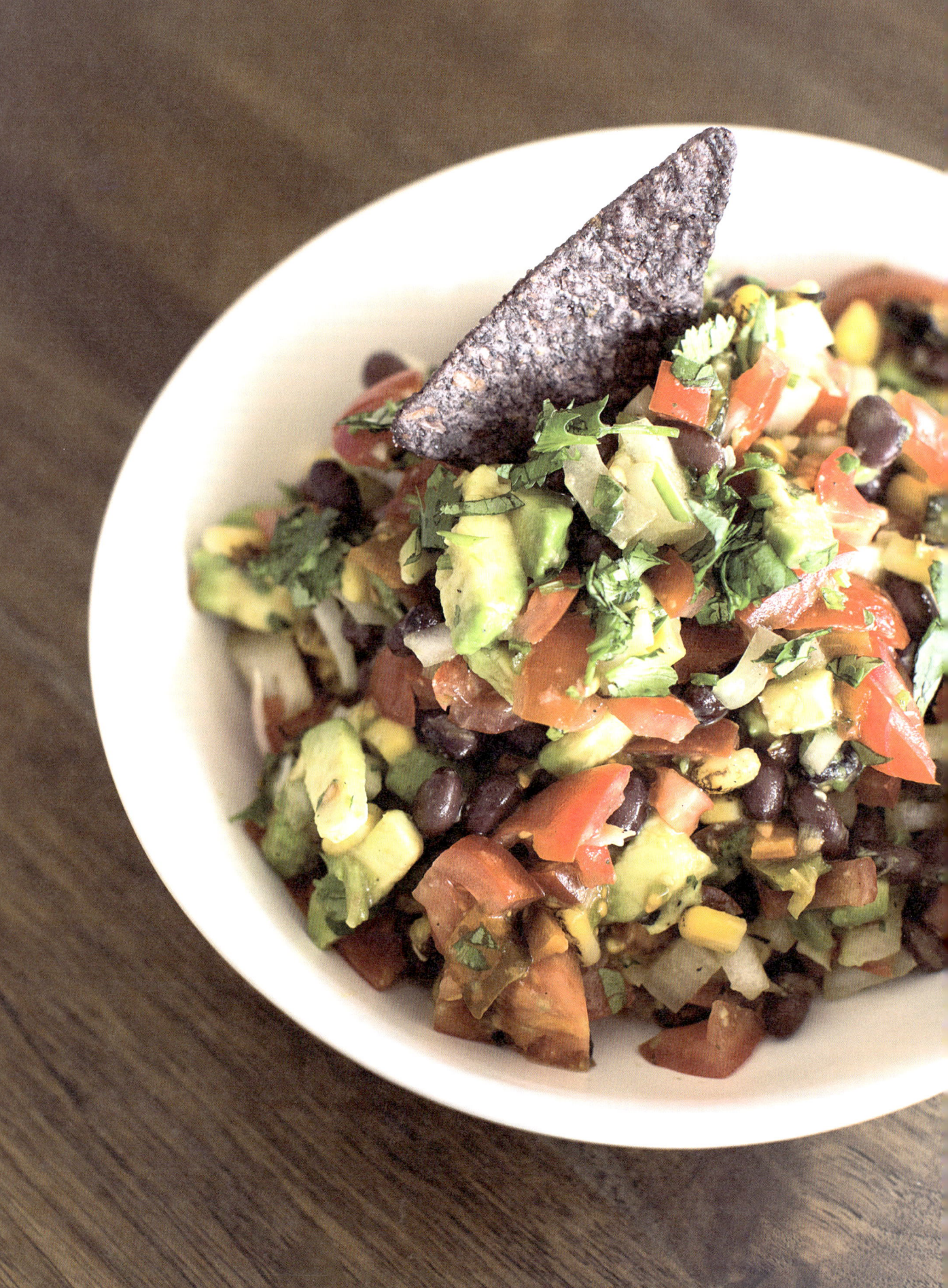

summer salsa

AS SOON AS SUMMER TOMATOES ARE RIPE I make salsa at least weekly for crowds at the lake. Hot and spicy at times or with peaches or mango for seafood. It's a given condiment in the house, until the tomato season ends and summer is over, which is a pretty sad day! Of all the vegetables, tomatoes are one that should only be consumed in season. I often make a quick pico de gallo for tacos but this version is more of my crowd-pleasing combination for munching with fresh tortilla chips.

4 large ripe tomatoes, cored and diced

1 medium sweet onion, diced

1 serrano pepper, roasted and finely chopped

1 medium poblano pepper, roasted and finely chopped

1 can of organic black beans, rinsed and drained

½ bag of roasted corn, steamed and cooled, or 2 fresh cooked ears of corn, cut off the cob

½ diced ripe avocado

juice of 1 lime

sea salt to taste

½ cup fresh cilantro, chopped

1. Combine all ingredients in a bowl, mix gently, adding salt to taste.
2. Serve with fresh tortilla chips or use for topping on Mexican dishes.

Enjoy!

MBK'S TIPS

Roast the peppers before use for added flavor. Roasting can be done over a flame, if you have a gas stove in your kitchen.

NUTRITION EXTRAS

This is a light appetizer that does not ruin an appetite, but satisfies a pang of hunger.

Loaded with vitamins and very low in fat.

GF
DF
V
LS

roasted carrot hummus

THIS IS ADAPTED FROM GLADA DE LAURENTIS' RECIPE. I loved the idea that not all hummus needs to have tahini in it to be called hummus. I've tweaked the roasting process and added less garlic. Adding a touch more lemon adds a bit of tartness to go along with the sweet carrots and olive oil. I have made several varieties of hummus over the years but this one I really love of late. You can serve it with raw vegetables or veggie chips and it is a light and healthy appetizer.

MBK'S TIPS

Make ahead of time and keep refrigerated. This will last 10 days, but best when eaten soon after it's made.

- 8 ounces of carrots, peeled and cut into 1-inch pieces
- 2 tablespoons plus ⅓ cup extra virgin olive oil
- 2 garlic cloves
- sea salt
- 1 - 15-ounce can garbanzo beans, drained and rinsed
- 3 tablespoons fresh lemon juice
- ¼ cup water
- ⅛ teaspoon cayenne *(more if you prefer spicy)*
- 1 teaspoon cumin

NUTRITION EXTRAS

Full of vitamin A and C, along with the fiber rich vegetables. Plant-based protein from the beans.

GF
DF
V

1. Preheat oven to 425° convection. Line a baking pan with parchment paper.
2. Toss carrots with 2 tablespoons olive oil, garlic, and 1 teaspoon salt. Spread evenly on parchment-lined pan.
3. Roast in the oven for 15 minutes or until vegetables are soft and starting to caramelize. Remove from oven and cool.
4. In a food processor, pulse the roasted carrots and garbanzo beans until combined.
5. Add lemon juice, olive oil, water, cayenne, cumin and additional salt if necessary *(¼ - ½ teaspoon)* and puree until smooth. *(If dry, add ¼ cup water and extra lemon juice if necessary).*
6. Serve with desired accompaniments.

Enjoy!

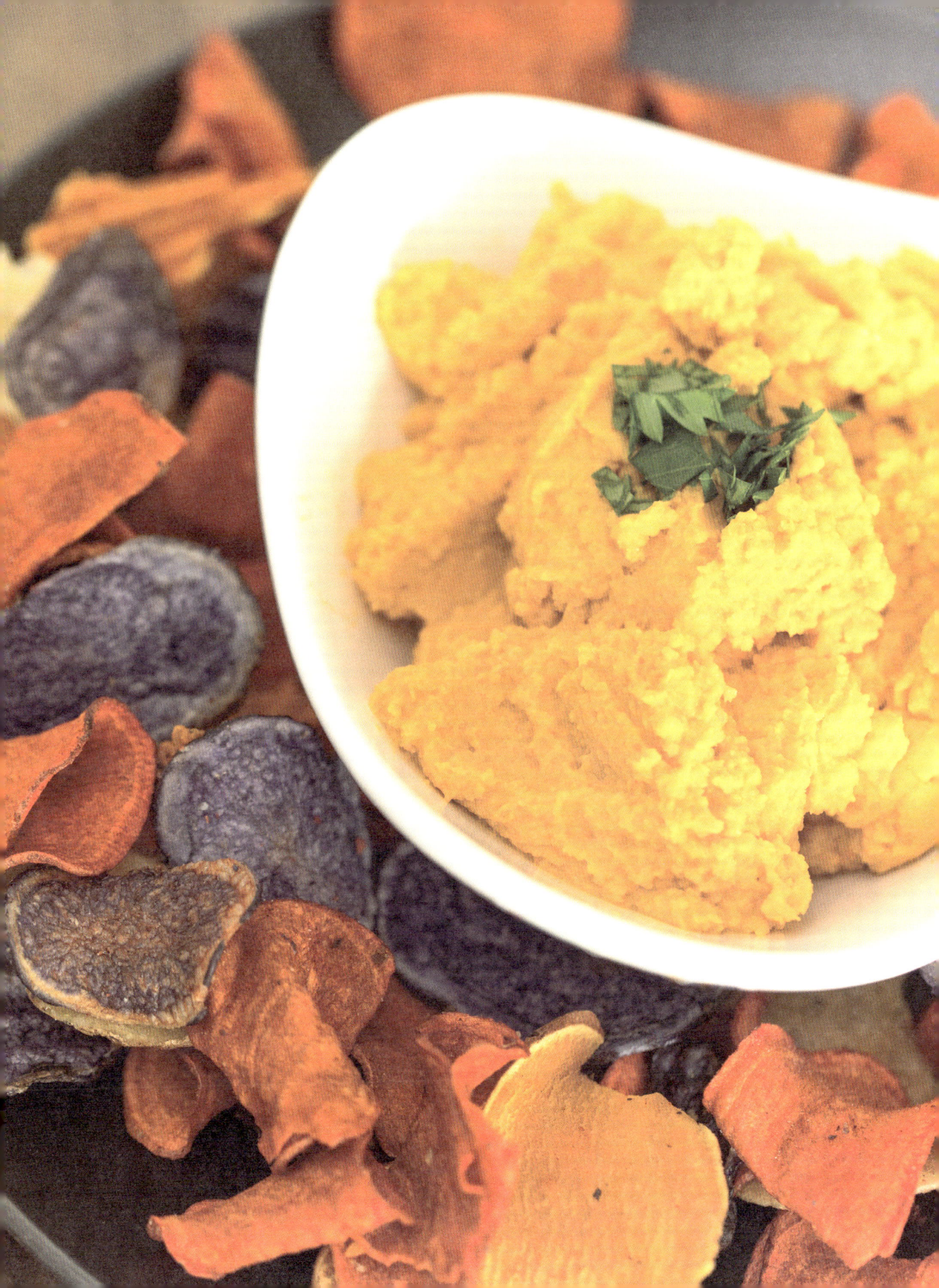

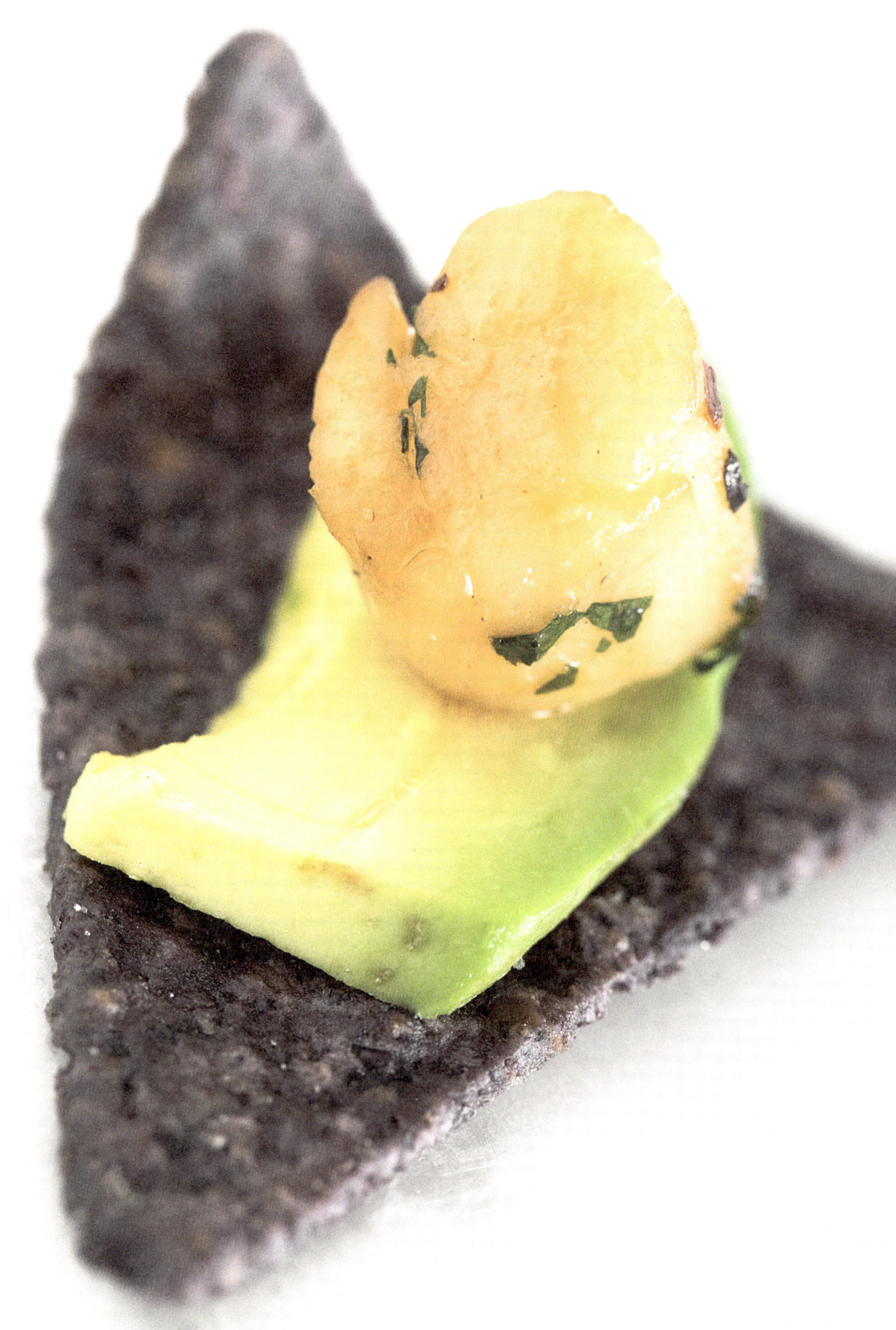

lime & avocado sea scallops

THE COMBINATION OF THIS DELICATE SCALLOP and avocado is somehow a perfect little bite. It goes well with a Mexican themed get together and looks beautiful once plated.

- 1 pound sea scallops
- ¼ cup olive oil
- ¼ cup cilantro, chopped
- 1 garlic clove, minced
- 2 teaspoons low-sodium soy sauce
- 1 teaspoon crushed red pepper flakes
- ½ teaspoon fresh black pepper
- tortilla chips
- small avocado slices
- lime wedges

1. In a medium bowl toss sea scallops with next 6 ingredients. Marinate for 20 minutes.
2. Using a slotted spoon remove scallops from bowl and grill on moderate to high heat until cooked, approximately 2 minutes per side.
3. Cut scallops in half and place on a tortilla chip with avocado underneath. Serve with a lime wedge on the side.

Enjoy!

MBK'S TIPS

Bay scallops work well with this, but the larger sea scallops are much tastier and easier to cook correctly.

NUTRITION EXTRAS

Gluten-free appetizer that is a healthy protein and fat combination. Pleasing to all pescatarians, with any type of diet proclivity.

GF
DF
LS

spicy shrimp

THIS RECIPE IS ADAPTED FROM A RECIPE BY GIADA DE LAURENTIS that I find easy to pull together and has loads of flavor. Everyone loves shrimp at a party! You can have these made in advance, cook when guests arrive and serve at room temperature.

- 1 pound large shrimp, peeled and deveined, tail intact
- 2 teaspoons chili paste
- ¼ teaspoon dried oregano
- ⅓ cup grated Parmigiano Reggiano
- 1 tablespoon lemon juice, freshly squeezed, from ½ lemon
- 2 tablespoons olive oil
- ¼ teaspoon salt
- 1 teaspoon lemon zest from 1 lemon

NUTRITION EXTRAS

Great protein that is low in calories and high in Iron and B12.

Shellfish are close to the top of the food chain when it comes to nutrients.

GF
LS

1. Preheat oven to 425°.

2. In a medium bowl whisk together all the above ingredients except lemon juice, then gently mix in the shrimp.

3. Spread shrimp evenly on a rimmed baking sheet, lined with parchment paper, and bake for 8 to 10 minutes or until shrimp are pink and opaque.

4. Remove from oven and while still hot, squeeze lemon over shrimp and they are ready to serve!

Enjoy!

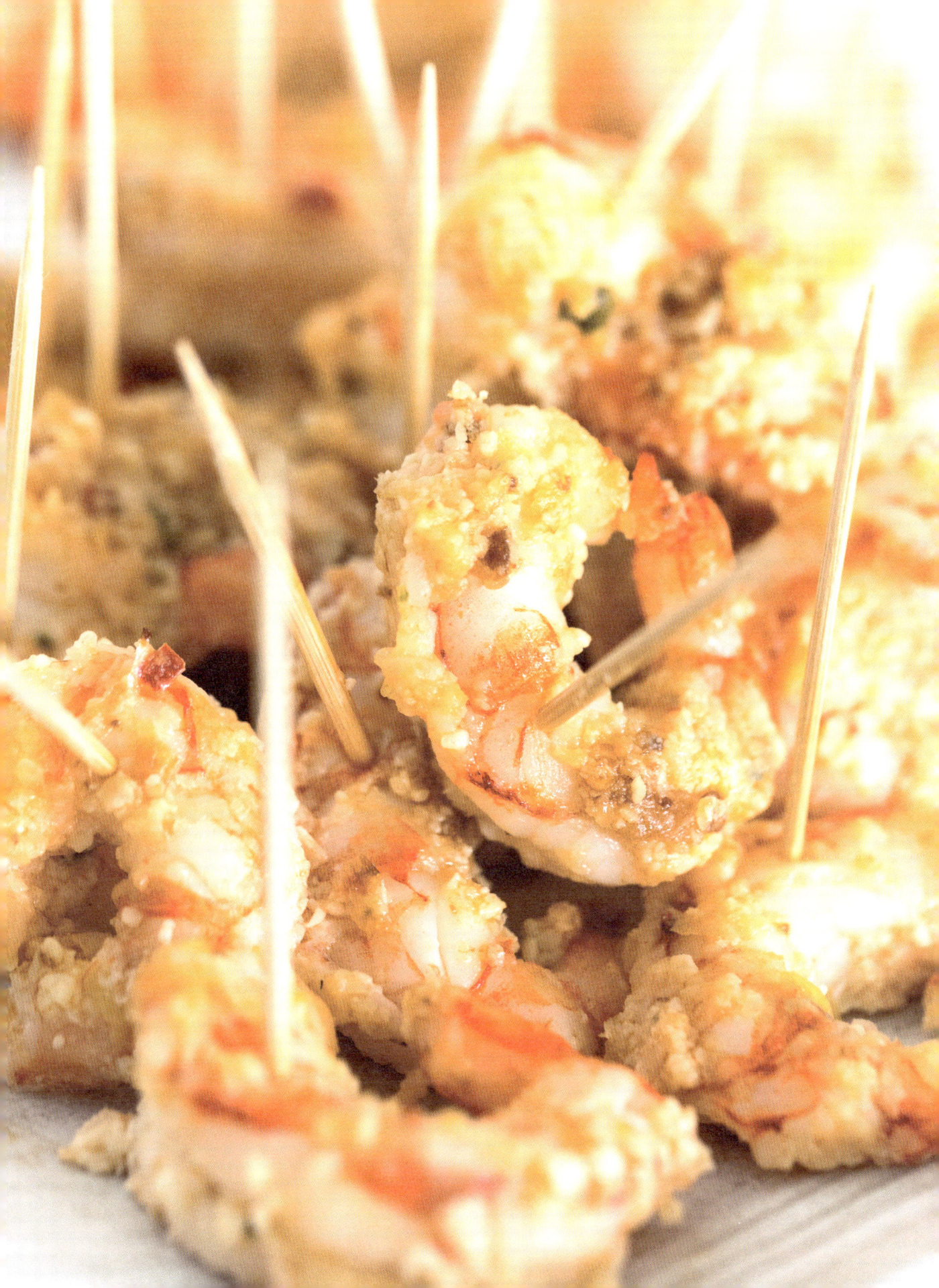

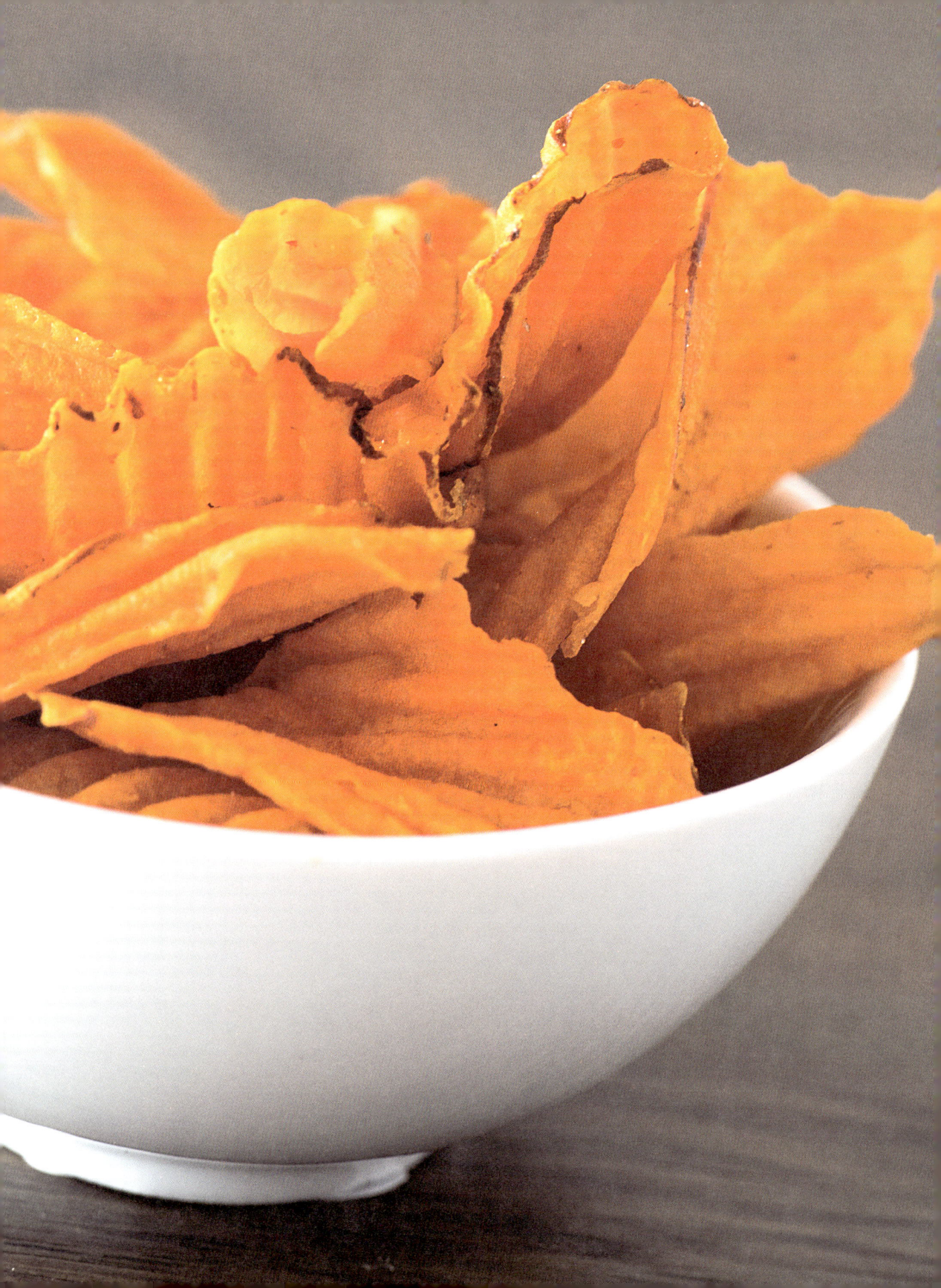

sweet potato chips

THESE CHIPS LOOK MUCH BETTER WHEN YOU USE a mandolin, but I have made them many times by simply slicing by hand. The trick is to keep the cut uniform so the chips cook evenly. They will taste just like you opened a fresh bag of chips, once you let them dry.

1 medium sweet potato, peeled and sliced paper-thin *(if using a mandolin set to ⅛ inch)*

3 tablespoons extra virgin olive oil

fine sea salt and fresh pepper to taste

1. Preheat oven to 275°.
2. Set up two cookie sheets with drying racks inserted.
3. In a bowl toss potato, oil, salt and pepper. Arrange in a single layer on racks.
4. Bake for 45-50 minutes, rotating once during the cooking process and baking until chips are deeply golden. Chips will crisp as they cool.

Enjoy!

MBK'S TIPS

Keep the chips on the large size *(silver dollar)*, as they tend to shrink in the process.

NUTRITION EXTRAS

Sweet potato chips are delicious with hummus and other appetizers and much healthier than your typical crackers, that usually sit on a cheeseboard.

They are high in fiber, loaded with vitamin A and are low glycemic carbohydrates.

GF
DF
V
LS

baked tequila lime chicken drumsticks

I HAVE CHANGED THIS RECIPE EVERY TIME I'VE MADE IT. However, I think I have it nailed down with the discovery of ancho chili powder. Drumsticks are always a hit, similar to chicken wings, but they have more meat. This version is crowd friendly and not too spicy. You can add or change this recipe to adapt to your taste and it's very forgiving when it comes to adding flavor.

MBK'S TIPS

If you do not have a convection oven, you can broil at the end of baking to crisp up the skin. Watch carefully; this will only take a minute. Let cool before serving.

NUTRITION EXTRAS

A healthy chicken snack that is not fried, yet still tastes decadent.

Be sure to buy quality organic poultry.

GF
DF

- 20-25 free-range, organic drumsticks
- ¾ cup tequila
- ¾ cup fresh lime juice *(about 8 limes)*
- ⅓ cup honey
- 1 jalapeno, diced
- 2 teaspoons ancho chili powder
- 1 teaspoon ground coriander
- 2 teaspoons dried oregano
- 3 tablespoons olive oil
- 2 teaspoons salt
- fresh pepper to taste
- fresh cilantro for serving

1. Mix all ingredients except chicken, until thoroughly combined.
2. Season chicken lightly with salt and pepper. Place chicken in a resealable plastic bag and pour marinade over chicken. Seal and refrigerate for up to 8 hours.
3. Preheat oven to 425° convection.
4. Pour liquid from a plastic bag into a small saucepan. Cook liquid on a low boil until reduced and thickened. Save for later use.
5. Place chicken in a single layer on a baking sheet. Be careful not to crowd the chicken. This may require a second baking sheet. Bake chicken for 45-55 minutes, turning occasionally and basting with reserved marinade, until chicken is crisp and cooked throughout.
6. Toss with desired amount of fresh cilantro before serving.

Enjoy!

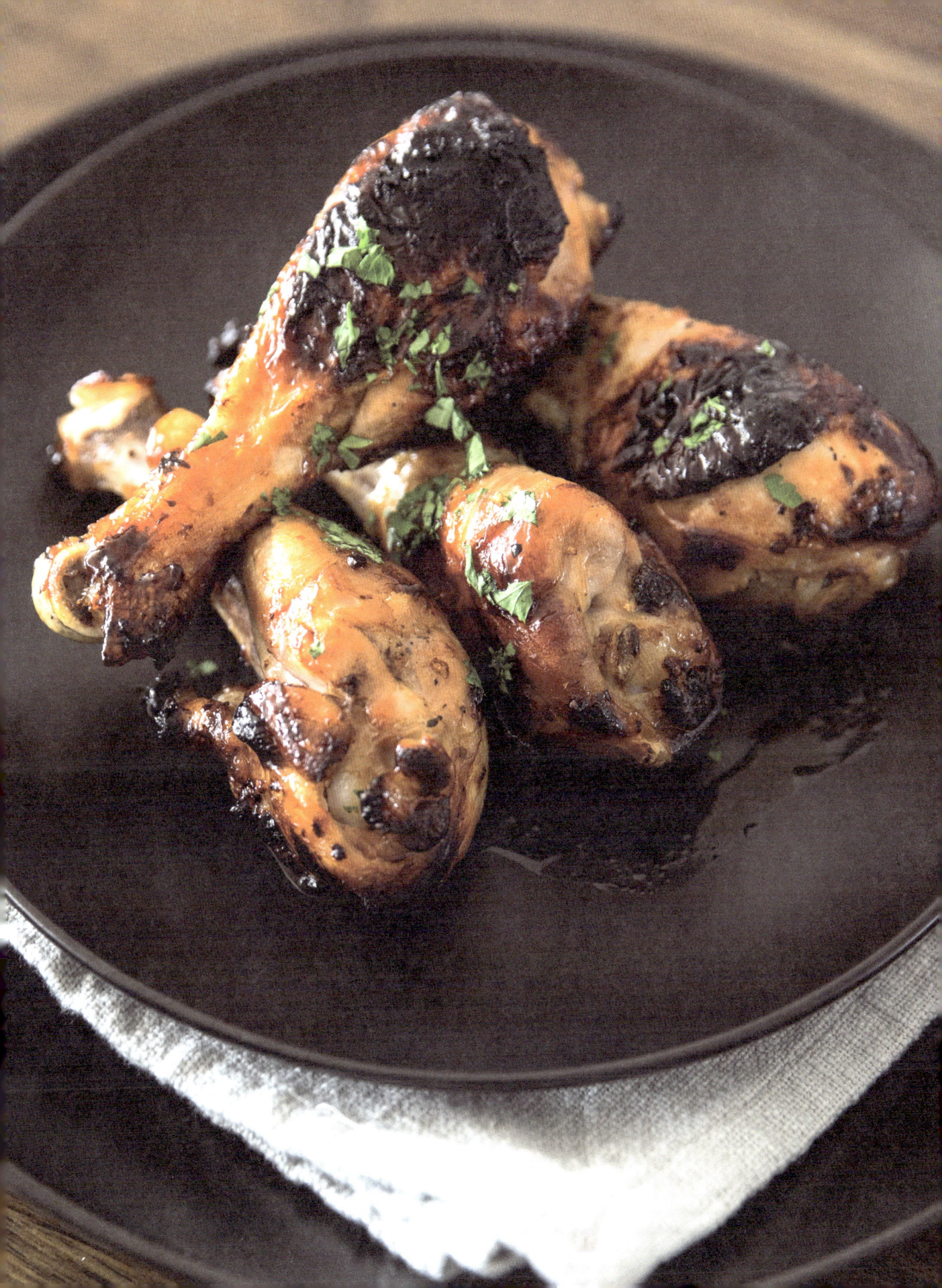

a touch of salt

It was my oldest sister Connie and her husband Pat who taught me many years ago that everything tastes better with salt, pepper and olive oil. You can turn any fresh protein or vegetable into a delicious roasted delight with very little prep and very little spice, as long as you have good quality olive oil and fresh cracked salt and pepper. If that's all a kitchen has to provide, such as a vacation or rental home, you can still make quick and tasty dishes.

When eating a whole foods diet you are rarely consuming processed foods. Salting your food should never be a concern, as long as you have no health issues, such as high blood pressure. Salt has the power to bring out the best flavor of our food. It's also an essential element and crucial to our overall health.

I always keep several types of salts in my pantry. A few are kept on the counter in little dishes right next to the stove for quick access when cooking. I always have kosher iodized salt for baking, Himalayan sea salt for meats and vegetables and Maldon crystals for a finishing salt. In addition I may have salts from other regions of the world, even a smoked salt for the occasional recipe.

With each recipe that I say, "salt to taste," I mean to suggest that salting food is really a personal preference. There are those individuals that no matter how much salt is in a recipe always salt their food before eating. That's not my preference. I like to adjust the amount slowly as I cook, so it's not overdone. You can always add more salt, but once a dish becomes too salty it's very challenging to dilute the spice. Add with caution and always taste the progress. Practice makes perfect.

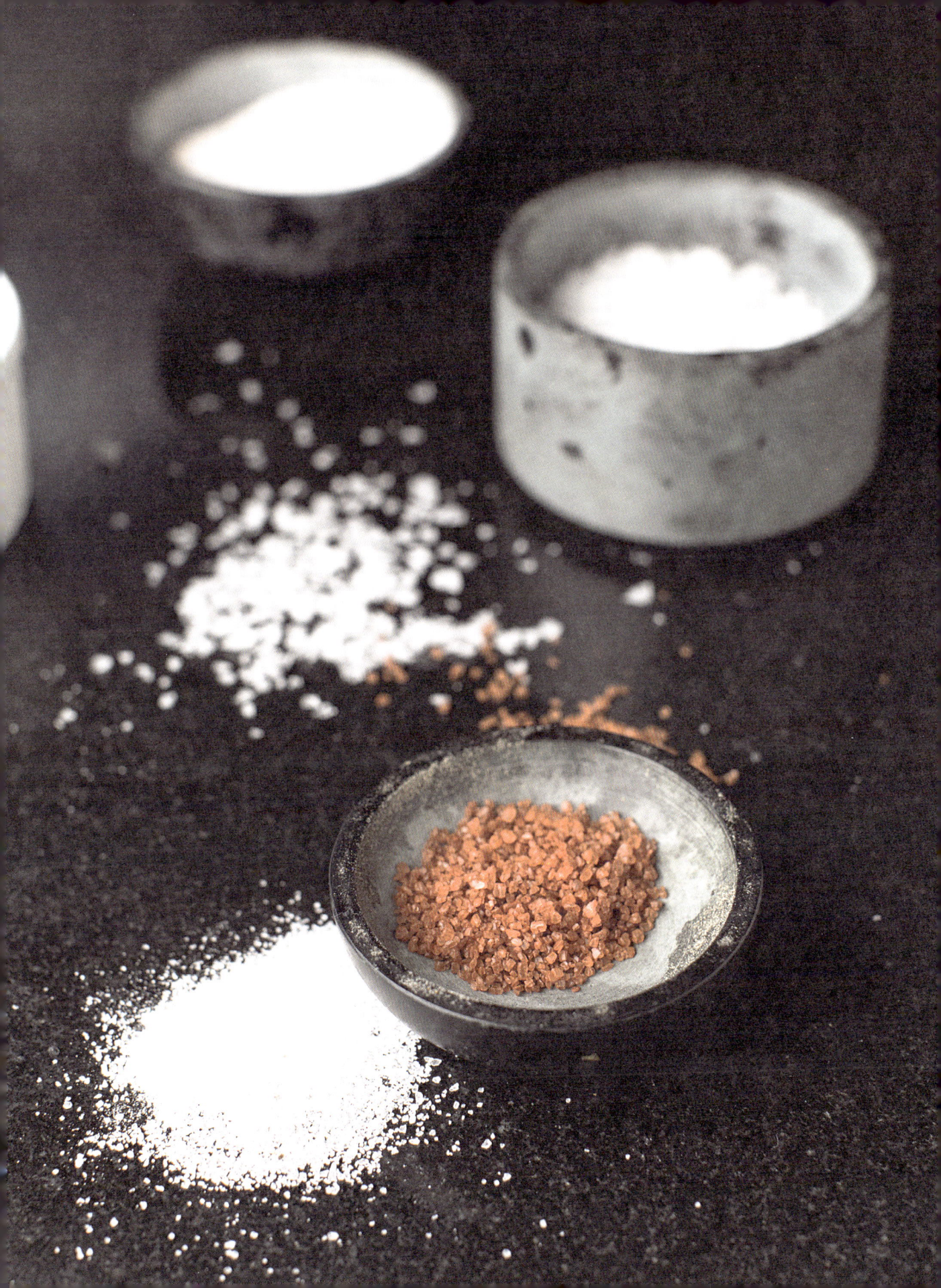

CHAPTER 3
soups

broccoli soup 58

butternut squash soup 61

creamy artichoke soup 62

easy chicken noodle soup 65

french onion soup 66

Megan's minestrone 69

Mexican tortilla soup 70

New Orleans gumbo with the works 72

pumpkin soup 75

asparagus soup 76

turkey chili 79

summer market corn chowder 80

turkey orzo soup 83

I'M RARELY WITHOUT A FRESH POT OF SOUP ON THE stove. From September through April and as long as the weather has a chill in the air, I have soup on the brain. I have hosted many lunchtime gatherings in my home over the years and have come to be known for many of those soup recipes that I served. I know many people will be happy to see their favorite in this book. I love them all and some are seasonal favorites for sure. Many of these recipes I have been making for twenty years and I have yet to tire of making, serving, and enjoying them with others.

Soup is so healthy, especially when you start with homemade broth. It can always be enjoyed, either as a quick lunch, a filling dinner or simply to replace a salad. There is no comparison of eating fresh soup to canned or boxed processed soups. By keeping the ingredients on hand in your freezer and pantry, it's easy to pull together a fresh pot!

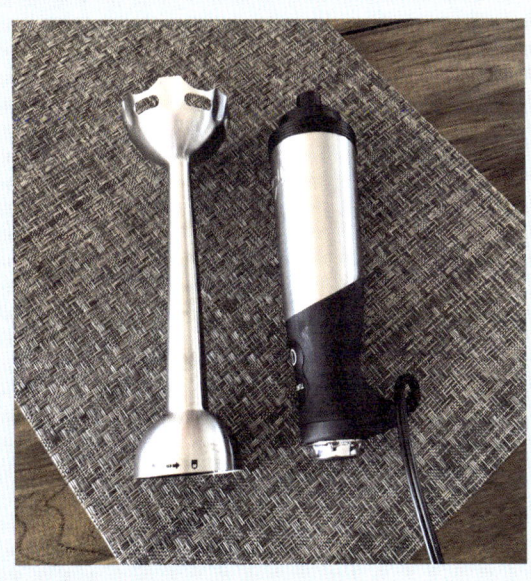

broccoli soup
4-6 Servings

THERE IS ONE THING YOU CAN ALWAYS SAY about broccoli and that is, it's always available fresh. If you are in need of some fiber and a soup rich in vitamin C and K this is a good choice. I can usually pull this together quickly, as I always have fresh broccoli on hand and it makes for a light lunch or a small side for dinner. You will love the rich taste of this soup, that feels restorative, with its substantial nutrient content.

2 tablespoons olive oil

1 large sweet onion

1 cup baby bella mushrooms, sliced

3 cups fresh organic baby spinach or baby kale

2 quarts chicken stock - 1 reduced-sodium, 1 regular

2 large heads of broccoli, including portions of the stems (*can use organic frozen broccoli florets - 2 to 3 bags depending on size*)

⅓ cup heavy cream

fresh salt and pepper to taste

NUTRITION EXTRAS

In addition to vitamins C and K, broccoli is rich in potassium and B9. It's a superfood among vegetables.

GF
LS

1. In a large soup pot saute onion, mushrooms and spinach, until onion is translucent and mushrooms have softened.

2. Add stock and broccoli and simmer on low-boil until broccoli has softened, approximately 20 minutes.

3. Puree soup with handheld mixer. Add half and half and seasonings to taste.

4. Serve with parmesan croutons.

Enjoy!

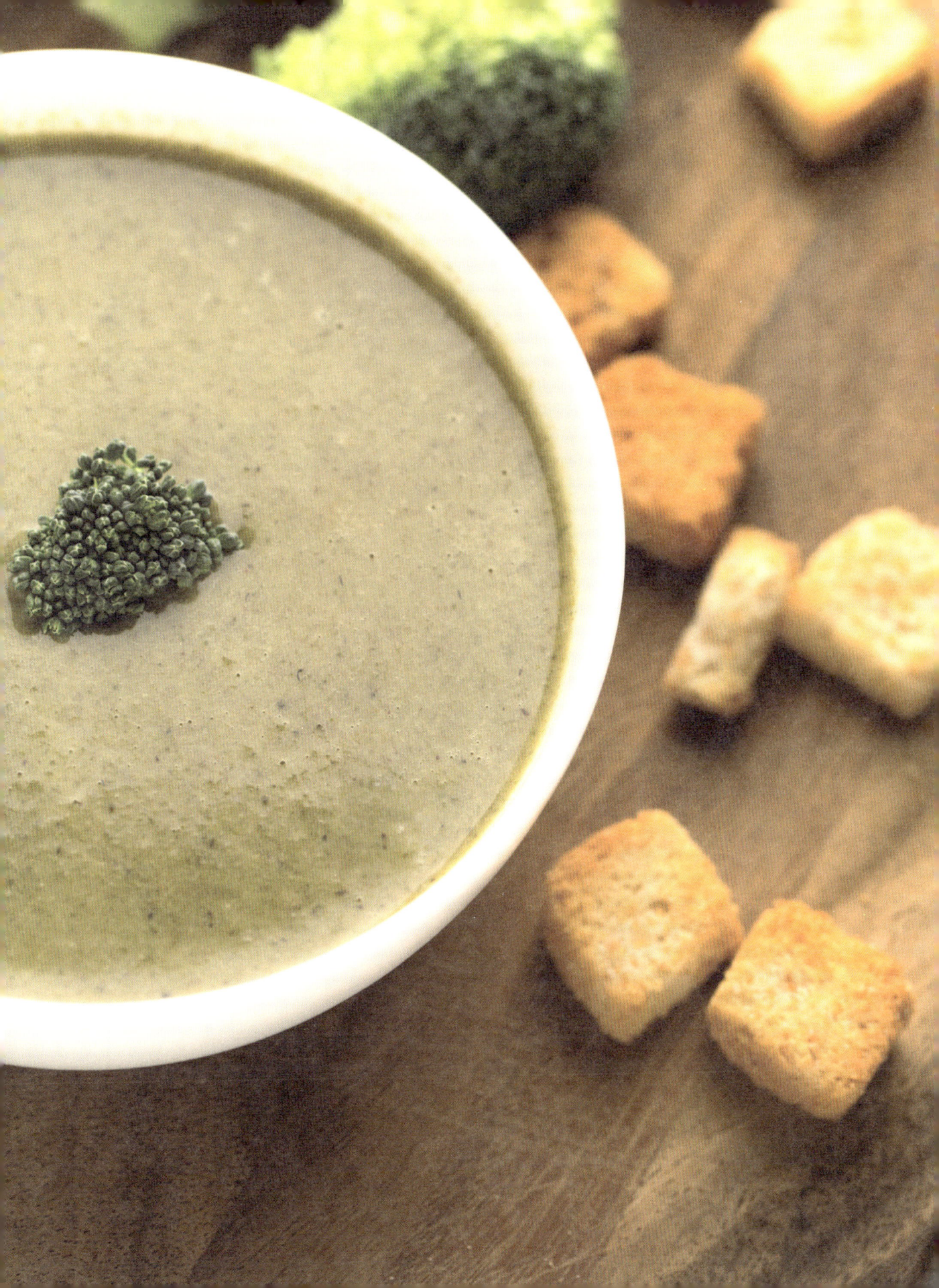

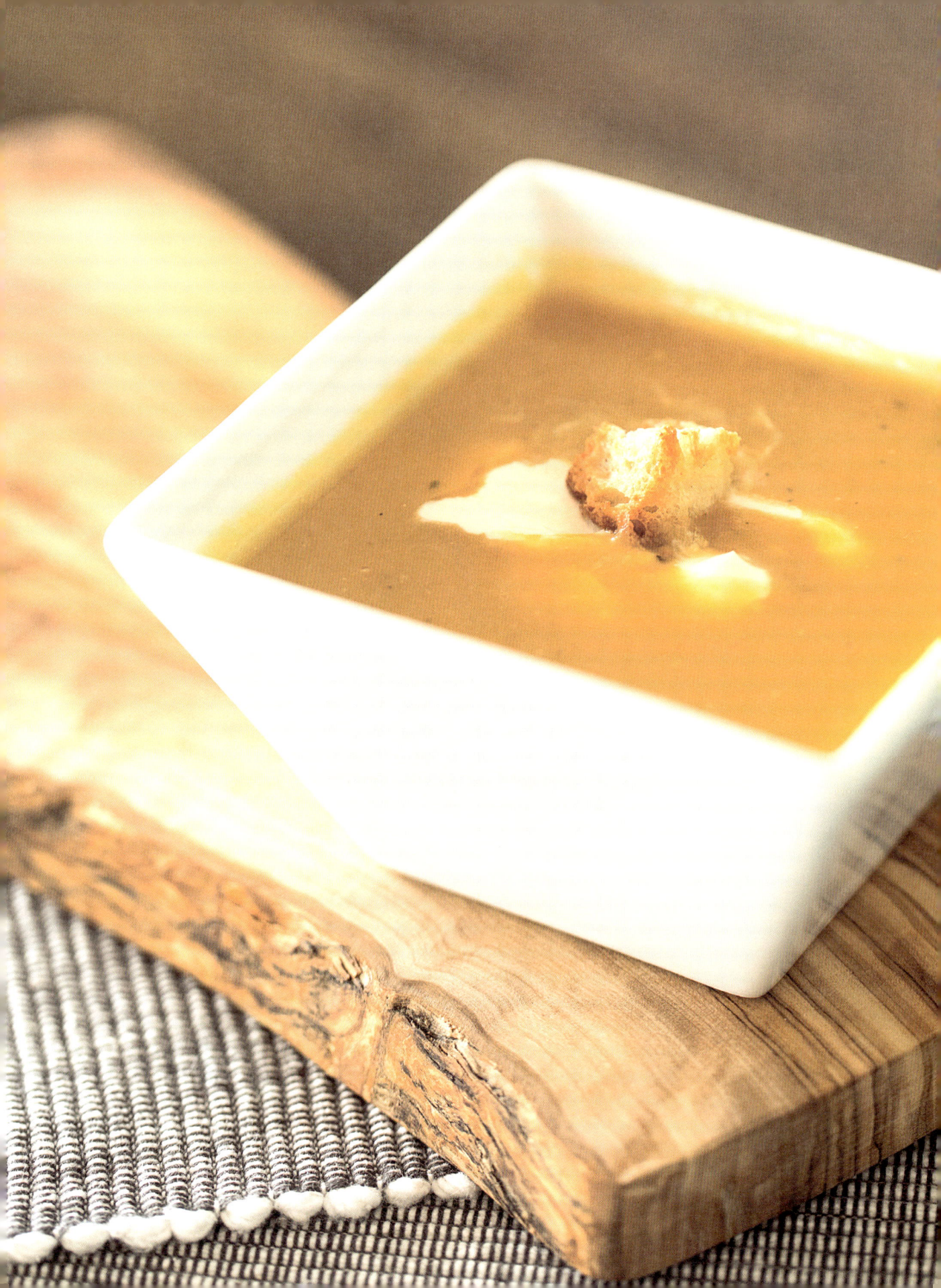

butternut squash soup

4-6 Servings

THIS IS ANOTHER ONE OF MY FAVORITE change of season soups. Early fall calls for this soup at least once or twice before the holidays. It's even better if you roast the fresh butternut squash. This adds an extra step, but it's well worth the effort. The buttery, nutty flavor of the soup intensifies with the roasting process. It's a light and delicious soup and the perfect lunch on a cold afternoon.

- 1 tablespoon unsalted butter
- 1 tablespoon olive oil
- 1 large sweet onion, chopped
- 1 large carrot, peeled and chopped
- 2 garlic cloves, minced
- 2 pounds or 4 cups butternut squash, cubed, cleaned, seeded, and peeled *(can be purchased already prepared)*
- 4 cups chicken or vegetable stock
- 3 tablespoons fresh sage, chopped
- fresh salt and pepper to taste

1. In large 8-quart stockpot, heat butter and oil together over medium heat.
2. Add onion and carrot, occasionally stirring. Cook for approximately 5 minutes, until onion is translucent.
3. Add garlic and cook for another minute.
4. Add squash, broth and sage and bring the mixture back to a low boil. Simmer until vegetables are soft, approximately 20 minutes.
5. Turn off heat and puree mixture with your immersion blender, until smooth.
6. Season with fresh pepper to taste. Keep warm on low heat until served.

Enjoy!

NUTRITION EXTRAS

Loaded with vitamin A and vitamin C. A great fresh vegetable to incorporate during winter, to help replace the plentiful fruits and vegetables of summer.

GF
LS

creamy artichoke soup

4 Servings

I GET CRAVINGS FOR THE ORIGINAL TASTE OF THIS SOUP because it tastes like no other soup that I make fresh. The ingredients are always in my pantry for when the yearning hits. I suggest doubling this recipe, as you will want leftovers for the week in the refrigerator.

MBK'S TIPS

Canned artichoke hearts are so easy to work with and keep for a long time in the pantry. You can also buy frozen ones and they are just as good.

NUTRITION EXTRAS

Low in calories with no fat. Artichokes are rich in potassium, vitamin C, magnesium, and dietary fiber.

This is a great easy way to eat a healthy artichoke.

GF
LS

- 2 tablespoons olive oil
- 2 leeks, white part only, cleaned and sliced
- 1 garlic clove
- 1 potato, peeled and chopped
- 1 can good quality artichoke hearts packed in water, drained *(Whole Foods or Trader Joes)*
- 3 cups chicken stock *(low or reduced sodium)*
- additional salt if necessary and fresh pepper to taste
- mascarpone cheese *(room temperature)*

1. Heat oil in a large pot over medium heat. Add leeks and garlic and stir.
2. Add potato and cook for 5 minutes, stirring often.
3. Add artichokes, stock, salt and pepper. Cook until vegetables are tender, approximately 20 minutes.
4. Puree with a handheld blender, then add 2 tablespoons of soft marscarpone cheese. Blend again.
5. Serve soup with a dollop of additional softened cheese.

Enjoy!

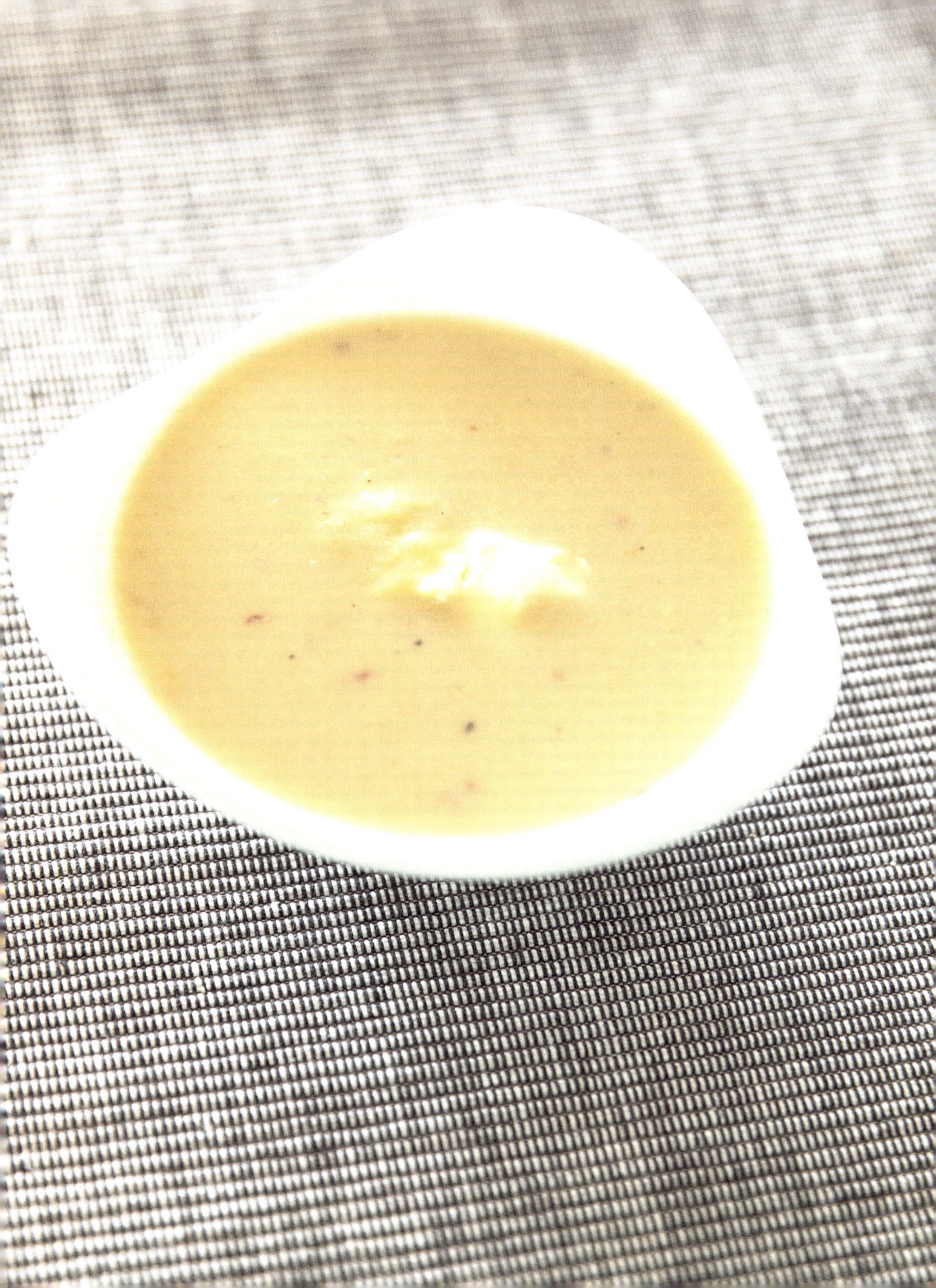

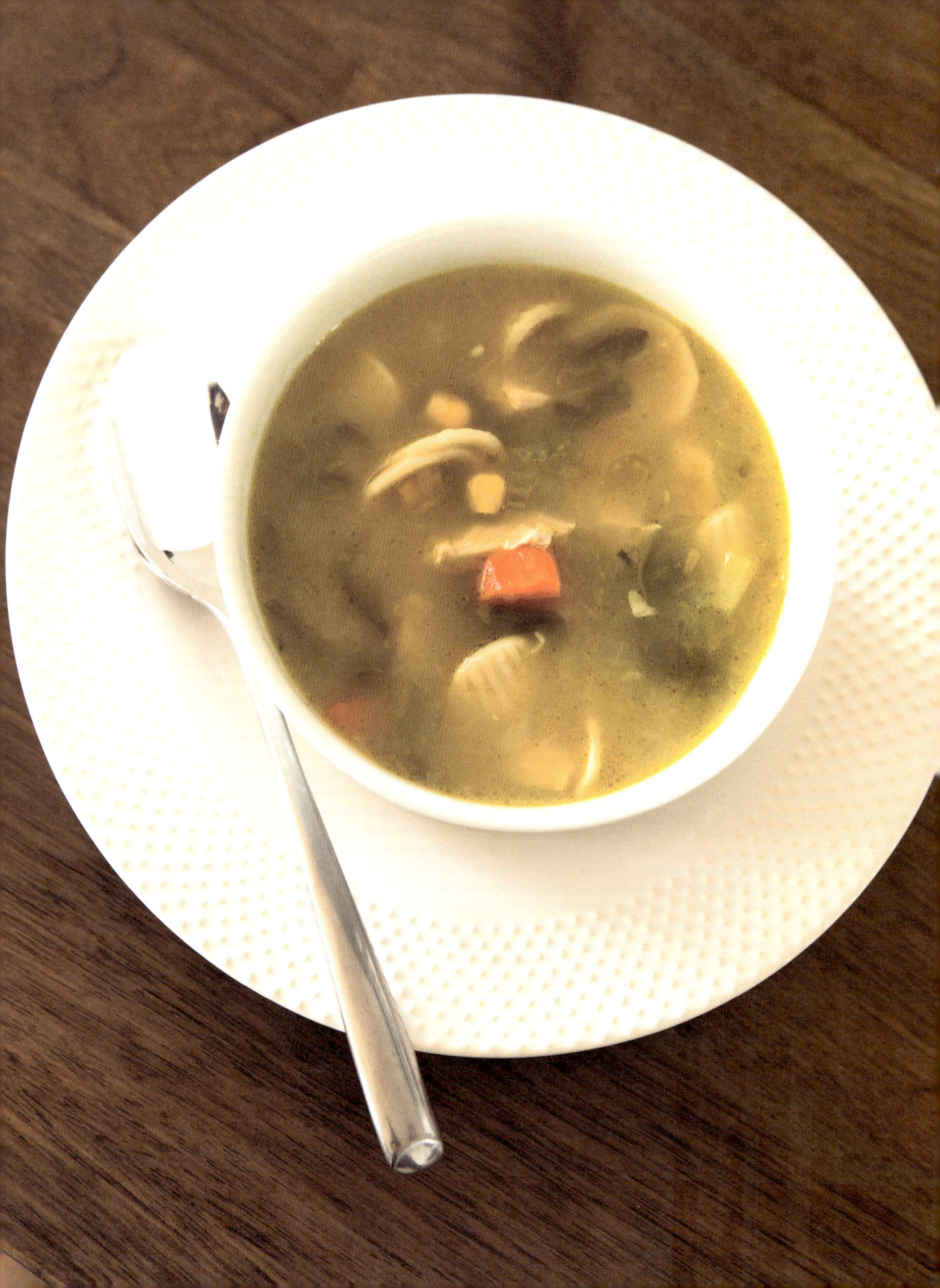

easy chicken noodle soup

4-6 Servings

THIS SOUP IS A CHEAT ON ALL ACCOUNTS. It does not stem from fresh stock. I did not start with roasting my chicken. However, it's just as delicious as if you started with the long process of making a homemade broth. These ingredients should be kept in your pantry and freezer to grab when you need a bowl of quick chicken soup. If you are sick, or your stomach is a little upset, this is just what the doctor ordered.

2 large chicken breasts with skin on

2 tablespoons olive oil for sautéing

1 large sweet onion

2 large fresh carrots

3 stalks of celery

2-quart boxes of chicken stock *(1 full sodium + 1 low sodium)*

3 cups fresh spinach

½ bag of frozen corn

Bay leaf or sage, if preferred

fresh pepper and additional sea salt to taste

8 ounces egg noodle *(pasta of choice)*

MBK'S TIPS

Always have stock and dried pasta in your pantry. The shelf life is long, and you don't want to have to go out, once you think about pulling this quick recipe together, especially if you are under the weather.

DF
LS

1. In a saucepan on low, poach chicken in 3 inches of water. Cook for approximately 45 minutes until done. Remove chicken and let cool.

2. Heat oil in a large soup pot. Add onions, carrots, and celery and cook until softened.

3. Add stock, spinach, corn and any additional seasonings that you prefer.

4. Add shredded poached chicken.

5. Once the soup has returned to a low boil, add pasta and cook for 15 minutes until pasta has finished cooking.

Enjoy!

french onion soup

6 Servings

THIS IS A CLASSIC SOUP that has been gracing the pages of cookbooks for countless years and the recipe usually does not change from one kitchen to the next. I've kept most of the same ingredients and made just a few changes to make it my own verson. Nothing beats a hearty bowl of french onion soup on a cold winter day.

4 tablespoons unsalted butter

5 large sweet onions, cut into rings

2 garlic cloves, minced

1 leek, white part only, cleaned and cut into rings

2 tablespoons flour

2 bay leaves *(to be discarded)*

1 bunch of fresh thyme *(to be discarded)*

2 cups dry white wine

1½ quarts (6 cups) chicken or vegetable stock *(1 full sodium + 1 low sodium)*

fresh pepper and sea salt to taste

fresh country bread rounds

grated gruyere cheese

NUTRITION EXTRA

Onions and any vegetable in the allium family (3 in this recipe) will ward off infections. Getting lots of these vegetables in your diet will powerfully support your immune system.

1. Preheat oven to 450°.

2. Heat butter in a large non-stick soup pot. Add onions, garlic and leeks and saute on medium heat until onions are translucent and starting to brown, approximately 15 minutes.

3. Sprinkle flour evenly on cooked onions. Add thyme and bay leaves and stir for 2 minutes.

4. Add wine and reduce liquid for approximately 5 minutes.

5. Add stock and any additional salt and pepper to taste and boil for 15 minutes on medium-low. Discard thyme and bay leaves.

6. Ladle soup into oven-proof dishes and top with country bread. Cover surface with grated gruyere cheese. Place in oven until bubbly and just starting to brown *(broiling is also an option)*.

Enjoy!

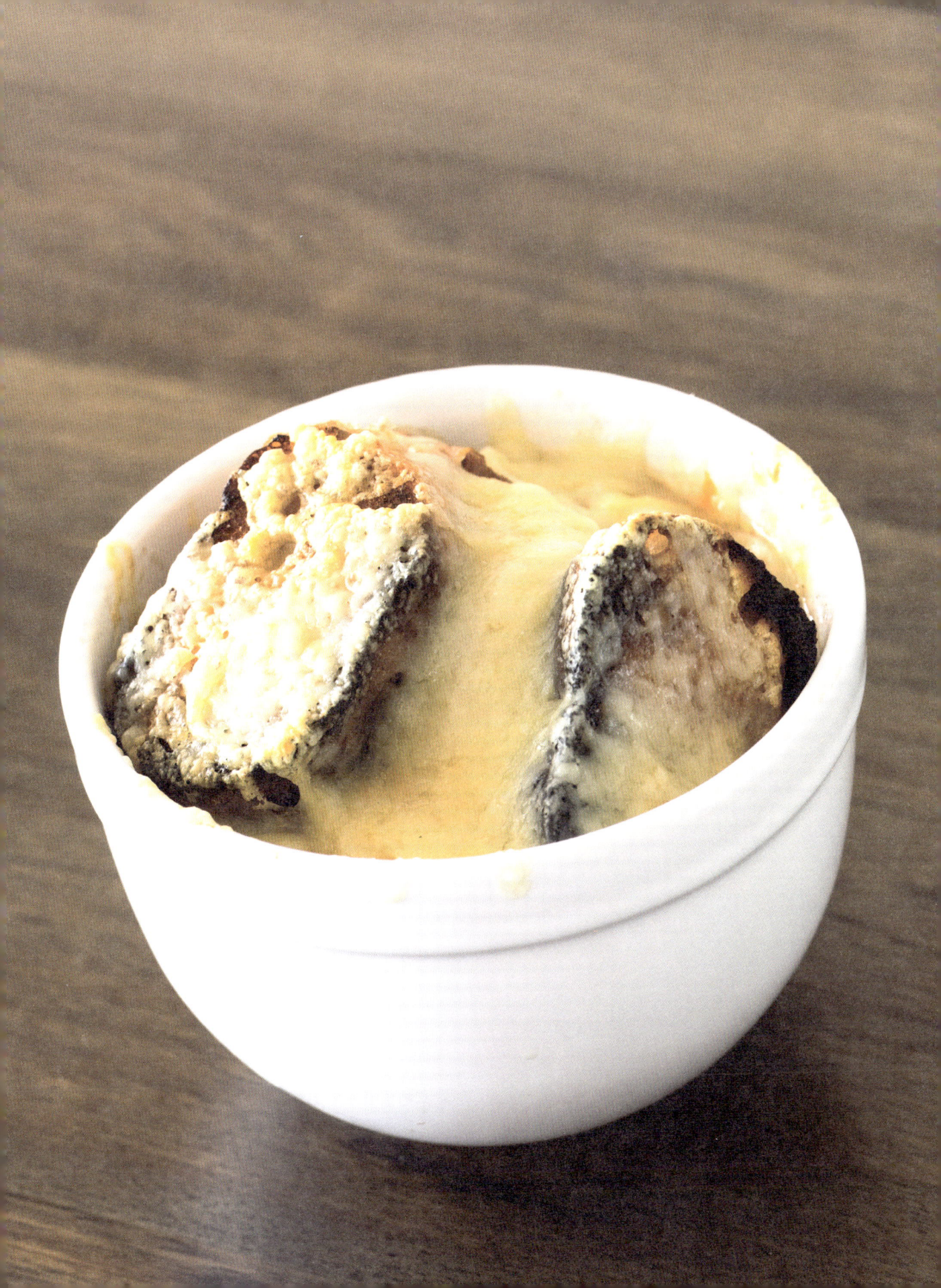

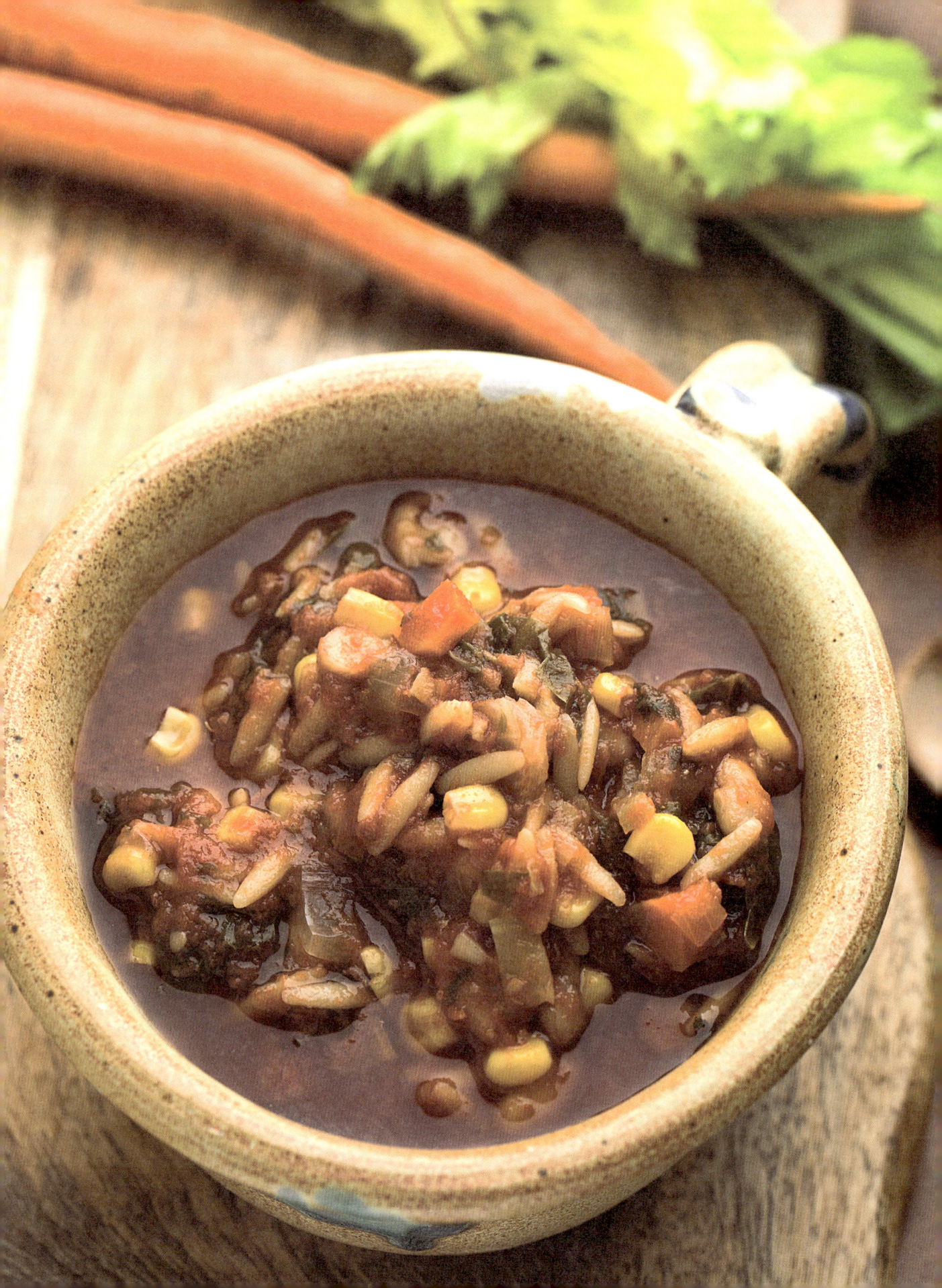

megan's minestrone

8 Servings

THIS SOUP WAS NICKNAMED MEGAN'S MINESTRONE by the crowds who have enjoyed it for many many years and hence the name stuck. The soups in this book are all my original versions, but this soup happens to be the one I have made for the longest amount of time. You want to be sure to make a fresh stock that is rich with flavor. I prefer beef bones but have used both ham and lamb bones as well.

- 2½ pounds of bones *(beef, ham or lamb)*
- 1 large can crushed San Marzano tomatoes
- 3 tablespoons tomato paste or 1 - 15-ounce can of tomato sauce
- 1 large russet potato, diced
- 1 large sweet onion, chopped
- 3 celery stalks, chopped
- 3 full-size carrots, chopped
- 1 bag frozen spinach or 8 ounces fresh spinach
- 1 bag of frozen corn
- 1 tablespoon dried thyme
- 1 tablespoon dried oregano
- 2 teaspoons dried basil
- ¾ teaspoon crushed red pepper
- fresh parsley, minced *(optional)*
- 6 ounces pasta such as orzo or bow tie *(can be gluten-free)*
- 1 can organic cannellini beans, rinsed and drained
- salt and pepper to taste

1. Fill a large stockpot or slow cooker full of water and simmer bones for 8-12 hours on low heat.
2. Drain fresh stock to use as the base for your soup, approximately 64 ounces *(8 cups)*. You can substitute 2 - 32-ounce boxed vegetable or beef stock, 1 full sodium + 1 low sodium.
3. Bring fresh stock to a low boil in a clean pot and add all the above ingredients, except pasta and beans.
4. Once the soup starts to boil, add pasta and cook on a low boil for 30 minutes, until the pasta has cooked and vegetables have softened.
5. Add beans and adjust salt and pepper to taste. Add an additional 2 cups of stock if the soup is too thick. Top with fresh parsley if desired.

Enjoy!

MBK'S TIPS

If the soup is bitter add a tablespoon of brown sugar to cut the tomatoes' acidity. Always buy quality canned products and be sure the beans are organic. I puree whole San Marzano tomatoes in the Vitamix, before adding to the soup.

NUTRITION EXTRAS

This meal has plenty of plant-based protein to satisfy as a meatless meal. It's hearty and packed with nutrients and fiber, and all it needs is crusty bread and you have a meal.

GF*
DF
V *(OTHER THAN STOCK)*
LS

* *(option)*

mexican tortilla soup
8 Servings

THIS SOUP IS A MEAL IN ITSELF. Pick up fresh corn chips and tortillas at your local tortilleria and you have an authentic Mexican dinner. Arrange lots of toppings on your serving bar for guests to choose from such as sour cream, extra cilantro, cheese and fresh roasted chopped jalapeños.

3 tablespoons olive oil

5 corn tortillas, chopped

2 onions, chopped

2 jalapeño peppers, seeded and chopped

4 garlic cloves

2 tablespoons cumin

1½ quarts chicken stock *(3 cups full sodium + 3 cups reduced-sodium)*

2 - 28-ounce cans chopped tomatoes *(Muir-Glen fire-roasted preferred)*

1½ pounds raw chicken tenders *(breast meat)*, cut into bite-sized pieces

1 bag of roasted frozen corn

1 can organic black beans, drained and rinsed

1 tablespoon chili powder

¼ teaspoon black pepper

fresh cilantro, queso fresco and sour cream *(if desired)*

NUTRITION EXTRAS

The soup is loaded with chicken, so the protein component is there. Along with plenty of fiber from the beans and corn. You might want to serve a salad of dark greens to accompany the dish.

GF
LS

1. In large nonstick pot heat oil on medium heat. Add chopped tortillas, onions, jalapeños, garlic and cumin. Stirring occasionally, until the onions are translucent, approximately 5-8 minutes.

2. Add stock and tomatoes and bring it to a boil. Reduce heat and simmer for 30 minutes.

3. Puree soup with a handheld blender.

4. Bring soup back to simmer, then add chicken, roasted corn, black beans and spices. Cook for approximately 30 minutes until chicken finishes cooking.

5. Garnish with cilantro, queso fresco and sour cream *(if desired)*.

Enjoy!

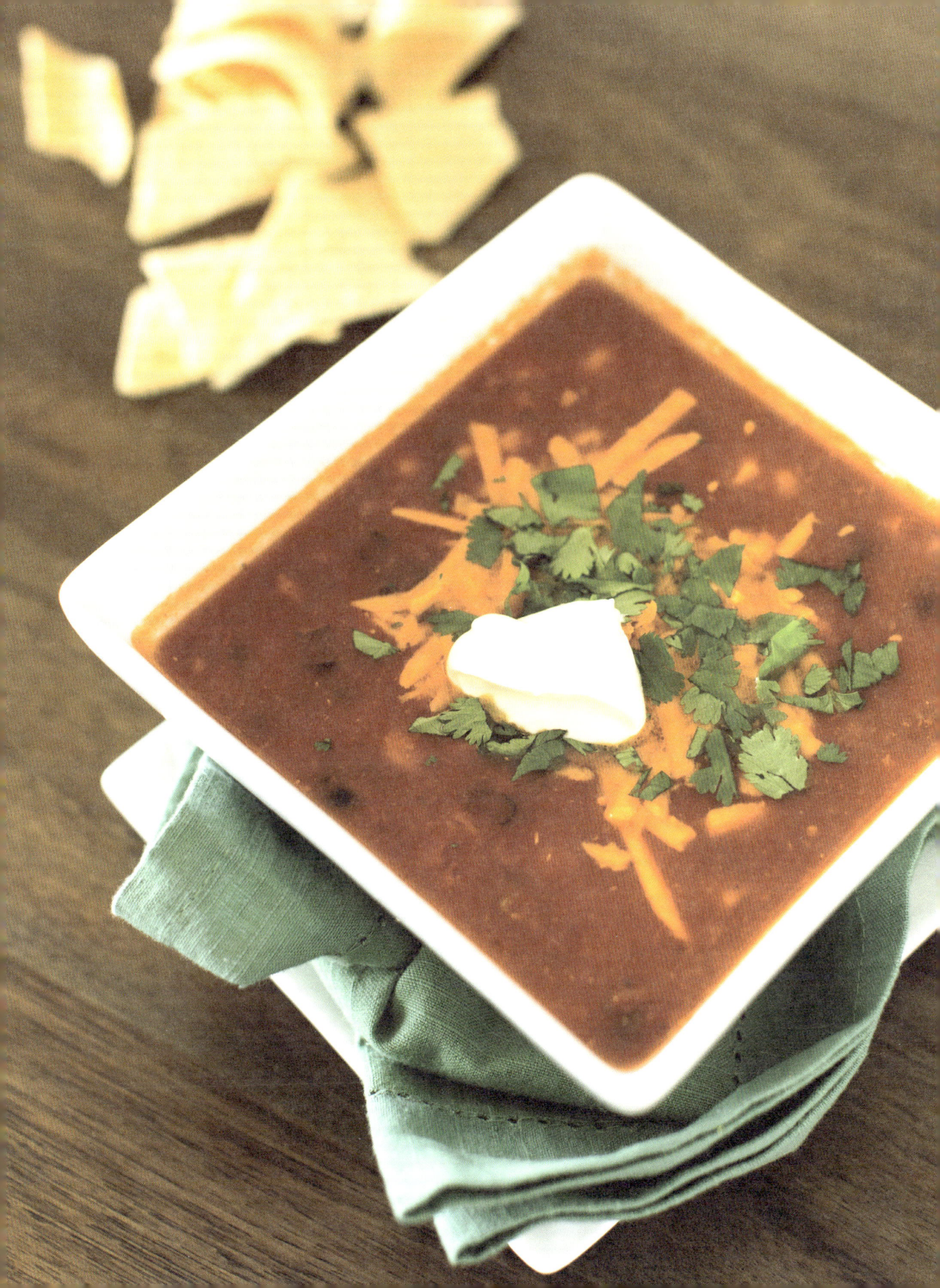

new orleans gumbo *with the works*

8 Servings

IT'S HARD TO CALL THIS A SOUP, as it is a full meal packed with protein, in a delicious broth that tastes like no other. I make this when I want to wow a guest or when my son Russell is in town for a visit from the west coast. His appetite is hard to fill, being 6'4" and very active. This recipe is one of his favorites! It takes some time and careful shopping to prepare for gumbo. Some of the spices are unique and the seafood needs to be fresh, but the result is worth the effort! Be sure to purchase authentic andouille sausage for the flavor permeates the gumbo when cooked. I love making large hearty meals where there are plenty of leftovers.

MBK'S TIPS

Don't forget the file powder, as it is a massive component to the flavor.

If you are unable to find fresh okra, look for the already cut frozen variety.

Be patient with the roux - it is the essence of gumbo.

NUTRITION EXTRAS

Loaded with fresh seafood and good quality protein. Oysters are also a great source of vitamin B12.

DF

- ½ cup all-purpose white flour
- ½ cup organic canola oil
- 2 medium sweet onions, chopped
- ½ tablespoon garlic, chopped
- 1½ cups celery, chopped
- 1 large green pepper, chopped
- 6 cups chicken stock
- 1 pound diced chicken breast tenders *(medium-size bites)*
- 1 pound andouille sausage, sliced into ½ inch rings
- 1 can of diced San Marzano tomatoes
- 1 to 2 cups okra, sliced
- 1 tablespoon + 1 teaspoon dried thyme
- 2 teaspoons white pepper
- 3 bay leaves
- 1 generous teaspoon cayenne pepper *(more or less depending on personal preference)*
- 2 teaspoons oregano
- 1 pound cleaned, deveined, raw shrimp
- 1 pound fresh oysters
- 2 tablespoons file powder
- additional salt and fresh pepper to taste
- rice of choice, prepared as directed

1. In a large heavy stock-pot stir together flour and oil until smooth. Cook over medium-high heat for 4 minutes, constantly stirring. Reduce heat to medium and continue to cook, stirring constantly, approximately 15 minutes or until roux is dark red-brown.

2. Add onion, garlic, celery and green pepper. Saute vegetables until softened, approximately 5-7 minutes.

3. Add chicken broth, chicken, sausage, tomatoes, okra and all spices and cook on a low boil for 1 hour.

4. Add seafood and file powder and cook for an additional 20-30 minutes. Cook until all flavors are combined and meat and seafood is cooked all the way through. Adjust seasonings to taste.

5. Serve over prepared rice of choice!

Enjoy!

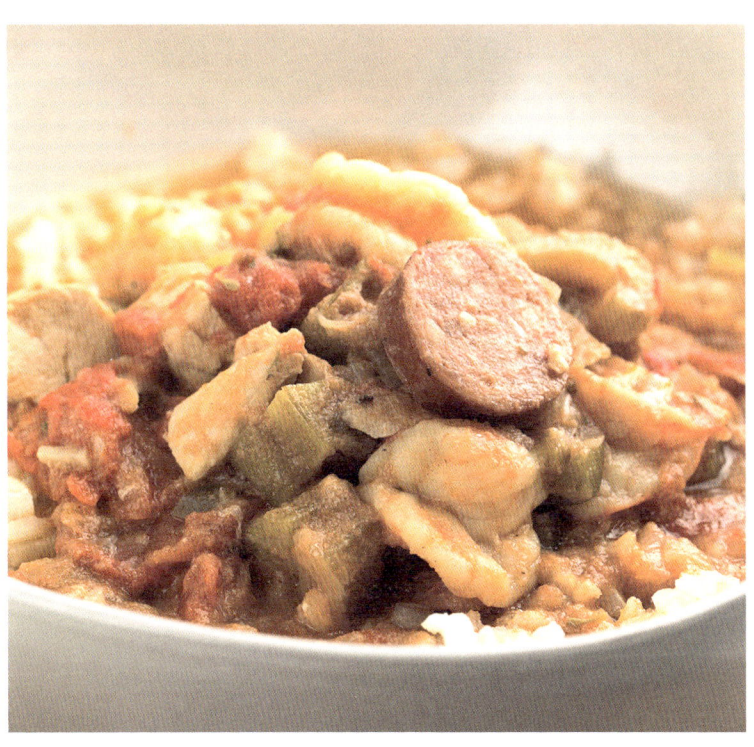

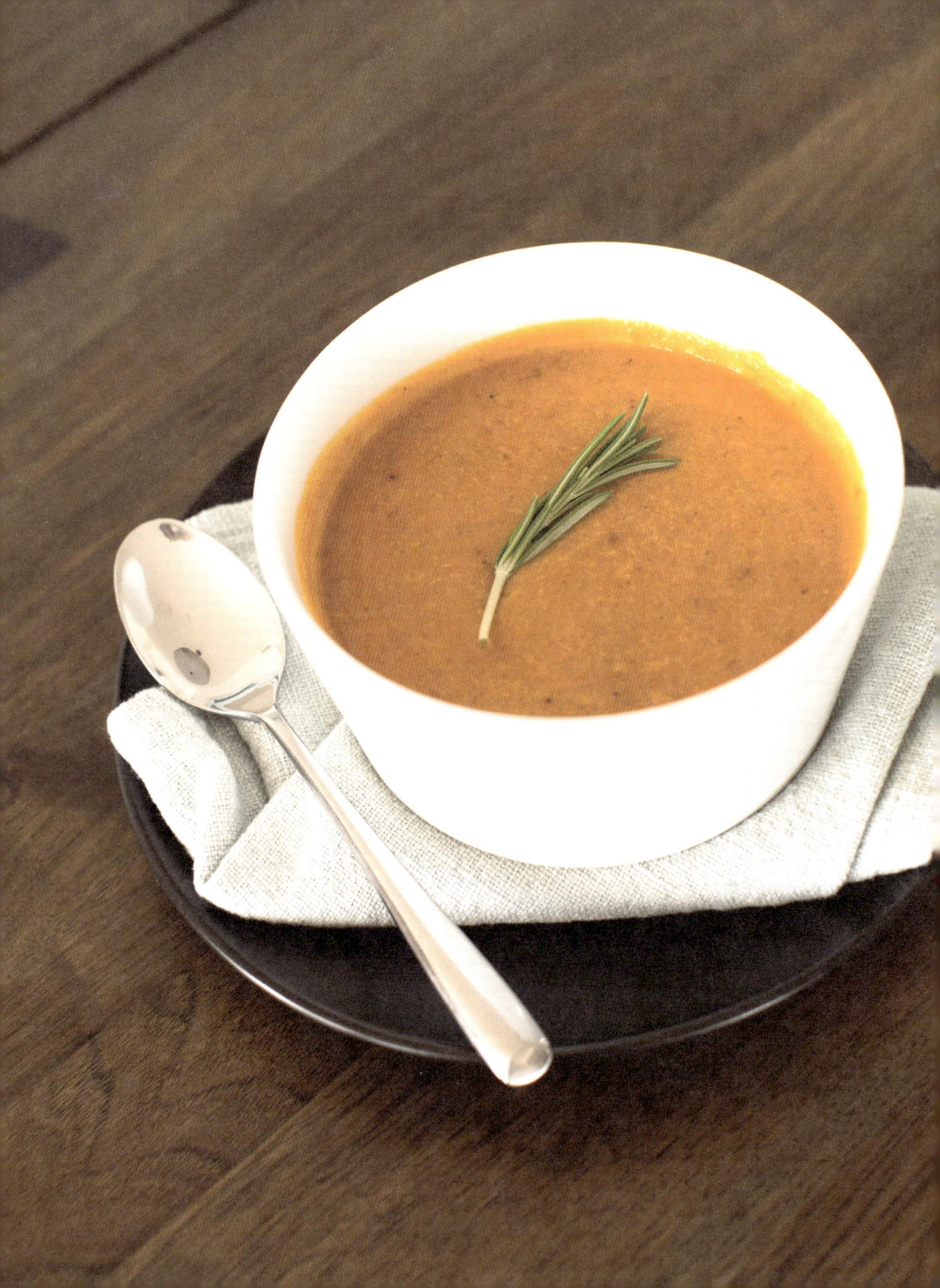

pumpkin soup
8-10 servings

EVERY FALL AROUND OCTOBER 1ST, when the weather in the mid-Atlantic starts to turn cold, I crave this soup without fail. My friend Ziba still talks about this soup that I used to serve at fundraiser meetings in which we were both involved. This soup and my chocolate covered graham's made her very happy *(recipe in the dessert section)*. During those years of hosting many meetings at my home, a hearty cheese plate with assorted crackers and a big bowl of soup made for a nice lunch.

- 4 slices nitrate-free bacon, chopped
- 3 tablespoons olive oil
- 2 large onions, chopped
- 2 medium carrots, chopped
- 2 celery stalks, chopped
- 8 cups chicken stock (4 full sodium + 4 reduced sodium)
- 2 - 16-ounce cans organic pumpkin puree
- 2 tablespoons fresh thyme, chopped
- 1 cup either half and half or evaporated fat-free milk
- ½ teaspoon ground nutmeg
- additional salt and ground pepper to taste

NUTRITION EXTRAS

Rich in vitamin A, vitamin C and potassium. Makes for a very nutritious bowl of soup.

Not very high in plant-based protein, so keep that in mind when serving as a meal.

GF *(omit croutons)*
LS

1. In a large heavy-duty soup pot saute bacon for approximately 8 minutes. Pour off drippings.
2. Add olive oil, onions, carrots, and celery to pan on medium high and saute vegetables until tender, approximately 15 minutes.
3. Stir in stock, pumpkin, and thyme and boil on a low boil for 20 minutes.
4. Puree soup with hand-held mixer, then add half and half and nutmeg. If the soup is too thick, add additional stock. Adjust seasonings to taste.
5. Serve with parmesan croutons.

Enjoy!

asparagus soup

6 Servings

ASPARAGUS IS OUR FIRST SIGN OF LIFE IN THE SPRING after a long winter of limited fresh vegetables. I usually cannot wait to make all things asparagus, including this soup. This soup is loaded with fiber and acts as a natural diuretic, so it is a wholesome detox for the body, which also feels right in the spring. If looking to have only soup for your lunch or dinner you can add fresh shrimp or scallops on top to complete the meal.

MBK'S TIPS

Snap the asparagus to rid the bitter ends from being added to the soup.

olive oil for sautéing
(2-3 tablespoons)

1 medium sweet onion, chopped

1 leek, white part only, cleaned and cut into ½ inch rings

2 garlic cloves, minced

2 pounds fresh asparagus, trimmed and cut into 2-inch pieces

½ cup fresh parsley, chopped

½ cup baby bella mushrooms, diced

5-6 cups good quality chicken stock *(reduced sodium)*

¼ cup half and half

additional water, if necessary

additional sea salt and ground pepper to taste

NUTRITION EXTRAS

Rich in vitamin A, C, K and folate and contains lots of fiber and small amounts of protein.

GF
LS

1. Heat oil on medium heat in a large non-stick soup pot. Add onion and leek to the hot pan, cooking until vegetables soften and start to caramelize, approximately 7 to 10 minutes.

2. Add garlic and continue cooking for 2 minutes.

3. Add asparagus, parsley, mushrooms and chicken stock and cook on low boil until vegetables are soft and can be blended.

4. Use your handheld blender and puree the soup.

5. Add half and half and adjust seasoning. If the soup is too thick add a half to a full cup of water. Adjust seasonings to taste.

Enjoy!

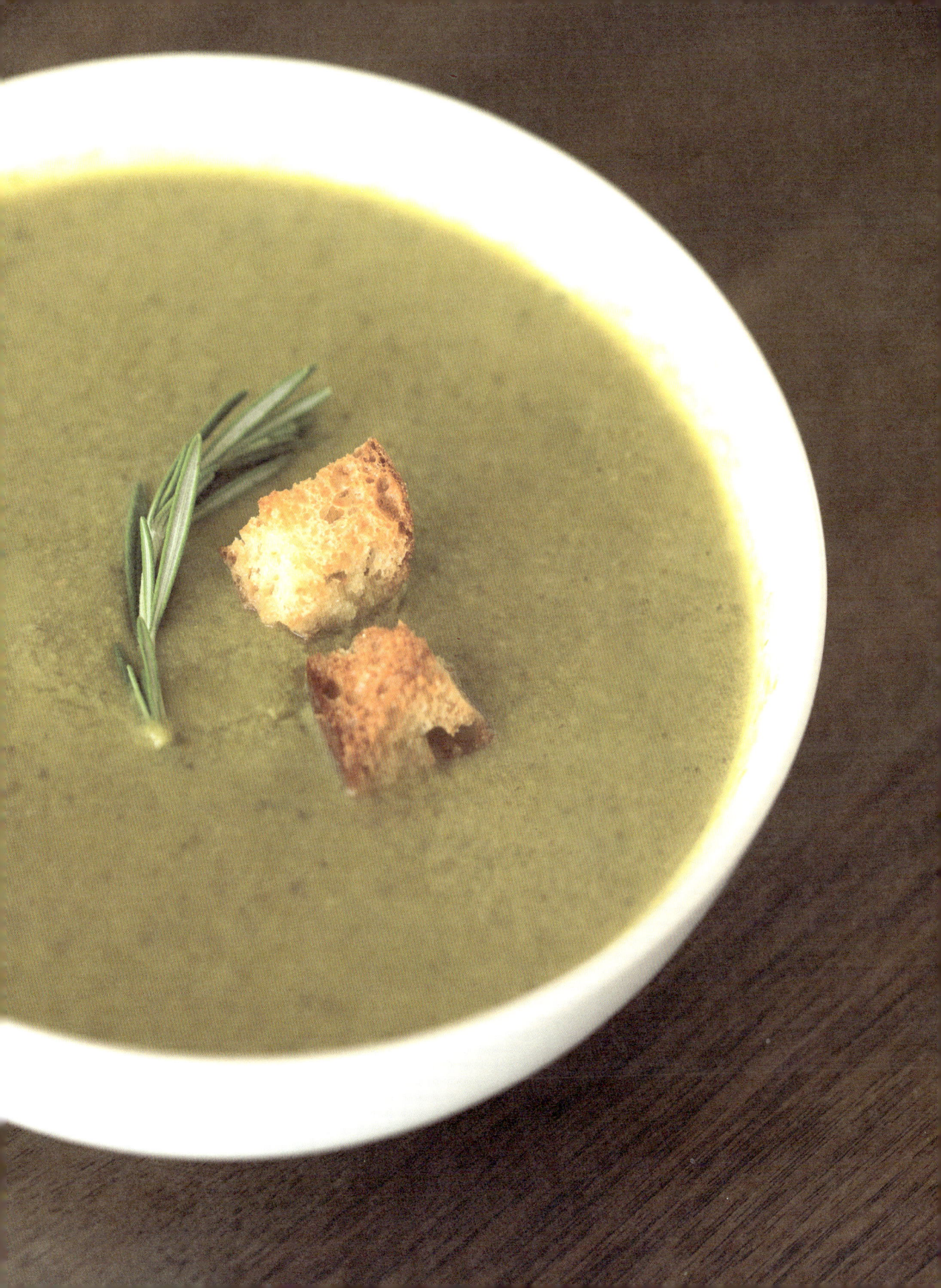

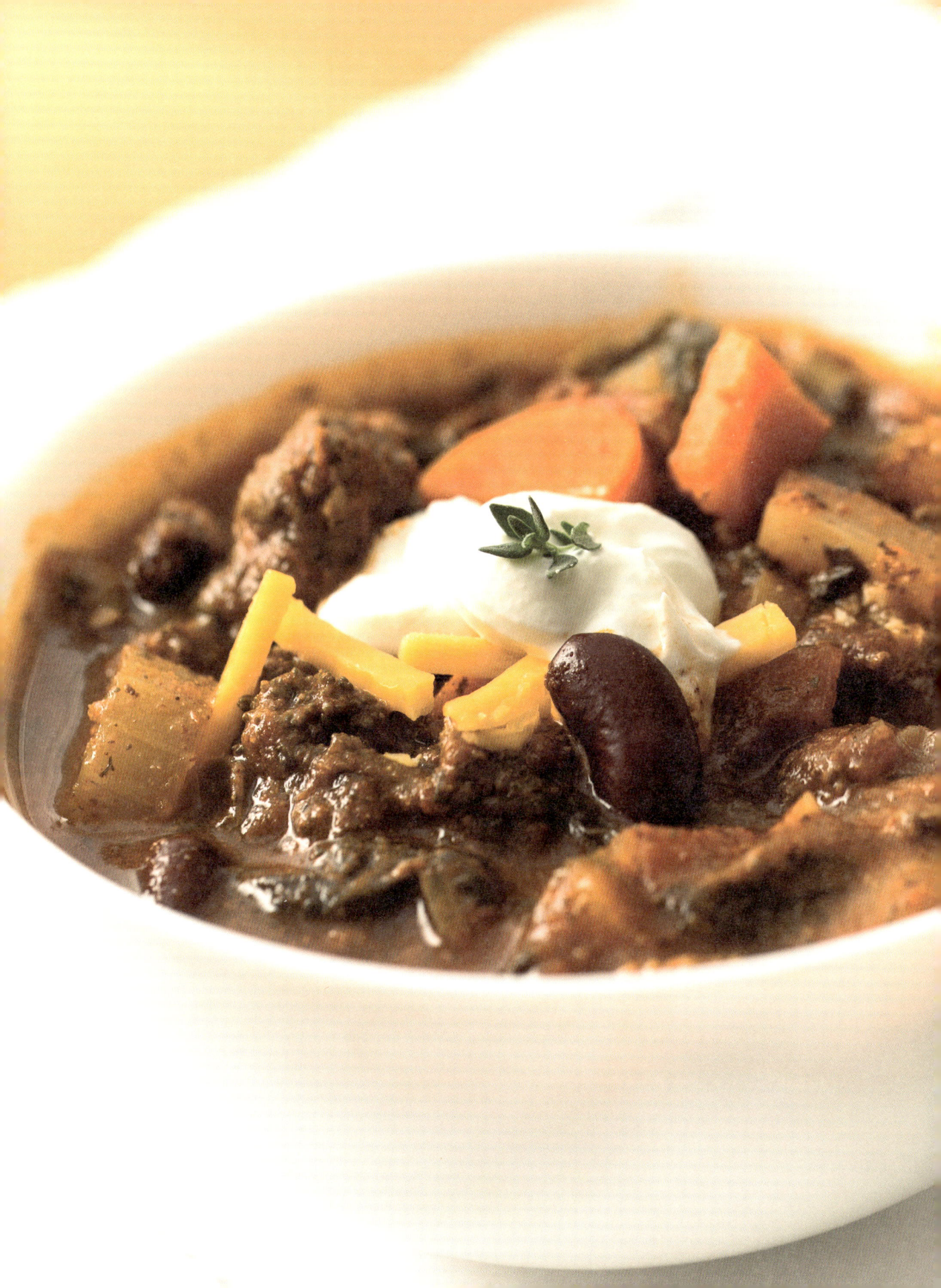

turkey chili

Serves a crowd
8 generous portions

THIS RECIPE IS THE MOST POPULAR REQUEST from my clients. Whether you are trying to lose weight or not, everyone loves a healthy version of a hearty bowl of chili. This recipe is loaded with vegetables, and eating a big bowl provides plenty of satisfaction and none of the guilt. It's a standard in my house during the cold winter months, and the leftovers are perfect for a quick lunch. Substituting any other ground meat, such as lamb, beef, or bison, works just as well. Test the spice and adjust according to your preference.

olive oil

1 pound ground turkey

½ pound turkey sausage

1 large onion diced

2-3 celery stalks diced

3 carrots, diced

1 pound bite-size broccoli florets *(can be frozen)*

½ bag frozen spinach

½ bag of frozen corn

1 - 28-ounce can of crushed tomatoes

1 - 15-ounce can tomato sauce + 1 cup water

¼ cup chili powder

1 tablespoon cumin

1 tablespoon dill

2 teaspoons oregano

1 teaspoons cayenne *(or more if you like heat)*

1 teaspoon tumeric

1 can red kidney beans, rinsed and drained

salt to taste

sour cream and shredded cheddar cheese, if desired

1. Heat 2 tablespoons olive oil in a large pot and brown meat, onion, celery and carrots. Drain fat.

2. Add all additional ingredients, except kidney beans and simmer on low for 30-40 minutes.

3. Add kidney beans 10 minutes before serving. Depending on canned tomato products, you may not need any additional salt. Taste before adding.

4. Top with a dollop of sour cream and shredded cheddar cheese, if desired.

Enjoy!

MBK'S TIPS

Add ancho chili powder for additional heat and spice.

NUTRITION EXTRAS

This meal has it all because it is loaded with fiber, protein, and packed with nutrient-rich vegetables. You can eliminate the cheese if you prefer dairy-free.

GF
DF*
LS

* *(option)*

summer farmer's market corn chowder
6-8 Servings

THE REASON THIS IS SUMMER CHOWDER is because of the delicious fresh corn that comes up half-way through the season in Maryland and is exquisite in every form. The rest of the ingredients are replaceable, depending upon what you have on hand. I love the flavor of poblano peppers, especially with the fresh corn, so I would not swap those out. I like to serve this hearty vegetable soup with a side of grilled shrimp and a fresh green salad. It tastes even better when eating outside on a summer night.

- 6 strips good quality nitrate-free bacon
- 2 tablespoons olive oil
- 1 large sweet onion, chopped
- 2 garlic cloves, pressed
- 6 ears of corn, cut raw off the husk
- 2 celery stalks, diced
- 2 poblano peppers, seeded and chopped
- 4 cups of vegetable stock
- 2 large or 4 medium yukon potatoes, cut into small cubes
- 1 bay leaf
- 1 can condensed milk
- 1 cup organic whole milk
- salt and pepper to taste
- fresh thyme or dill, if desired

MBK'S TIPS

To avoid having kernals flying all around your kitchen when cutting the corn from the cob, place the corn in a large, deep bowl with a flat bottom surface.

GF

1. Saute bacon in a soup pot until crisp and fat has been rendered. Remove from pan for later use.

2. Use rendered fat and additional olive oil to sauté onion, garlic, corn, celery and peppers. Cook until softened and just starting to brown on the bottom of pot, approximately 7 minutes.

3. Add stock, potatoes, bay leaf, condensed milk and milk and simmer until potatoes are soft and flavors have developed, approximately 20 minutes.

4. Adjust seasoning with salt and fresh pepper to taste. Ladle soup and top with reserved bacon and fresh herbs of choice.

Enjoy!

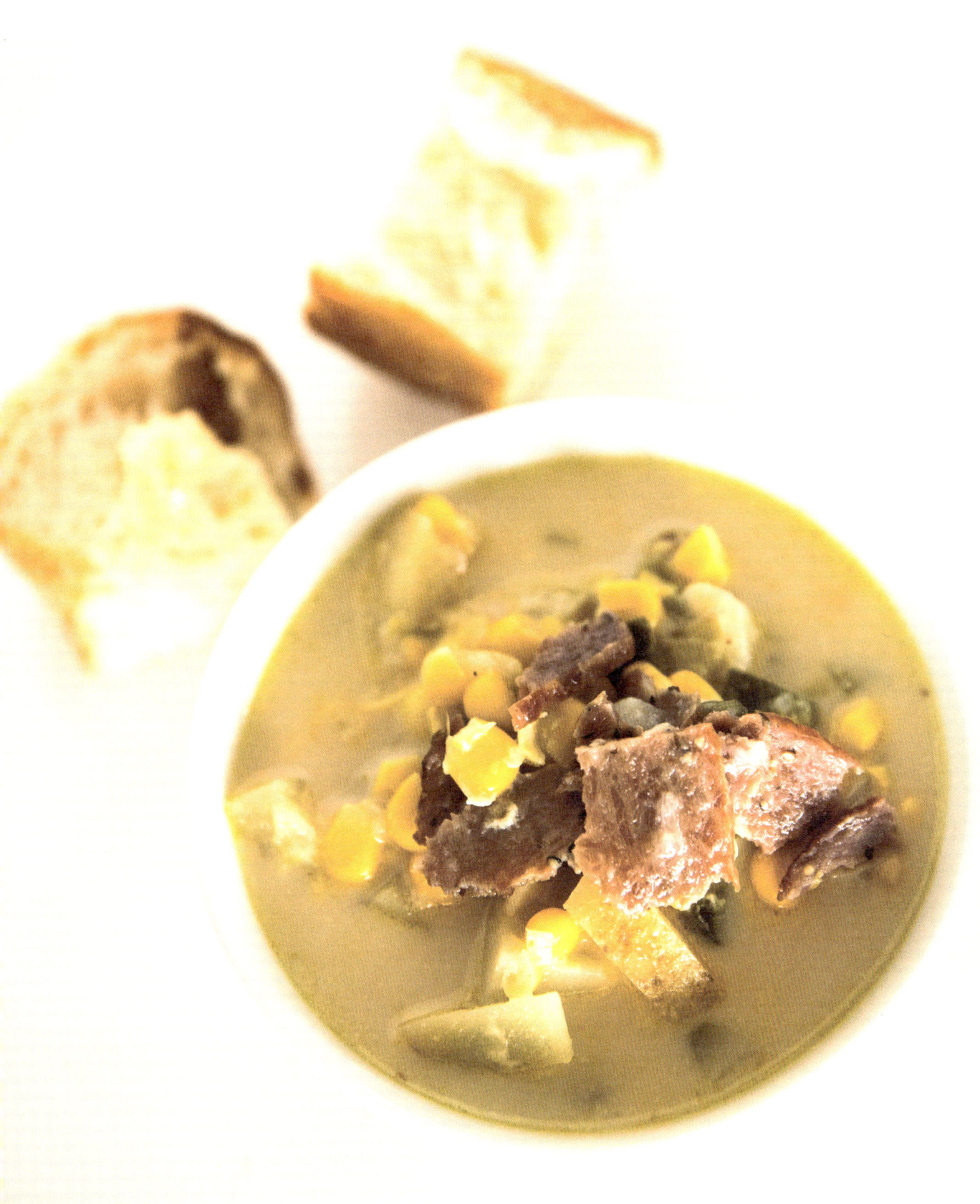

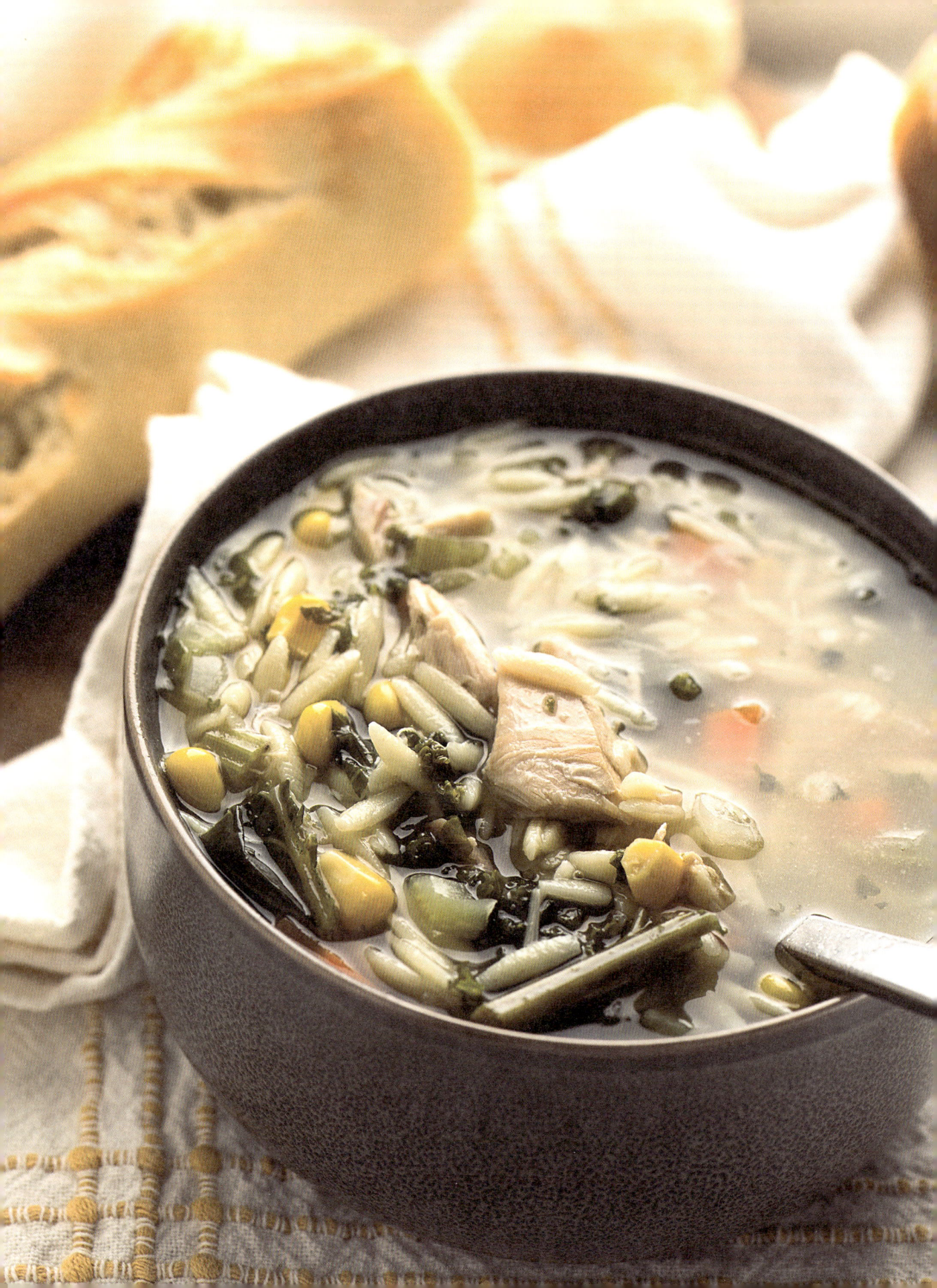

turkey orzo soup

Serves a crowd
8 generous portions

THIS SOUP IS A LABOR OF LOVE, only because it takes all day to cook the leftover turkey carcass from your Thanksgiving bird. Your home will smell like the holiday all over again, as the broth permeates the indoor air. I find this soup to be vibrant with flavor and always wonder why I wait until Thanksgiving to make it. If the stock is evaporating too quickly, add more water as needed throughout the day. It will keep for a good week in the refrigerator and makes for delicious leftovers if you have lingering holiday guests.

STOCK
leftover turkey bones

SOUP
- 1 large sweet onion, diced
- 3 carrots, diced
- 3 full celery stalks, diced
- 2 cups frozen sweet corn
- 2 cups fresh or frozen spinach, chopped
- 2 cups leftover turkey, diced
- 2 teaspoons dried thyme
- 1 cup dried orzo
- salt and pepper to taste

1. Cook turkey bones in a covered slow cooker or large dutch oven for 6+ hours on low heat. You may want to add vegetables such as onion, carrot and celery or aromatic herbs for additional flavor, while stock is simmering.

2. Drain stock into a clean soup pot yielding approximately 3 quarts of liquid *(you can use good quality boxed turkey bone broth as a substitute)*.

3. Add all soup ingredients, except orzo, and boil on low for 20 minutes.

4. Add orzo and continue to cook on a low boil, until the pasta has finished cooking.

5. After 30 minutes, adjust seasonings if needed.

Enjoy!

MBK'S TIPS

Don't worry if your bird has stuffing in the carcass, it just adds to the flavor of the stock.

I may throw in some leftover sage and a whole onion, while the turkey bones simmer.

Drain with a very fine sieve when you are ready to make the soup.

NUTRITION EXTRAS

Collagen from bone broth is good for our hair, skin, and nails. It is the most abundant protein in the human body.

DF

CHAPTER 4
salads & dressings

summer caprese salad 87

quinoa with black beans and nectarine 88

white bean and farro salad 91

quinoa with kale, mixed vegetables, and garbazo beans 92

white bean and tuna salad 95

southwest quinoa salad 96

celery and fennel salad 99

broccoli and mushroom salad 100

with shrimp 103

kale and shaved brussels sprouts salad with cranberry vinaigrette 104

basic balsamic vinaigrette 107

basil lemon vinaigrette 107

fajita marinade 108

MIXED GREENS ARE A STAPLE ON MY TABLE ALMOST daily. I start with a variety of fresh lettuces, add some purple cabbage and chopped celery, and build from there. The best foods for optimal health are colorful fruits and vegetables. I can't imagine a better way to get a large variety of vitamins and nutrients than a large bountiful salad, either for lunch or dinner. I don't have this salad in a recipe, because it changes daily, but you get my point.

These recipes provided add more options to the daily ritual. My basic dressings, located at the end of the chapter, are always made fresh and kept in the refrigerator for up to 4 weeks. Having your dressings made ahead of time, makes pulling a quick lunch or dinner together, that much easier.

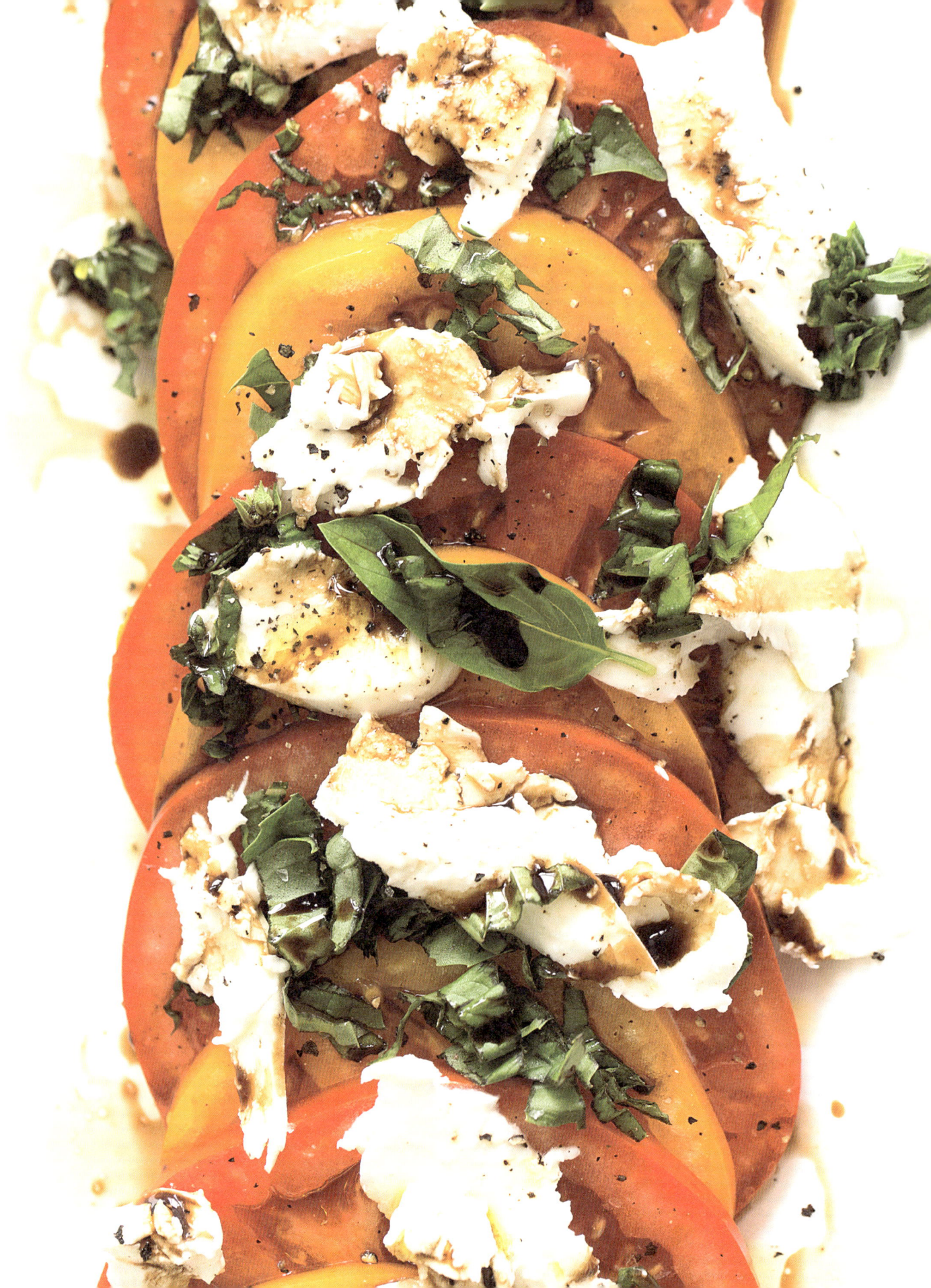

summer caprese salad

THIS SALAD IS A STAPLE IN MY HOUSE when fresh tomatoes are in season. During the summer, fresh basil is always in my kitchen and tomatoes and basil call my name from mid-July, through August. The two are an excellent food combination that never gets old. Be sure to have good crusty bread to dip up all the extra balsamic vinaigrette.

2-3 large summer tomatoes

4 ounces shaved fresh mozzarella

¼ cup fresh basil rolled and cut into ribbons

3 tablespoons aged balsamic vinegar

2 tablespoons extra virgin olive oil

salt and fresh pepper to taste

NUTRITION EXTRAS

Be sure to buy a high quality balsamic vinegar that is from Modena. You want the richness and the sweetness from a thick aged vinegar to pair with rich organic olive oil.

GF

1. Slice and layer tomatoes, cheese, and basil in a symmetric pattern.
2. Drizzle with balsamic then olive oil. Sprinkle with sea salt and pepper.
3. Serve with crusty bread.

Enjoy!

quinoa with black beans
4-6 servings
& nectarine

THE REASON I HAVE THREE RECIPES FOR QUINOA in the book, is to showcase this grain's incredible versatility *(which is a pseudo-cereal and not considered a grain at all)*. I love having this salad ready in the refrigerator, either eating alone or in combination with other salads. This dish is a great post-workout snack or quick bite when hungry between meals.

NUTRITION EXTRAS

This plant-based protein packs a punch with 9 grams of protein per one-cup serving. It's also a good source of antioxidants and minerals such as manganese, phosphorous, and copper.

GF
DF
V
LS

- 1 cup cooked quinoa, prepared according to package directions
- 2 tablespoons extra virgin olive oil
- 2 tablespoons white balsamic vinegar
- 1 tablespoon red or champagne vinegar
- juice of 1 lime
- sea salt and fresh pepper to taste
- 1 can organic black beans, drained and rinsed
- 1 nectarine, pitted and diced
- ½ red bell pepper, seeded and diced
- ½ cup radishes, chopped
- ½ cup cilantro, chopped

1. Cook quinoa according to directions, let cool.
2. Mix oil, vinegar, lime, salt and pepper in a medium-size serving bowl.
3. Add all additional ingredients along with the cooked quinoa into the vinaigrette. Mix well and refrigerate for several hours, until desired temperature.

Enjoy!

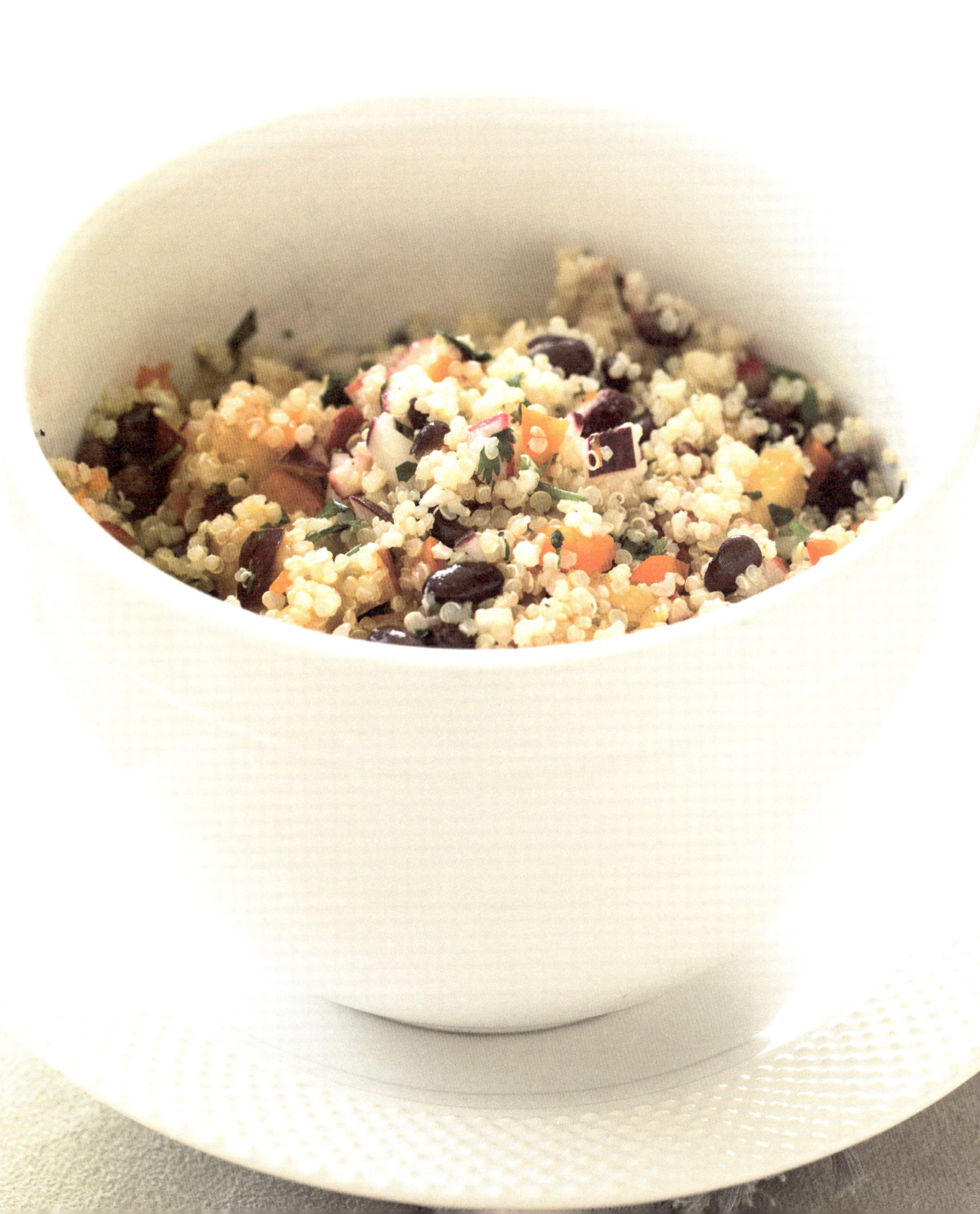

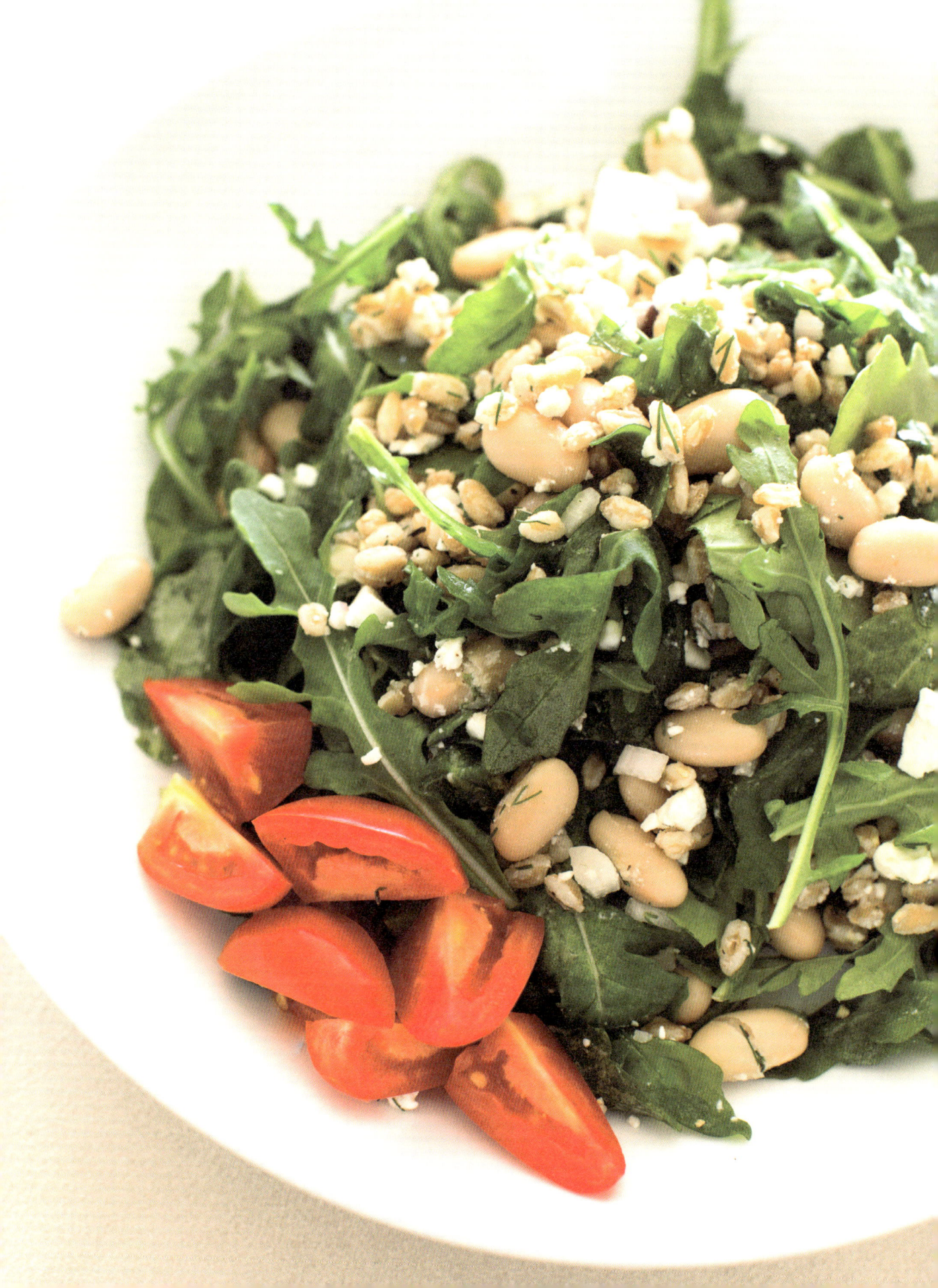

white bean & farro salad

4 servings

THIS SALAD IS A GREAT VEGETARIAN DISH *(providing cheese is allowed)* that supplies lots of fiber-rich protein in a tasty vinaigrette, along with peppery arugula. The combination is so satisfying and plenty filling. I keep lots of varieties of beans in the pantry for quick salads and lunch alternatives. The fresh dill pulls it all together.

- 1½ cups cooked farro
- 1 - 15-ounce can organic cannellini beans, drained and rinsed
- 1 small shallot, thinly sliced
- ¼ cup olive oil
- ¼ cup sherry vinegar
- ½ teaspoon seal salt and pepper to taste
- 5 ounces baby arugula
- 4 ounces feta cheese, crumbled
- 3 tablespoons fresh dill, chopped

1. Cook farro according to directions, drain, rinse and allow to cool.
2. Toss farro, beans, shallot, oil, vinegar, salt and pepper in a large bowl.
3. Let stand for 15 minutes before adding arugula and feta.
4. Toss gently and top with fresh dill.

Enjoy!

MBK'S TIPS

Partially processed farro is easy to keep in your pantry and cooks up relatively quickly. Check your direction before purchasing, if you are looking for the quicker version.

NUTRITION EXTRAS

Farro is an ancient whole grain, famous for its use in Middle Eastern and Italian cuisine. It has a beautiful chestnut hue, especially when the bran and husk are left intact. Farro is loaded with fiber, protein and vitamin B3.

LS

quinoa with kale
mixed vegetables & garbanzo beans
8 servings

THE REASON I HAVE THREE RECIPES FOR QUINOA in the book is to showcase this grain's incredible versatility *(which is a pseudo-cereal and not considered a grain at all)*. I love having this salad ready in the refrigerator, either eating alone or in combination with other salads. It's a great post-workout snack or quick bite when hungry between meals.

MBK'S TIPS

This recipe is a hefty serving and should be made when you need to serve a big group. Quinoa only stays fresh for a few days, so cut the recipe in half if you are making this for two people.

NUTRITION EXTRAS

This plant-based protein packs a punch, with 9 grams of protein per one-cup serving. It's also a good source of antioxidants and minerals such as manganese, phosphorous and copper.

GF
DF
V
LS

- 2 cups dry quinoa, rinsed and prepared as directed
- 2 cups chopped fresh kale, stems removed
- 1 cup purple cabbage, shredded
- ½ seedless English cucumber, peeled and diced
- 3 stalks of celery, diced
- 6 cherry tomatoes, diced
- ½ avocado, peeled and diced
- 1 can organic garbanzo beans, drained and rinsed
- 2-3 lemons, juiced
- ¼ cup olive oil
- salt and pepper to taste
- 3 tablespoons fresh herbs *(parsley, thyme, or tarragon)*

1. Make quinoa, let cool.
2. Add all remaining ingredients to large bowl along with cooled quinoa.
3. Mix and refrigerate.

* *If salad gets dry on second or third day, add more lemon. Adjust seasoning.*

Enjoy!

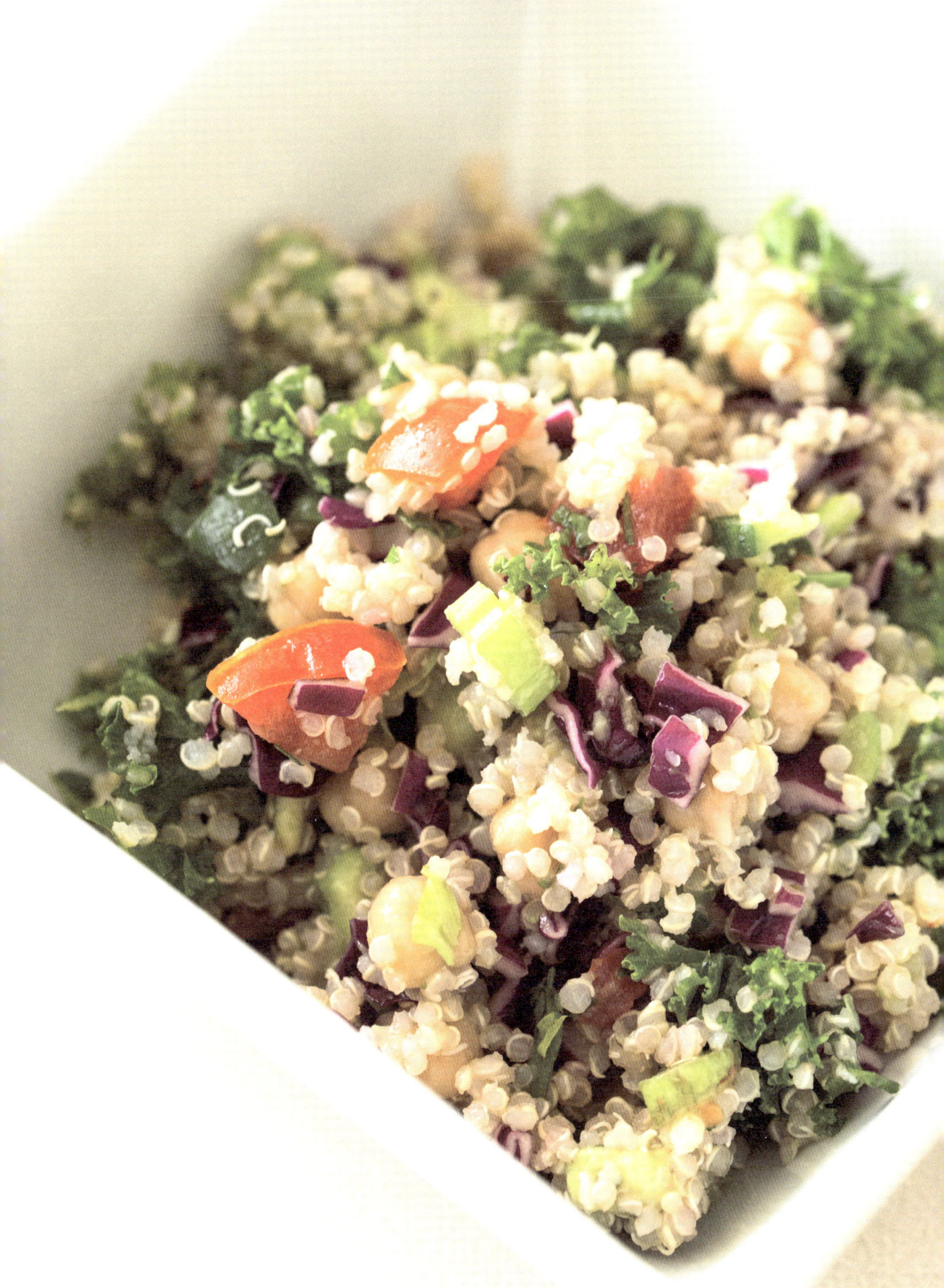

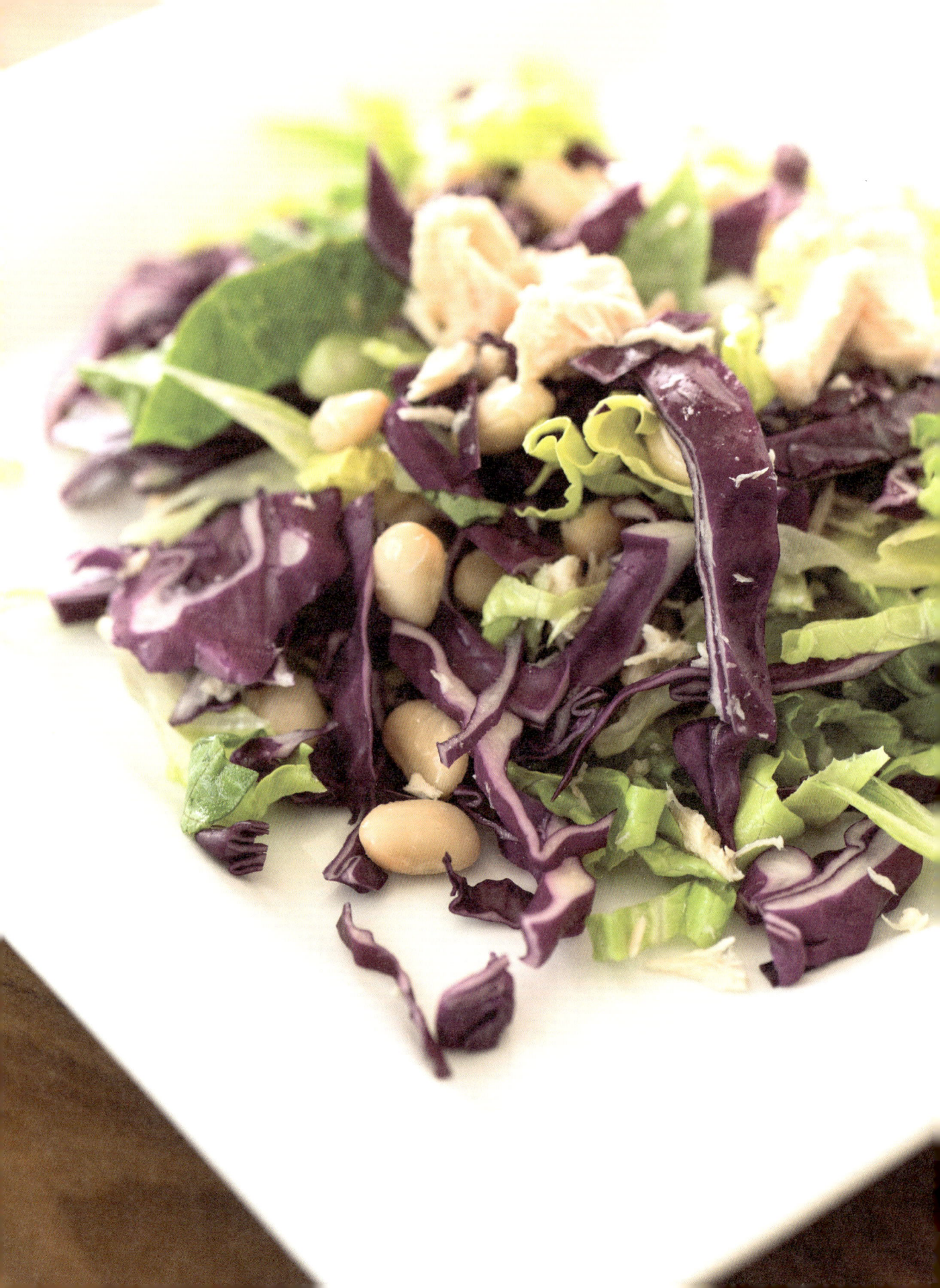

white bean & tuna salad
4 servings

THIS SALAD DOES NOT ONLY PRESENT WELL with its colorful display, it's also delicious. It's easy to pull together and looks impressive if you are serving guests. Boston lettuce is buttery and mild and works well with the cabbage and celery, which are much more robust in flavor.

- 1 half of medium head of purple cabbage, cored and shredded
- 1 head of Boston lettuce or other leafy green, shredded
- 1 - 15-ounce can cannellini beans, drained and rinsed
- 2 celery stalks, thinly sliced on a diagonal
- 1 can good quality tuna, drained and broken into large pieces
- fresh parsley for garnish

LEMON VINAIGRETTE DRESSING:
combine the following and whisk until emulsified

- $\frac{1}{3}$ cup olive oil
- 3 tablespoons fresh lemon juice
- 1 tablespoon champagne vinegar
- 1 garlic clove, crushed
- salt and pepper to taste

MBK'S TIPS

Keep plenty of sustainable good quality canned tuna in your pantry. When the refrigerator is running low you always have a high-quality protein that you can turn into several quick dishes.

NUTRITION EXTRAS

Loaded with protein from the beans and tuna. Great post-workout lunch that is not too filling.

GF
DF
LS

1. Combine first five ingredients and toss lightly with vinaigrette.
2. Top with fresh parsley.

Enjoy!

southwest quinoa salad
4-6 servings

THE REASON I HAVE THREE RECIPES FOR QUINOA in the book is to showcase this grain's incredible versatility *(which is a pseudo-cereal and not considered a grain at all)*. I love having this salad ready in the refrigerator, either eating alone or in combination with other salads. It's a great post-workout snack, or quick bite when hungry between meals.

NUTRITION EXTRAS

This plant-based protein packs a punch, with 9 grams of protein per one-cup serving.

It's also a good source of antioxidants and minerals such as manganese, phosphorous and copper.

GF
DF
V
LS

1 cup quinoa, prepared as instructed

juice of 2-3 fresh limes

4 tablespoons good quality olive oil

1 can of organic black beans, drained and rinsed

1 medium tomato, diced

1 ripe avocado, diced

⅓ cup fresh cilantro, chopped

1 jalapeno, diced

sea salt and fresh black pepper to taste

1. Prepare quinoa, fluff with a fork and let cool.
2. Add all ingredients and mix well.
3. Serve immediately at room temperature or refrigerate for 2 hours.

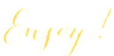

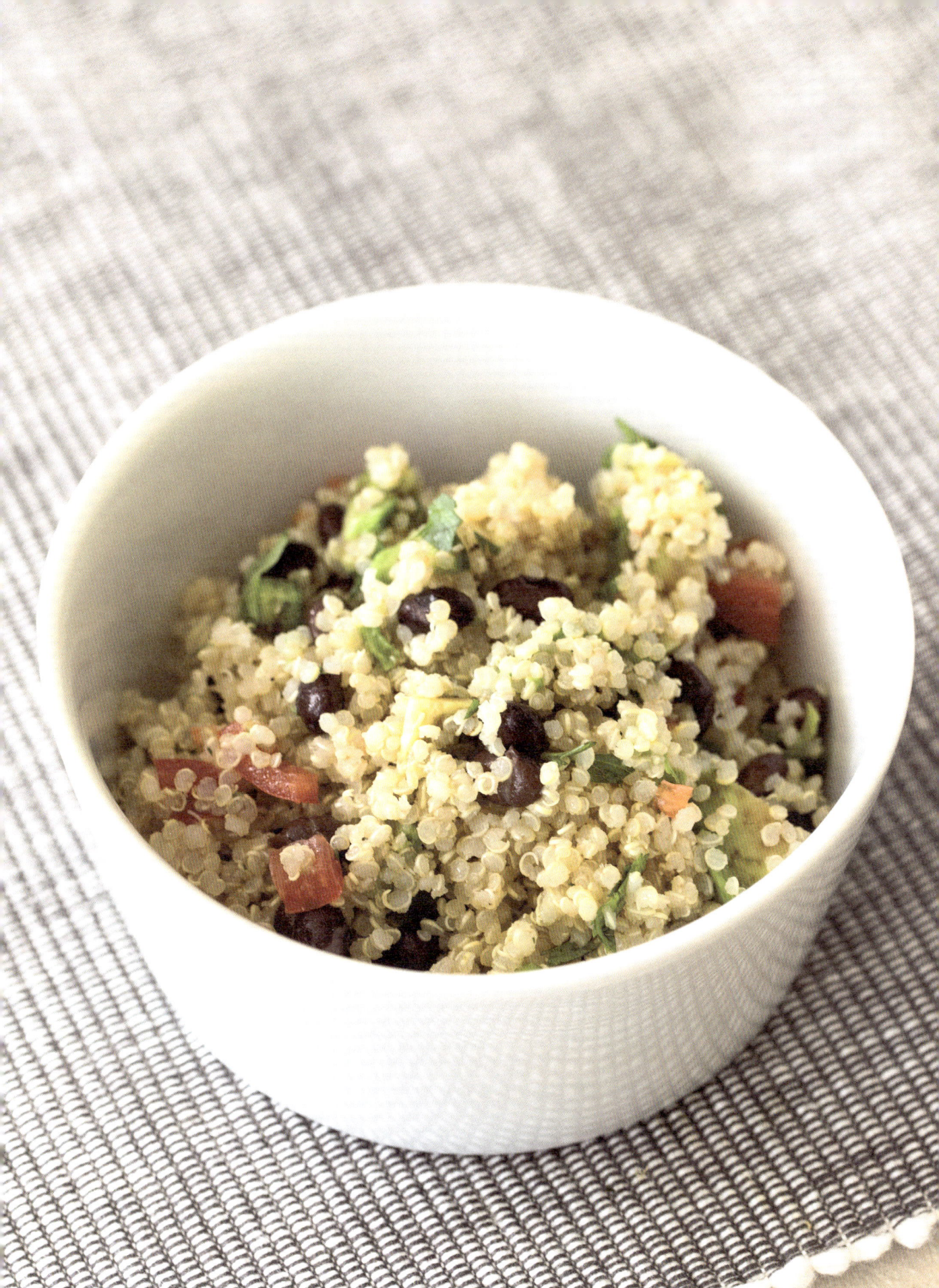

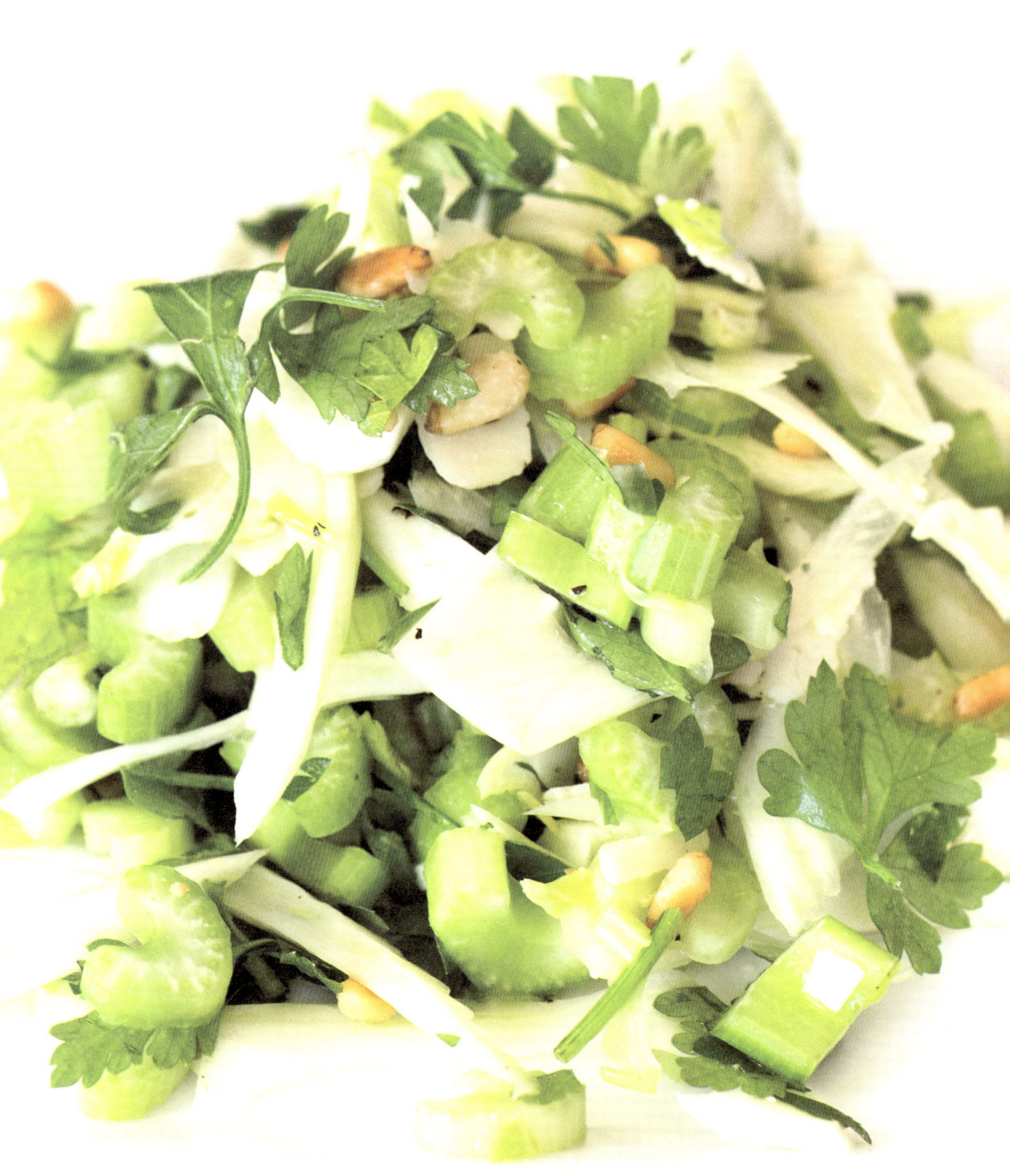

celery & fennel salad

Serves 4

THIS IS A LIGHT SALAD THAT IS NOT MEANT TO BE a meal in itself. It makes a beautiful tart side dish. Raw fennel tastes completely different than roasted fennel and brings a subtle licorice flavor to the salad. Be sure to mix the dressing well before tossing with the vegetables and adjust seasoning - this will ensure that it's not too lemony and strong, as that will only bring out a bitterness to the fennel. This salad is crunchy and delicious and goes perfectly with grilled prawns.

MBK'S TIPS

It's best to use a mandolin to slice the vegetables as thin as possible, but if you do not have access, a sharp knife also works well.

- 1 large fennel bulb, trimmed and very thinly sliced
- 6 celery stalks, very thinly sliced
- ½ cup fresh flat-leaf parsley leaves with tender stems
- 3 tablespoons fresh lemon juice, mixed thoroughly with 5 tablespoons of olive oil
- 3 ounces parmesan, shaved
- ¼ cup pine nuts, toasted
- sea salt and fresh pepper to taste

NUTRITION EXTRAS

Celery is high in vitamin A and vitamin C, along with fiber, magnesium and potassium. Fennel has some natural sugars.

GF
LS

1. Toss all ingredients in a large serving bowl. Season with salt and pepper.

Enjoy!

broccoli & mushroom salad

6 servings

THIS DISH WAS BROUGHT TO ME BY A GOOD FRIEND, Nancy Powell, who I started a book club with over 20 years ago. We have shared many meals and even established a dinner club together that continued for many years. I love that this recipe can be made ahead of time and is an excellent addition to a buffet. If you enjoy these two vegetables, you will be surprised how good this crunchy marinaded salad will taste.

MBK'S TIPS

You can transfer the salad to a heavy ziplock bag and refridgerate a day ahead of intended use.

- ⅓ cup olive oil
- ⅓ cup apple cider vinegar
- 2 teaspoons sugar
- sea salt and fresh pepper to taste
- 1 head broccoli, cut into bite-size florets
- 10 ounces mushrooms of your choice, sliced
- ½ red onion, thinly sliced
- 1 tablespoon of any fresh herbs of your choice

NUTRITION EXTRAS

Eating the broccoli raw, does not destroy the vitamin C. It's loaded with both vitamin C and K, along with folate and Iron.

1. In a large bowl whisk together the first four ingredients.
2. Add broccoli, mushrooms, onion and herbs. Toss and marinate for at least 8 hours. Serve cold.

Enjoy!

GF
DF
V

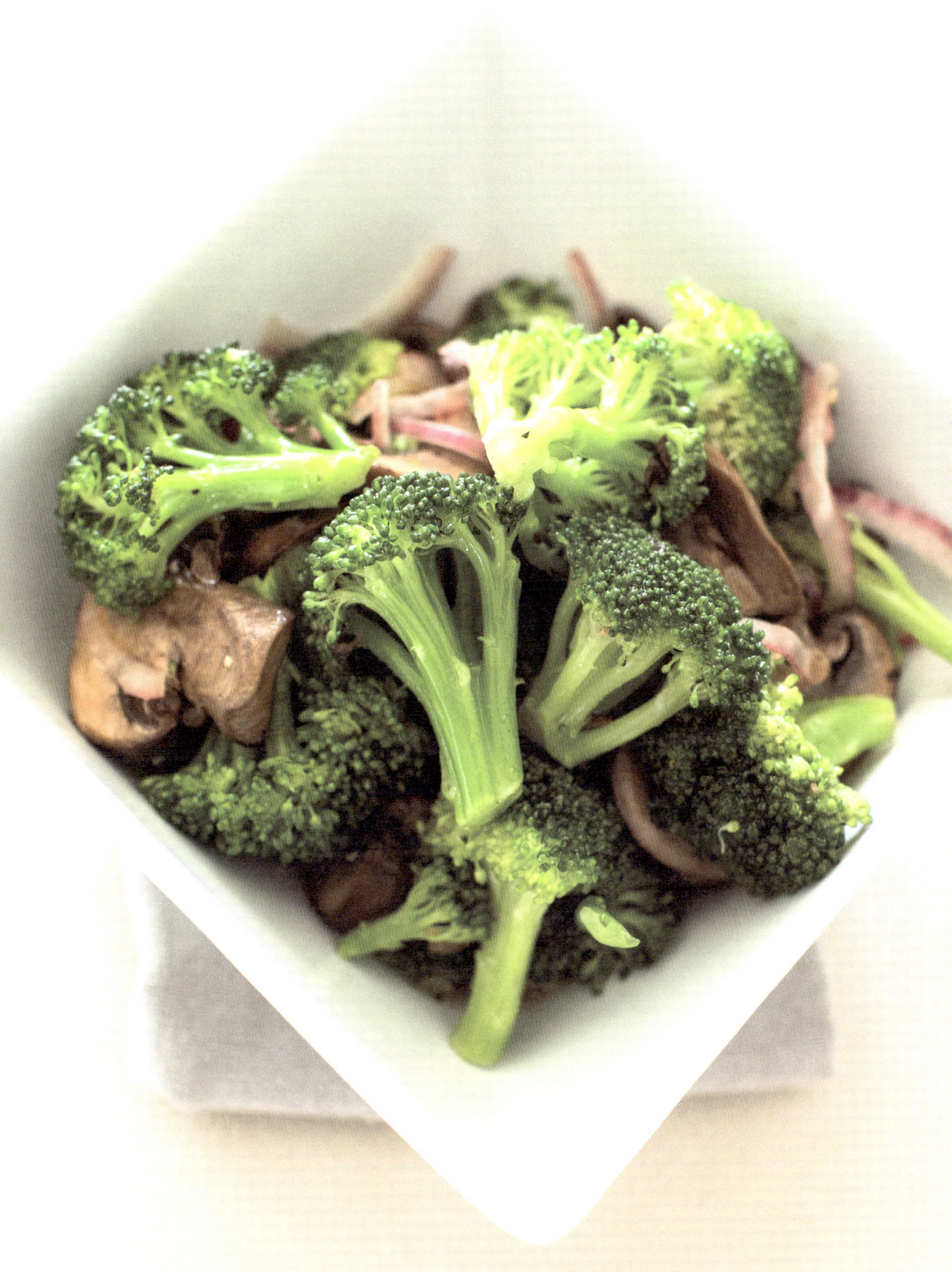

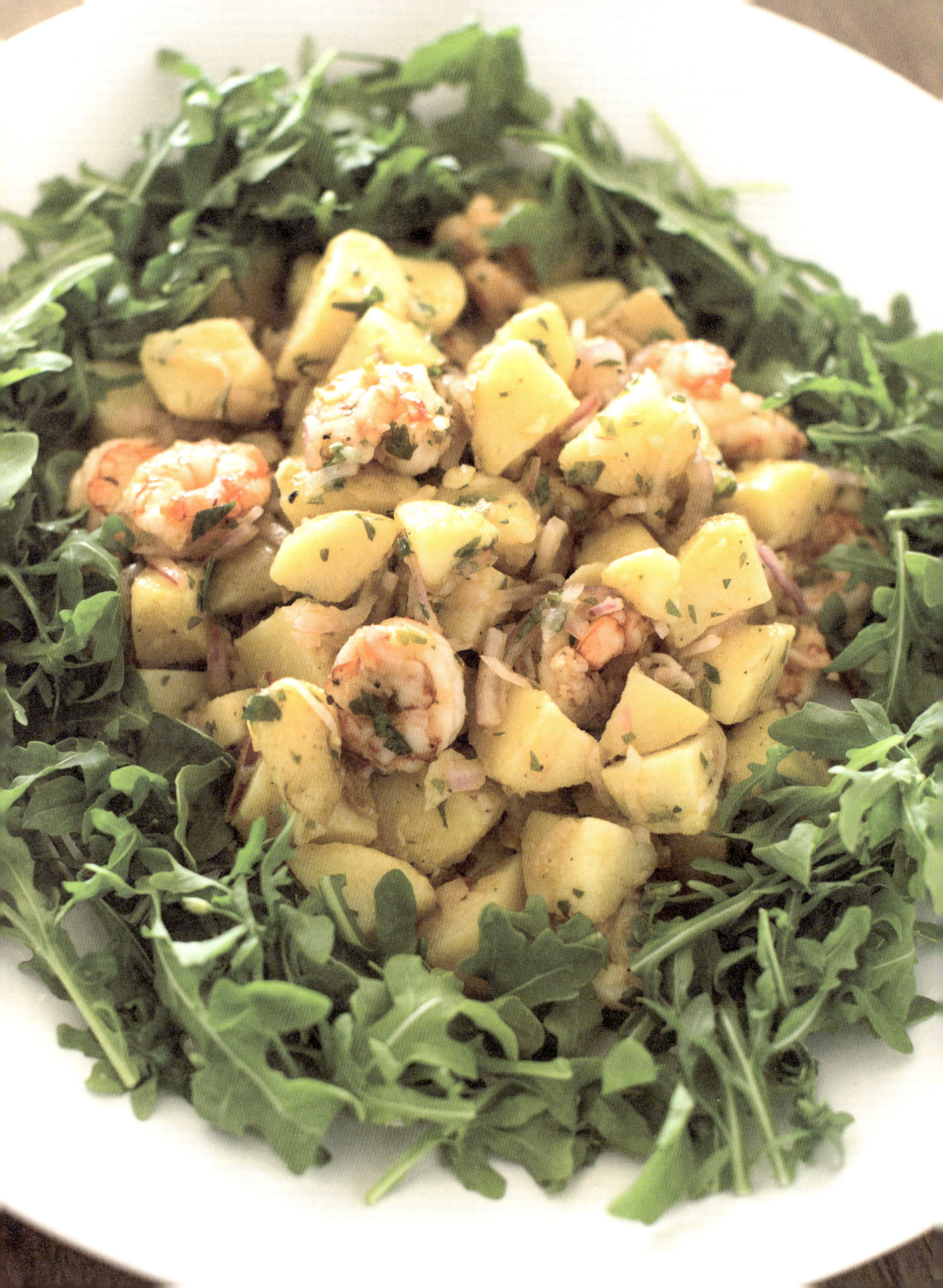

potato salad with shrimp

4-6 servings

THIS POTATO SALAD IS A LOT LIGHTER than the typical dish that is served in many restaurants and backyard BBQ's. I have made many varieties of this recipe, including bacon and parsley and one with wilted greens. This recipe here is simple and loaded with fresh, wild-caught shrimp. It's a great party dish for a large summer gathering.

- 1½ pounds yukon gold potatoes, not peeled *(about 5 medium potatoes)*
- ¼ cup red wine vinegar
- ½ teaspoon sugar
- ½ red onion, thinly sliced
- ¼ cup extra virgin olive oil
- 2 tablespoons fresh Italian parsley, chopped
- 1 pound fresh gulf shrimp, cleaned and deveined
- sea salt and fresh pepper to taste

MBK'S TIPS

Always buy wild-caught fish that you prepare yourself. It's ok if it is frozen, make sure it is not pre-cooked. My favorite is gulf shrimp.

1. Cook potatoes in a large pot of salted water until tender, about 30 minutes.
2. Drain and let cool to touch, then peel the potatoes.
3. Slice potatoes in ¼ inch slices and place in a large bowl.
4. In a small bowl stir red wine vinegar and sugar, until sugar is disolved. Drizzle mixture over potatoes and toss to coat.
5. Mix in onion and season with salt and pepper to taste. Let cool to room temperature.
6. Add olive oil, parsley and shrimp. Mix thoroughly and adjust seasoning if necessary.
7. Refrigerate for 2 hours before serving.

Enjoy!

NUTRITION EXTRAS

Shrimp is low in calories and loaded with nutrients, high in protein, selenium, zinc, B12 and Iron.

GF
DF

kale & shaved brussel sprouts salad with *cranberry vinaigrette*

6 servings

THIS IS THE SALAD I MAKE, WHENEVER I WANT TO IMPRESS A CROWD or convert a non-brussels sprouts eater into loving this vegetable raw. I find myself craving this salad if I have not had it in a while - it's that good! The leftovers are even better the next day, as the sprouts and kale hold up very well overnight in the refrigerator. It's a robust salad that pairs very well with grilled fish.

MBK'S TIPS

Make this way ahead of time, so you are not shaving brussels sprouts while entertaining.

Keep the dressing room temperature and mix right before tossing.

NUTRITION EXTRAS

Lots of vitamin C, vitamin A and vitamin K in both greens.

GF

Ingredients

- ⅓ cup olive oil
- 1 shallot, peeled and thinly sliced
- 1 clove garlic, coarsely chopped *(optional)*
- ½ cup dried cranberries
- 2 tablespoon red wine vinegar
- 2 teaspoons honey
- juice and zest of half a lemon
- ⅛ tsp. salt
- ⅛ tsp. pepper
- 1 bunch of kale, very thinly sliced
- 2 cups raw brussels sprouts, shaved
- ½ cup sliced toasted almonds
- ¼+ cup crumbled blue cheese

Instructions

1. Mix first nine ingredients in dressing cruet until well combined.
2. Let dressing stand at room temperature; do not refrigerate.
3. In a large salad bowl mix kale, brussels sprouts, almonds and blue cheese.
4. Add dressing and mix until well combined.

Enjoy!

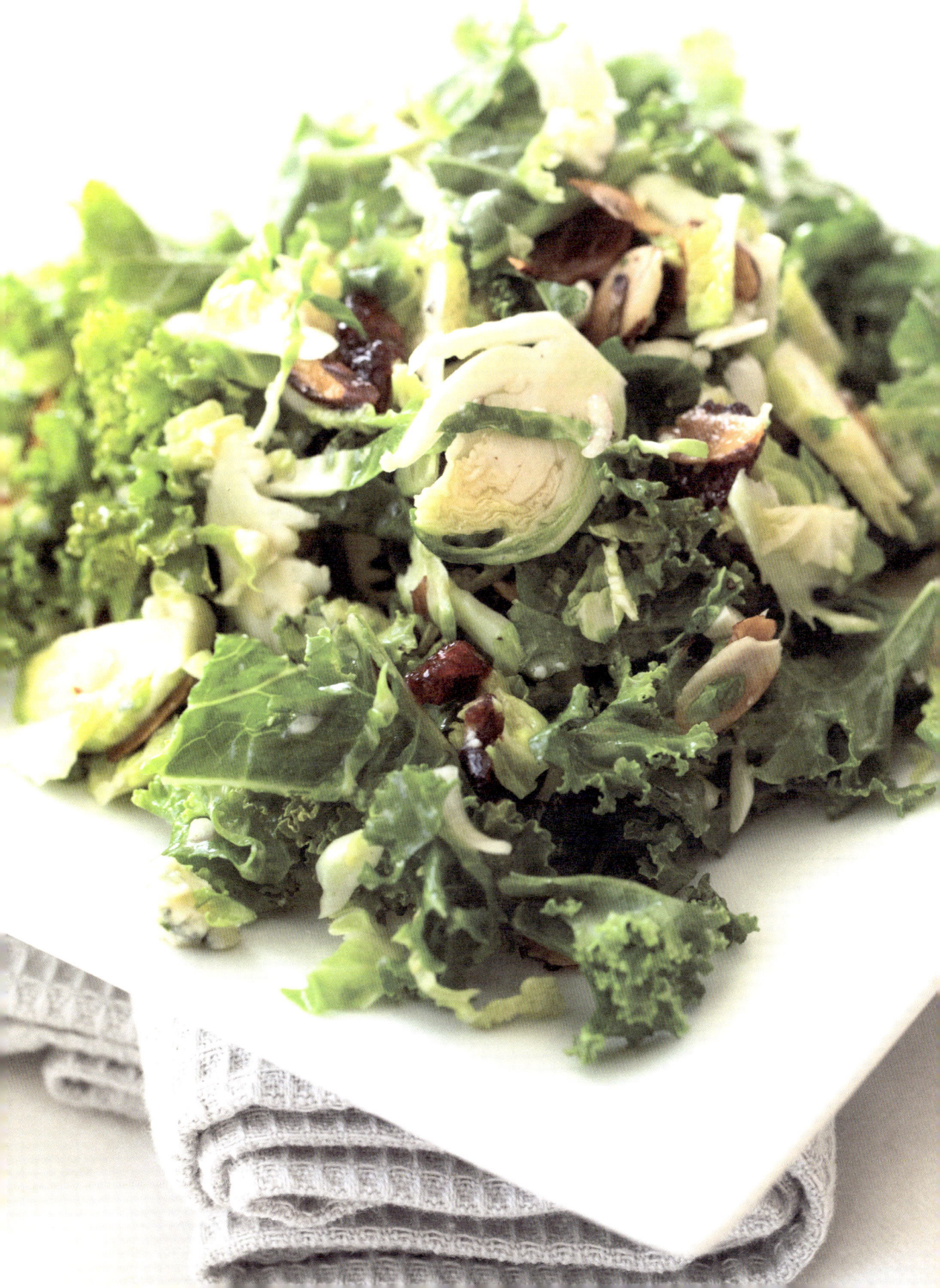

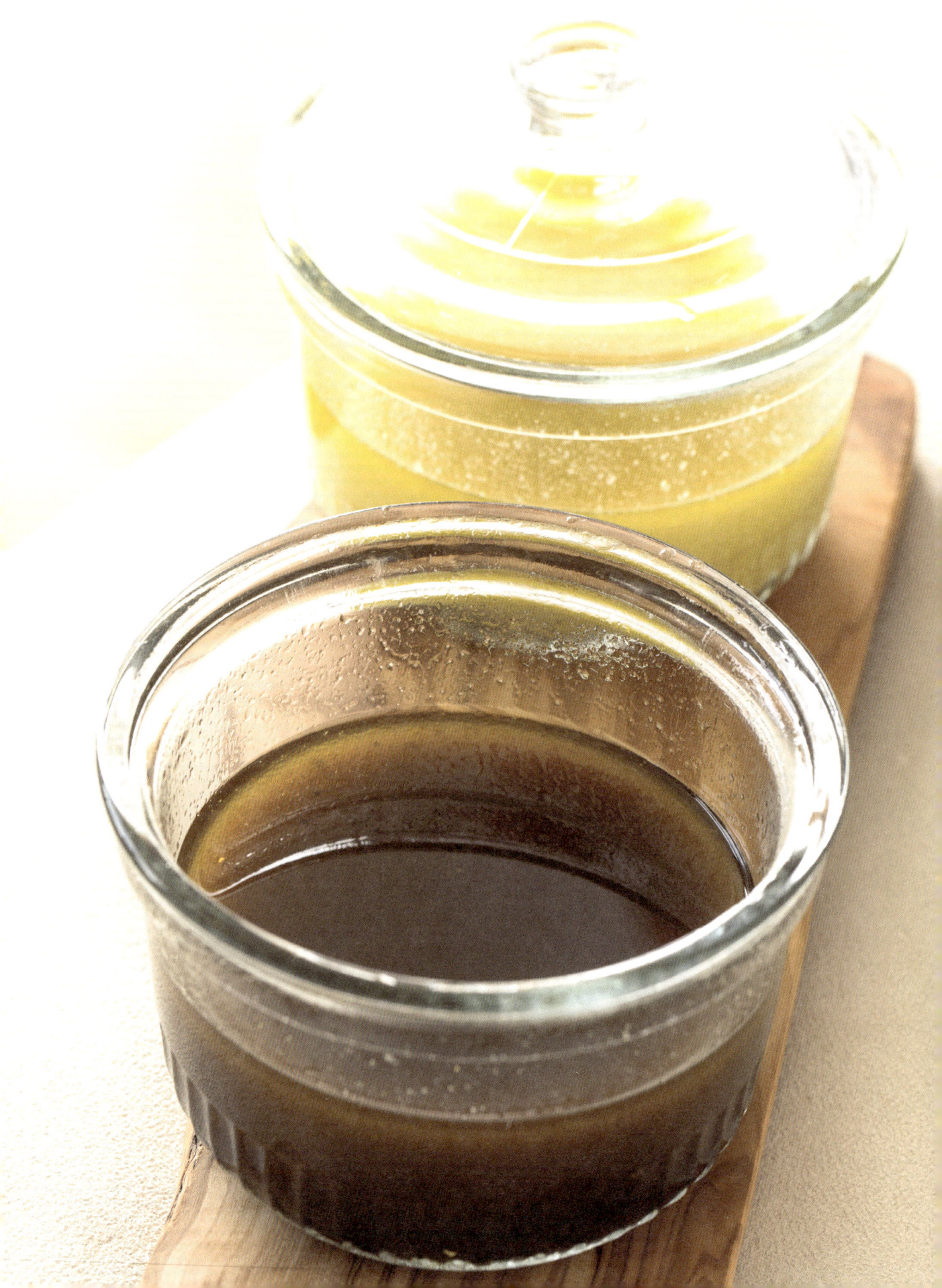

basic lemon vinaigrette

I OFTEN USE A WIDE VARIETY OF VINEGAR AND CITRIS JUICES when making dressings and these two are the standards that I always have in my fridge. I usually make them in large quantities, as my husband and I eat salads almost daily.

- 6 tablespoons extra virgin olive oil
- 2½ tablespoons fresh lemon juice
- 1 teaspoon lemon zest
- 1 teaspoon dijon mustard
- sea salt and fresh pepper to taste

MBK'S TIPS

Don't be afraid to adjust the amount of oil to vinegar, to suit your taste, All you need is a mason jar and a small whisk and your dressing is made fresh to order.

1. Mix all ingredients in a deep bowl and blend using a whisk.
2. Transfer to a salad cruet to use and store in the refrigerator for up to 2 months.

Enjoy!

basic balsamic vinaigrette

- 1 cup extra virgin olive oil
- ⅓ cup white balsamic or sherry vinegar
- ⅓ cup aged balsamic vinegar
- 1 teaspoon dijon mustard
- 1 teaspoon honey *(optional)*
- sea salt and fresh cracked pepper to taste

NUTRITION EXTRAS

Bottled dressings often have added sugars, loads of sodium and unnecessary water. Getting in the habit of making your dressings is so simple and easy to adapt.

1. Mix all ingredients in a small mason jar stirring with a whisk until well blended and has started to thicken. Salad dressings need very little salt, so keep the seasoning optional.
2. Refrigerate for use up to 2 months.

Enjoy!

fajita marinade
for 2 pounds of flank steak

THIS IS ONE OF THE MANY MEAT MARINADES YOU CAN use to tenderize a tough piece of meat. I like this combination if I am making Mexican food. The lime component is a delicious pairing with salsa and spicy peppers.

¼ cup soy sauce

¼ cup lime juice

¼ cup olive oil

⅛ cup brown sugar

2 teaspoons cumin

2 teaspoons black pepper

1 tablespoon chili powder

2 garlic cloves, diced

MBK'S TIPS

Place meat between two pieces of parchment paper and pound with a meat tenderizer or rolling pin. This will ensure that the meat absorbs all of the flavor.

1. Placed meat in a heavy-duty ziplock plastic bag.

2. Mix ingredients well in a mixing bowl, then pour it over meat and rerefrigerate for 8-24 hours.

3. Grill on high heat to sear in the flavors. Serve with your choice of toppings and warm tortilla shells.

Enjoy!

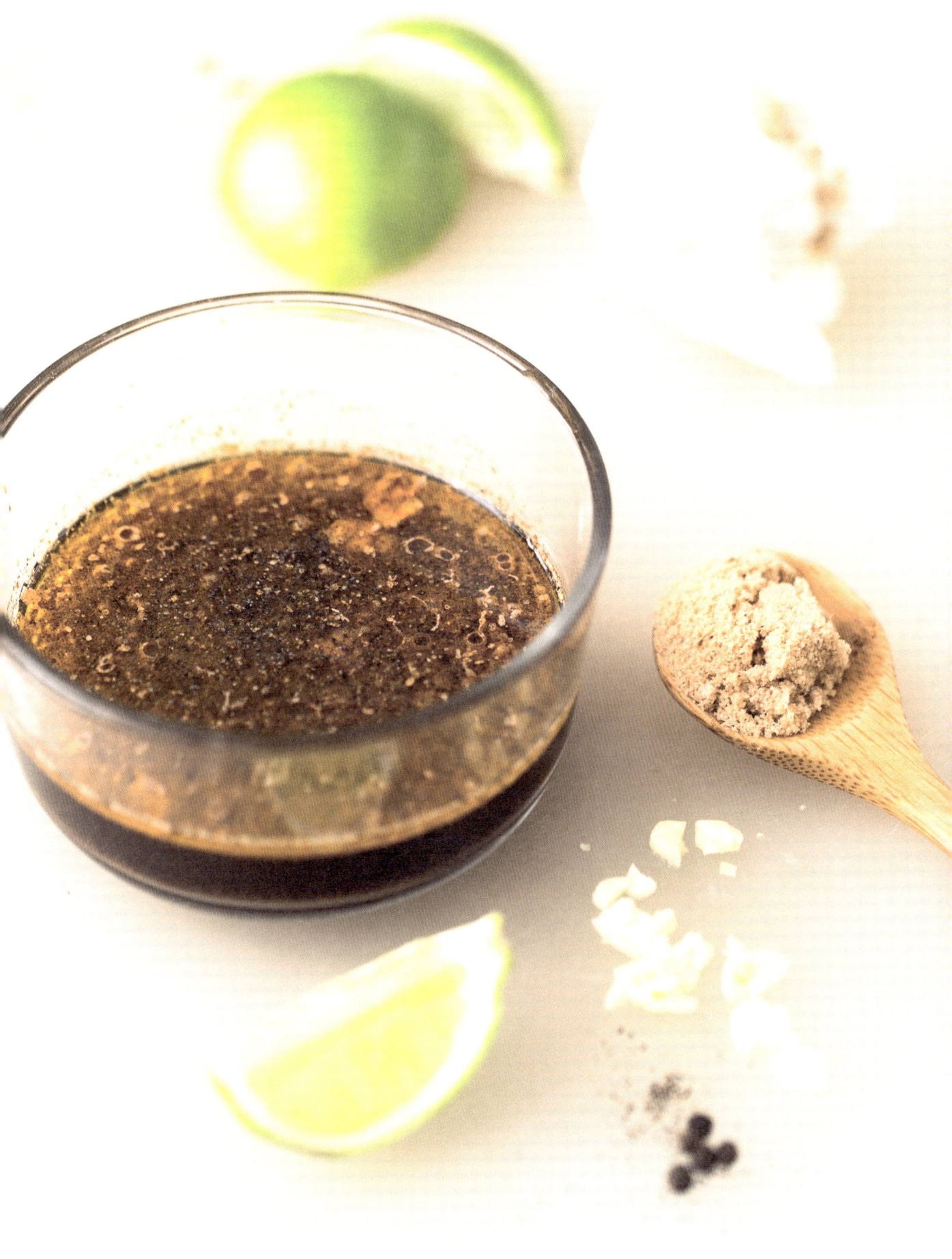

allium family of vegetables

The group of vegetables from the allium family includes garlic, leeks, onions, shallots, scallions and chives. These powerful vegetables, when consumed, have demonstrated significant protective effects of many types of cancer. A little know fact in Vidalia Georgia, where Vidalia onions come from, the death rate of stomach cancer is 50 percent lower than nationally. Onions contain potent antioxidants that are anti-inflammatory, antibiotic and antiviral. This reason alone is why my house is never without these basics to start many of my recipes.

In was found in a study in the European Journal of Clinical Nutrition, that vegetables from the allium family are part of a select group of foods, that when combined, are found to reduce mortality from coronary heart disease. This is by an impressive 20 percent (*the others included broccoli, tea, and apples*). These are called whole foods, real foods and good for you foods. As always, buy organic and local when possible.

I love the smell of cooking onions, sometimes with garlic, as a start to a beautiful soup or dish. You know good things are yet to come! I have long given credit to the wonder of these vegetables in aiding my robust immune system. I tell my clients to get them in their diet whenever possible.

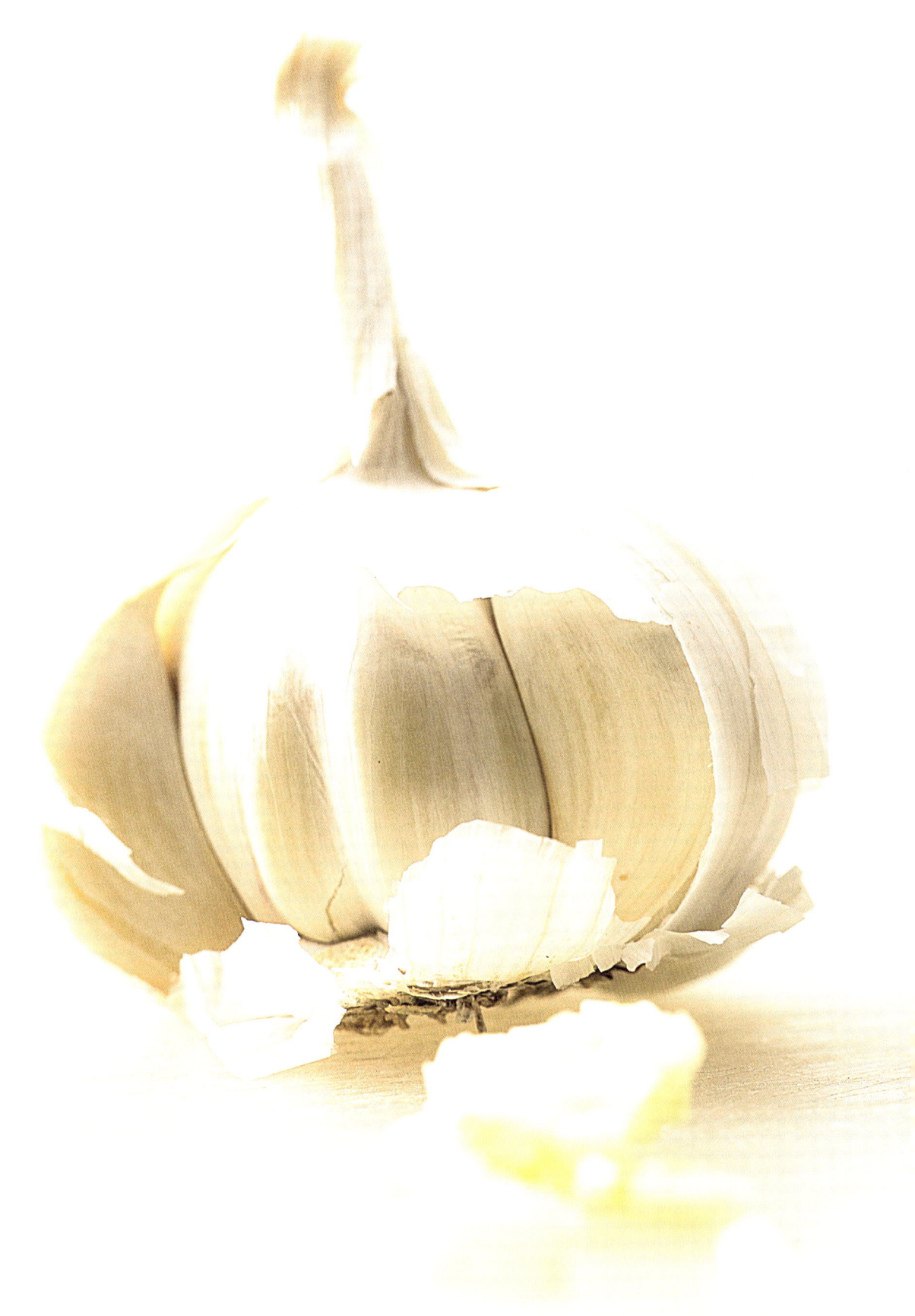

CHAPTER 5
main courses

beer-braised brisket 115

slow-cooked ribs 116

tagliatelle with bacon and leeks 119

taco meat 120

chicken cacciatore 123

pasta with shrimp and mixed vegetables 124

baby back ribs for the barbecue 127

pasta and spinach sauce 128

healthy chicken stir-fry 131

roast leg of lamb with crispy tomatoes 132

spring green risotto 135

grilled rosemary lamb chops 136

coconut chicken 139

fresh tomato sauce 140

meatballs 143

SOME OF THE RECIPES IN THIS COLLECTION GO BACK TO MY COLLEGE DAYS when I first started reading cookbooks and magazines. The iconic Bon Appetit magazine sparked my interest in the hobby of cooking in my early twenties and my passion has continued to this day. My heart remains in my kitchen!

These recipes have been edited, improved upon and updated along the way, as my eating habits have been modified over the years. I always say, "ages and stages" with food and in this collection there is a recipe for every stage.

Many of these dinners are our family favorites that once fed our very hungry family of six and are now getting a second go-around with the new generation. I love to see my children and grandchildren sitting around the table - hungry, and ready to be fed!

crab cakes   144

shrimp and grits with chorizo and kale   147

post-thanksgiving shepherd's pie   149

roasted chicken with vegetables   151

eggplant parmesan   152

fresh pizza dough   155

fresh pizza with the works   156

pasta with kale and tuna   159

chicken piccata   160

chicken parmesan   163

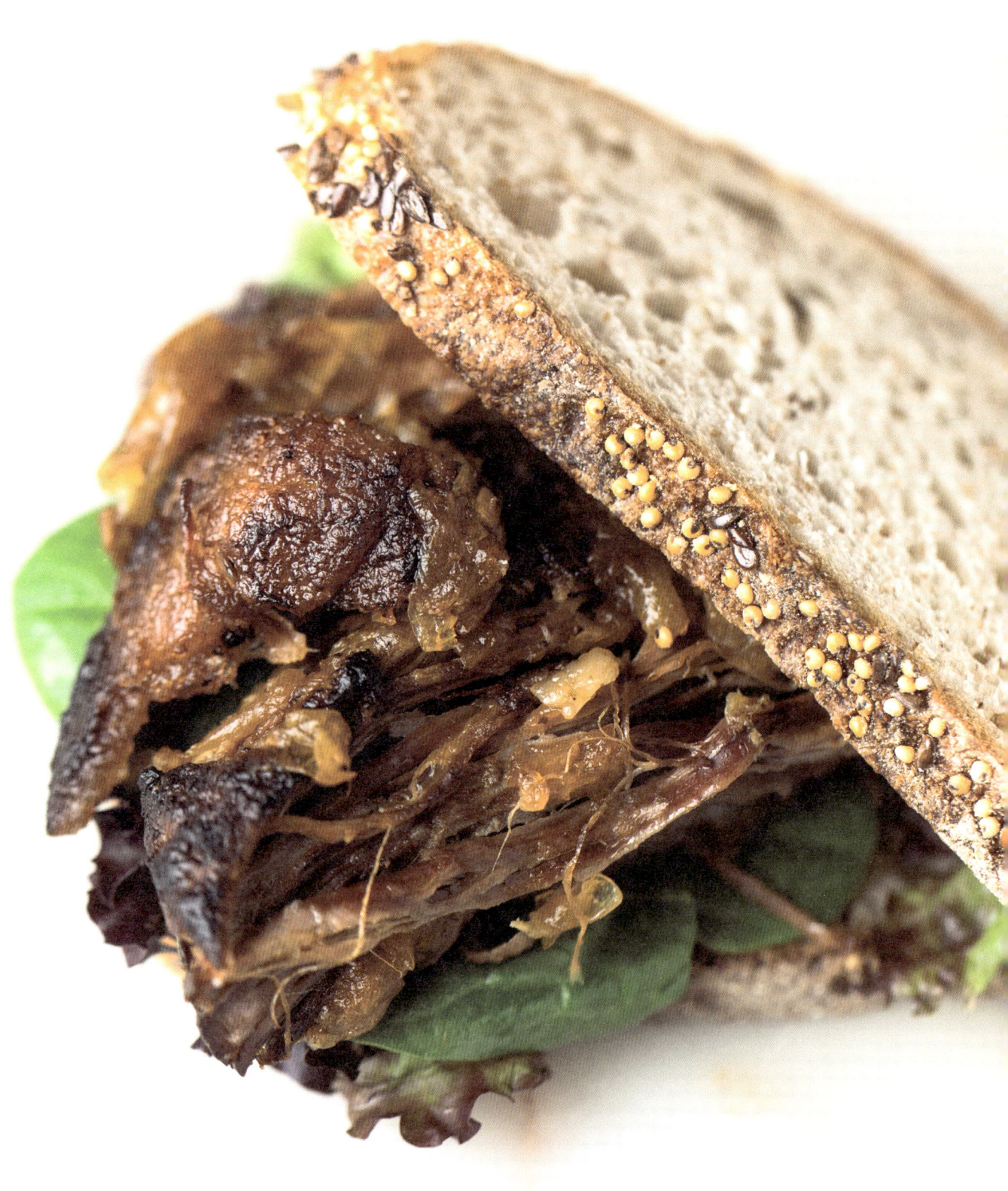

beer-braised brisket
12 servings

I MADE THIS FOR A FOOTBALL PARTY YEARS AGO after finding this recipe in Food and Wine and was wowed with the flavorful delight. I remember going out that Sunday and left the meat simmering for a few hours. When I returned, the house smelled so delicious and I could not wait to try it. It was such a hit that I have since gone back to it several times when cooking for a crowd on a lazy Sunday afternoon. I serve it with buttermilk biscuits, purple cabbage coleslaw and a large green salad. This recipe is a large piece of meat that feeds a big crowd. Don't wait until St. Patrick's Day to purchase a brisket!

- 6 garlic cloves
- 2 tablespoons brown sugar
- 2 tablespoons dijon mustard
- 2 tablespoons olive oil
- 1 tablespoon freshly ground black pepper
- 1 tablespoon ground cumin
- 1 tablespoon paprika
- 1 teaspoon cayenne
- ¼ cup fine sea salt
- 1 - 8 pound untrimmed flat front brisket
- 2 large onions, sliced
- 1 - 12-ounce can lager beer

1. Finely chop garlic in a food processor. Add the next eight ingredients and pulse until smooth. Rub over entire brisket and wrap meat in plastic. Refrigerate for at least 24 hours.

2. Preheat oven to 325°. Bring meat to room temperature for at least 1 hour before cooking.

3. In a large roasting pan scatter onions. Set brisket on top, fat side up, then cover with beer. Cover with foil or use the lid to your roasting pan and cook for 6 hours.

4. Remove from oven and heat broiler. Broil brisket uncovered, until the top is browned and crisp, 5-10 minutes. Let brisket cool slightly, then shred the meat.

5. Remove onions with a slotted spoon and mix into the brisket. Taste and moisten with some of the cooking liquid.

Enjoy!

MBK'S TIPS

This meat is marinated for 24 hours, so making this meal takes some planning ahead. You need to bring the meat to room temperature before cooking for 6 hours, so pull the marinaded meat from the refrigerator early.

DF

slow-cooked ribs

THESE RIBS ARE GREAT TO MAKE IF YOU HAVE A LARGE CROWD coming for dinner and the weather is not ideal for grilling. You can leave them in the oven to cook for hours and the meat will fall right off the bone.

5 pounds spare ribs or country ribs, cut into individual slabs

⅓ cup quality chili powder

2 tablespoons cumin

2 tablespoon brown sugar

2 tsp paprika

2 tsp ground white pepper

2 tsp cayenne pepper

1 tsp turmeric

2 tsp salt

1 tsp dried thyme

1½ cups of your favorite all natural barbecue sauce

MBK'S TIPS

I think there are plenty of tasty local natural bbq sauces to choose from these days. I prefer low sugar and no corn syrup. Check your ingredients.

Be sure to buy meaty quality ribs.

GF
DF

1. Preheat oven to 225° or turn the slow cooker on low.

2. Mix all of the dry ingredients in a bowl and evenly coat all sides of the ribs.

3. Place ribs in a large covered roasting pan or on a cookie sheet covered with foil and cook for 1 hour.

4. Remove from oven and drain fat. Return to oven and cook for an additional hour. If using a slow cooker, this process may take an additional hour.

5. Remove from oven and drain fat. Spread barbecue sauce evenly onto partially cooked ribs. Return ribs to oven and increase the temperature to 275°. Cook for an additional hour.

6. If you desire a crisp finish, place under broiler for 1 minute. Remove from oven... they should melt right off the bone!

Enjoy!

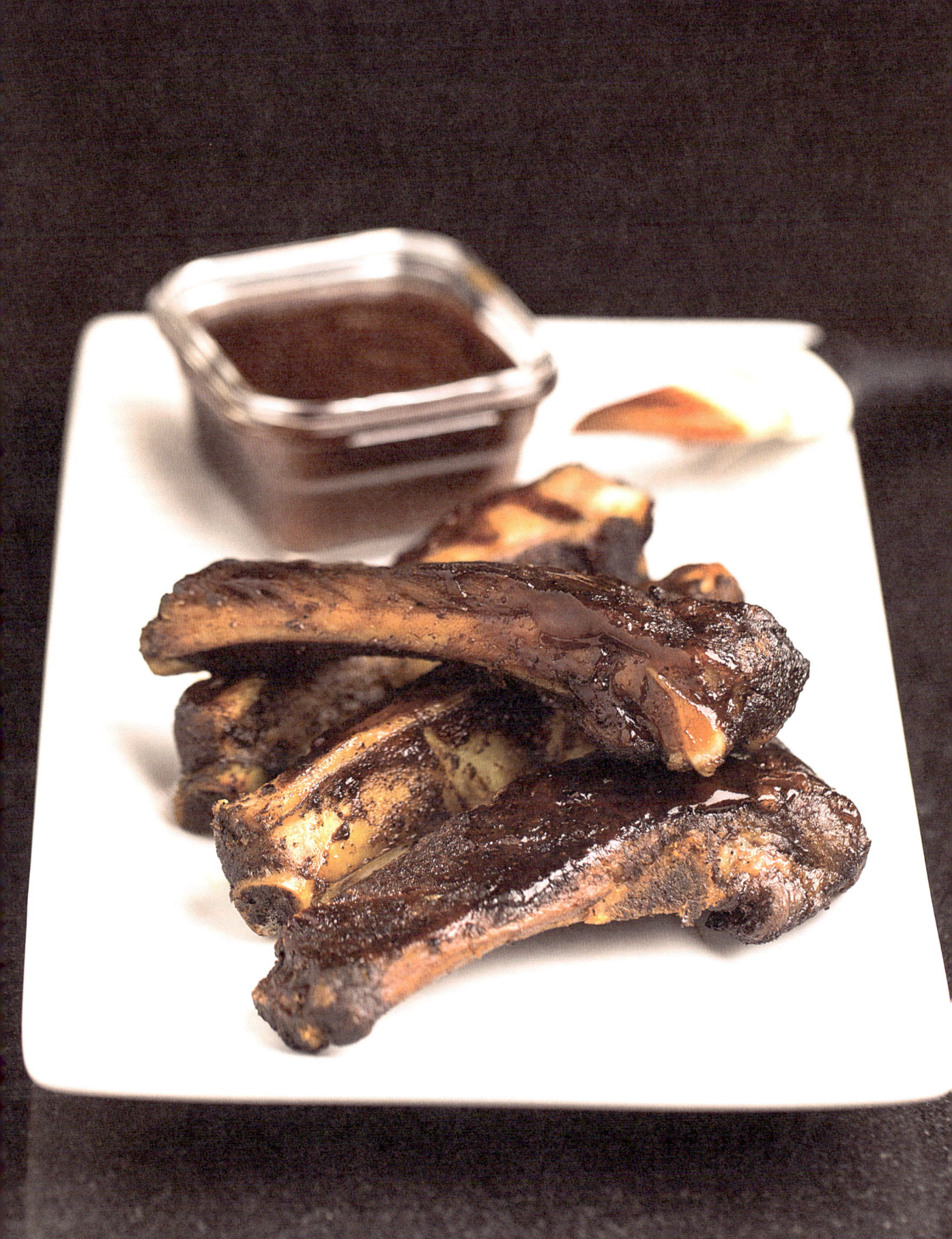

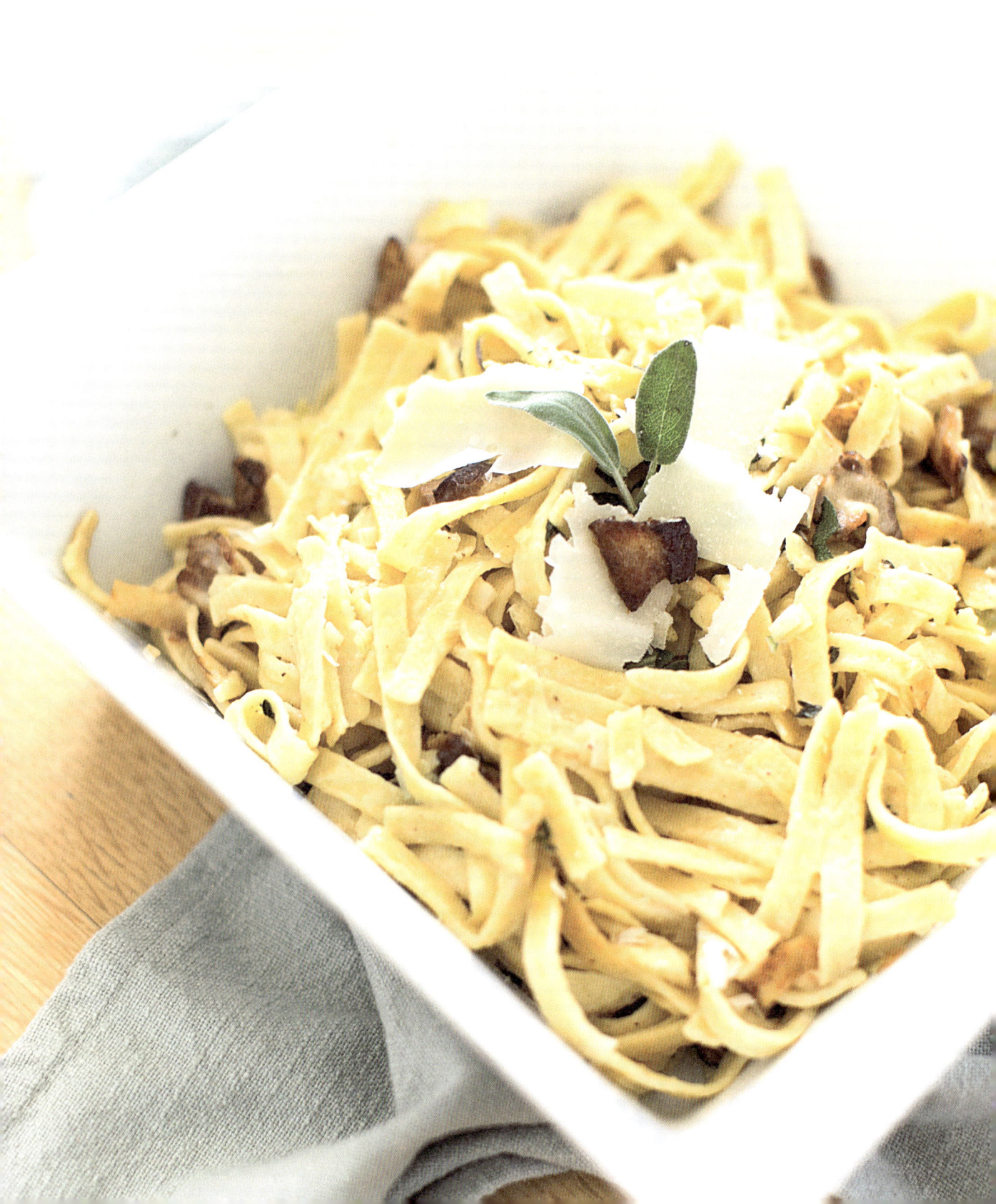

tagliatelle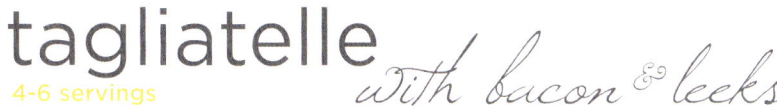

4-6 servings

THIS PASTA IS RICH AND DELICIOUS. With the smokiness of the bacon, along with the buttered leeks, it's a decadent treat. It makes a wonderful side dish next to roasted meat. I have served this dish, alongside both lamb and beef and it compliments either nicely - an enjoyable winter meal when you are hungry.

- 4 slices thick-cut nitrate-free bacon, chopped into bite-size pieces
- 2 tablespoons olive oil
- 1 tablespoon unsalted butter
- 2 medium or 1 large leek, *(white and pale green parts only)* cleaned, rinsed, then sliced into ½ inch rings
- 1 cup heavy cream
- 2 teaspoons fresh thyme
- 1 pound tagliatelle pasta, reserve 2 cups pasta water
- 1 cup + 2 tablespoons grated parmesan cheese
- salt and pepper to taste

1. In a non-stick cooking pan over medium heat cook bacon, until bacon is crisp. Drain excess fat.

2. Add olive oil, butter, and leeks and cook for an additional 5 - 6 minutes, until leeks are just starting to brown.

3. Add cream, thyme and ½ cup of water. Continue cooking until sauce has thickened and coats the back of a spoon, approximately 5-8 additional minutes.

4. Cook pasta in salted boiling water until pasta is al-dente. Drain pasta, reserving 2 cups of cooking liquid.

5. Combine pasta with cream sauce, adding 1-2 cups of reserved pasta liquid, just until desired creaminess occurs.

6. Add 1 cup grated parmesan. Adjust seasoning with additional salt and pepper if needed.

Enjoy!

MBK'S TIPS

After you have sliced the leeks, run them under water to be sure you have removed all the sand. You only need to make that mistake once, where grit is in your dish because you did not clean the leeks thoroughly!

taco meat
4-6 servings

THIS IS A BASIC TACO MEAT RECIPE that I would often make for my children when they were young. It was a standard when vacationing and often enjoyed after the beach or skiing. I could make this no matter whose house we were renting or where we were residing. I always doubled the recipe so we would have leftovers for quick nachos when the hungry, busy boys came through the door. You can substitute turkey or bison if you prefer. They all taste great with these spices added.

MBK'S TIPS

Be careful with cayenne if you have small children who cannot tolerate heat. Eliminate the spice if necessary.

NUTRITION EXTRAS

This recipe is a great high protein dinner that is light on carbs. Adding lots of fresh add-ons makes it a complete meal.

GF
DF
LS

Ingredients

- 1 tablespoon olive oil
- 1 sweet onion, diced
- 2 pounds ground beef or bison
- 3 tablespoons chili powder
- 2 teaspoons cayenne
- 2 tablespoons cumin
- 2 ounces tomato paste with 1½ cup water or 1 cup tomato sauce with ½ cup water
- salt to taste

Instructions

1. Saute onion in heated oil until translucent, approximately 5 minutes.
2. Add room-temperature beef or bison to the pan, breaking into small bits as beef cooks.
3. Once the meat is fully cooked, drain fat and add all the other ingredients.
4. Cook on medium to low heat for 15 minutes, until flavors have been incorporated.
5. Serve with your favorite toppings on warm tortillas.

Enjoy!

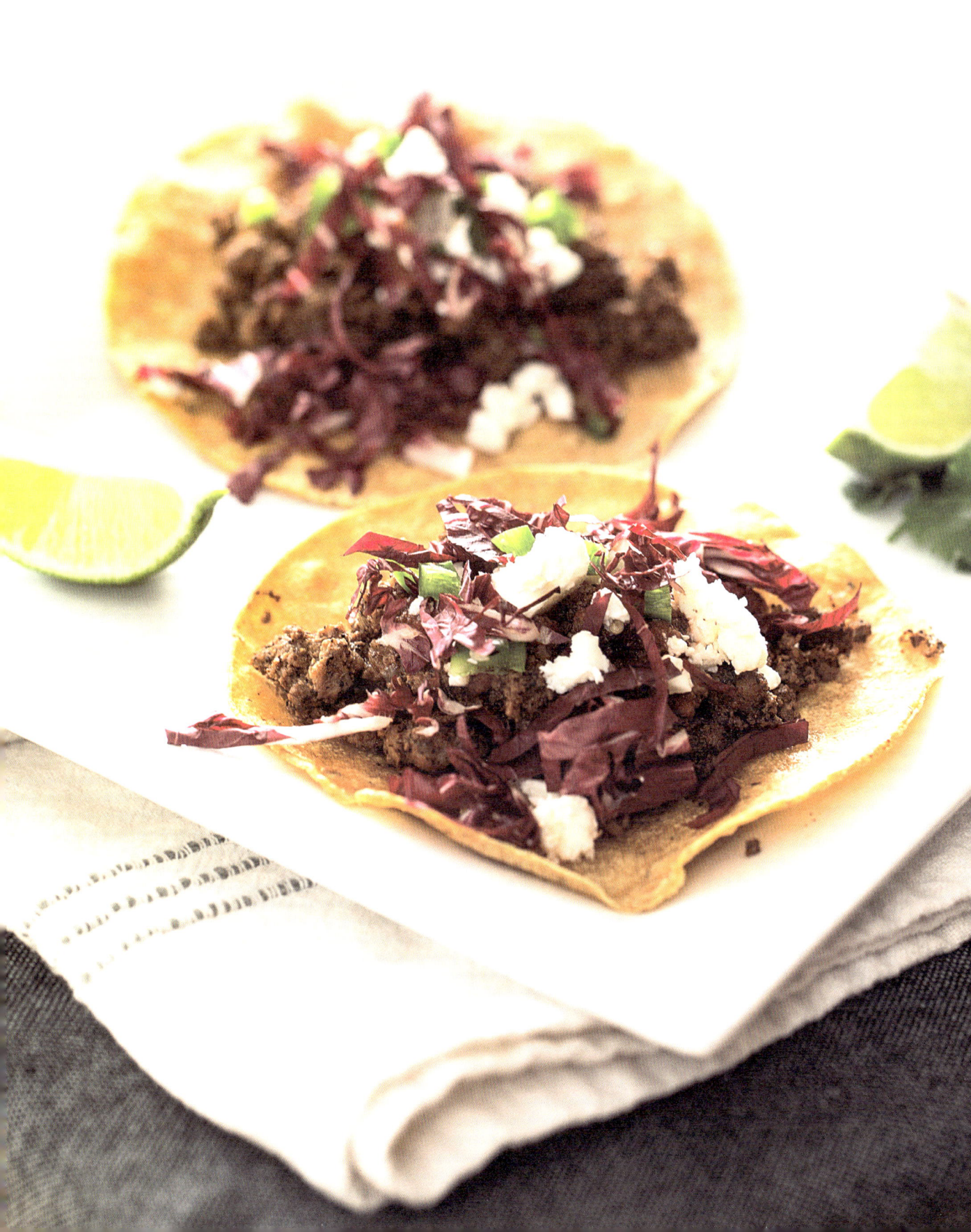

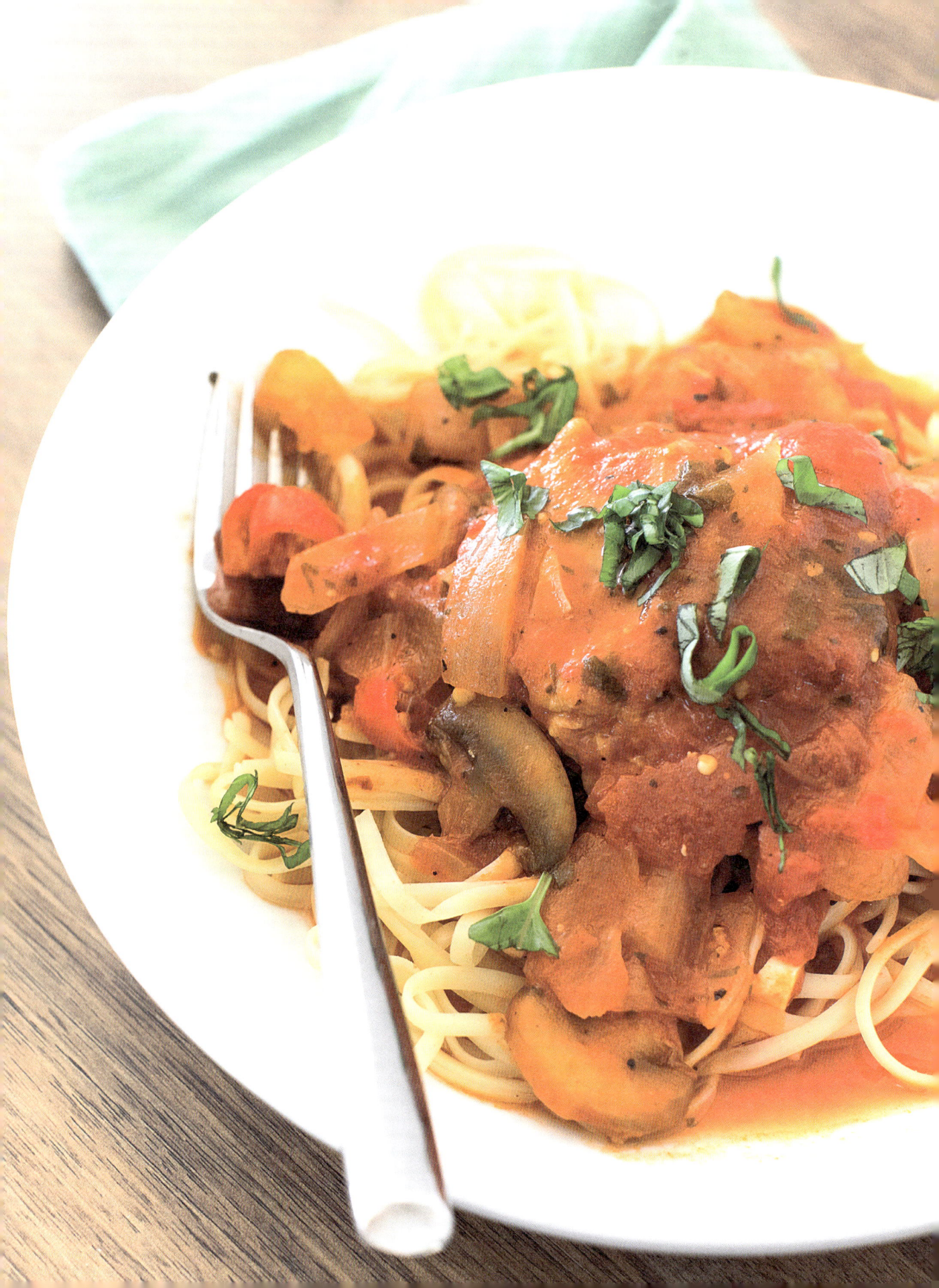

chicken cacciatore
4-6 servings

I LOVE MAKING THIS DISH, as I feel that it's a forgotten treasure these days. When I share this recipe with clients they react so positively, because it is an easy, one-pot dish that has it all. As this dish simmers on the stove, the aroma is so fragrant that it leaves your mouth watering. The chicken literally melts off the bone. Serve this with crusty bread to soak up the sauce!

- 4 bone-in chicken breast, skin attached
- 4 tablespoons olive oil
- 1 red pepper, coarsely chopped
- 1 large sweet onion, coarsely chopped
- 10 ounces mushrooms, sliced
- 3 garlic cloves, crushed
- 1 cup dry white or red wine
- 1 - 28-ounce can diced San Marzano tomatoes, with juice
- 1 small can tomato paste (3-4 ounces)
- 1 cup reduced-sodium chicken stock
- 1 tablespoon dried oregano
- ¼ cup fresh basil, chopped
- 1 teaspoon crushed red pepper
- salt and pepper to taste
- freshly grated parmesan, for topping

MBK'S TIPS

Pound the chicken, to tenderize the meat before you start to brown. You can also opt for chicken thighs if you prefer dark meat.

1. Sprinkle chicken with salt and pepper to taste.
2. In large, heavy dutch oven heat oil over a medium-high flame. Add chicken and brown, approximately 5 minutes per side. Transfer chicken to a plate and set aside.
3. In the original pan scrape brown bits off the surface, and add additional oil, if needed. On medium heat, add red pepper, onion, mushrooms and saute until vegetables are tender for about 5 minutes.
4. Add garlic and continue cooking for an additional 2 minutes..
5. Add wine and reduce liquid by half, approximately 3 minutes.
6. Return chicken to the pan and add all remaining ingredients. Simmer on a low boil, stirring often, for about an hour.
7. Serve chicken and vegetables over pasta of your choice or spaghetti squash. Top with freshly grated parmesan.

enjoy!

NUTRITION EXTRAS

Although pictured with traditional pasta, this can be a very light meal when served with roasted spaghetti squash. High in protein and loaded with vegetables

GF
eliminate pasta + bread

DF
eliminate parmesan

pasta with shrimp
4-6 servings
& mixed vegetables

A BIG PLATE OF PASTA WITH ALL THE FIXINGS goes a long way in feeding a crowd. This recipe is so easy to pull together after a fruitful trip to the farmer's market. I love the combination of vegetables here, but you can mix and match whatever vegetables you have on hand. It all tastes good with this light sauce and fresh shrimp.

[Handwritten note: okay to use 3/4# pasta. - add minced garlic - fresh herbs much better flavor]

MBK'S TIPS

If you have guests who don't want cheese with seafood, serve the parmesan on the side.

NUTRITION EXTRAS

With all these vegetables included this could stand alone for dinner, but also pairs well with a simple arugula salad.

Ingredients:

- 1 pound wide noodle pasta, *(fettuccine or pappardelle)* reserve ½ cup of pasta water
- olive oil
- 1 medium shallot, minced
- ½ pound sugar snap peas, cleaned, trimmed, and diced
- ½ pound asparagus, cut into 1-inch pieces
- 1 red pepper, cleaned, seeded, and chopped
- 1 cup low-sodium chicken stock
- ¼ cup heavy cream
- salt and pepper to taste
- 1 tablespoon unsalted butter
- 1 pound wild-caught shrimp, cleaned and deveined
- ¼ cup fresh herbs for finish, *(oregano, dill, sage, parsley or basil. Can use a combination of any two herbs)*
- freshly grated parmesan cheese

1. Cook pasta and set aside while reserving 2 cups of pasta water.

2. In a large non-stick saute pan heat 3 tablespoons oil over medium heat. Add shallots and cook for 2 minutes. Add snap peas, asparagus and red pepper and cook until tender and starting to brown.

3. Add chicken stock and cream. Let mixture come to a low boil, add pasta to the pan, mix well and adjust seasoning. Add more reserved pasta water, if necessary. Keep warm on low heat.

4. In a clean pan heat 2 tablespoons oil + 1 tablespoon butter. Add shrimp and cook for 2-3 minutes, on medium-high heat, just until they turn pink. *[Handwritten: - squeeze ½ lemon over shrimp]*

5. Add shrimp, herbs and fresh parmesan to the pan with pasta and vegetables. Toss gently and serve immediately.

Enjoy!

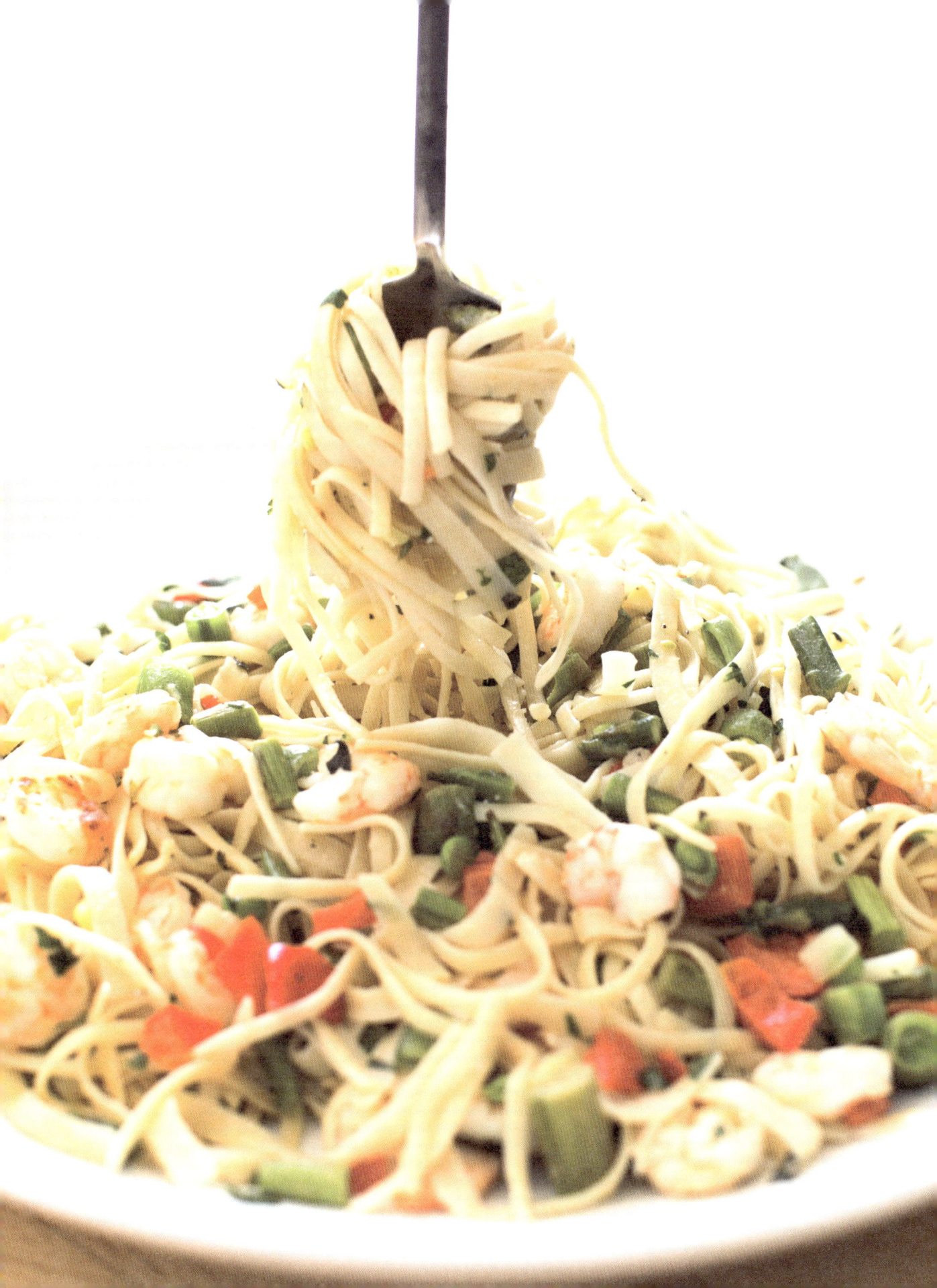

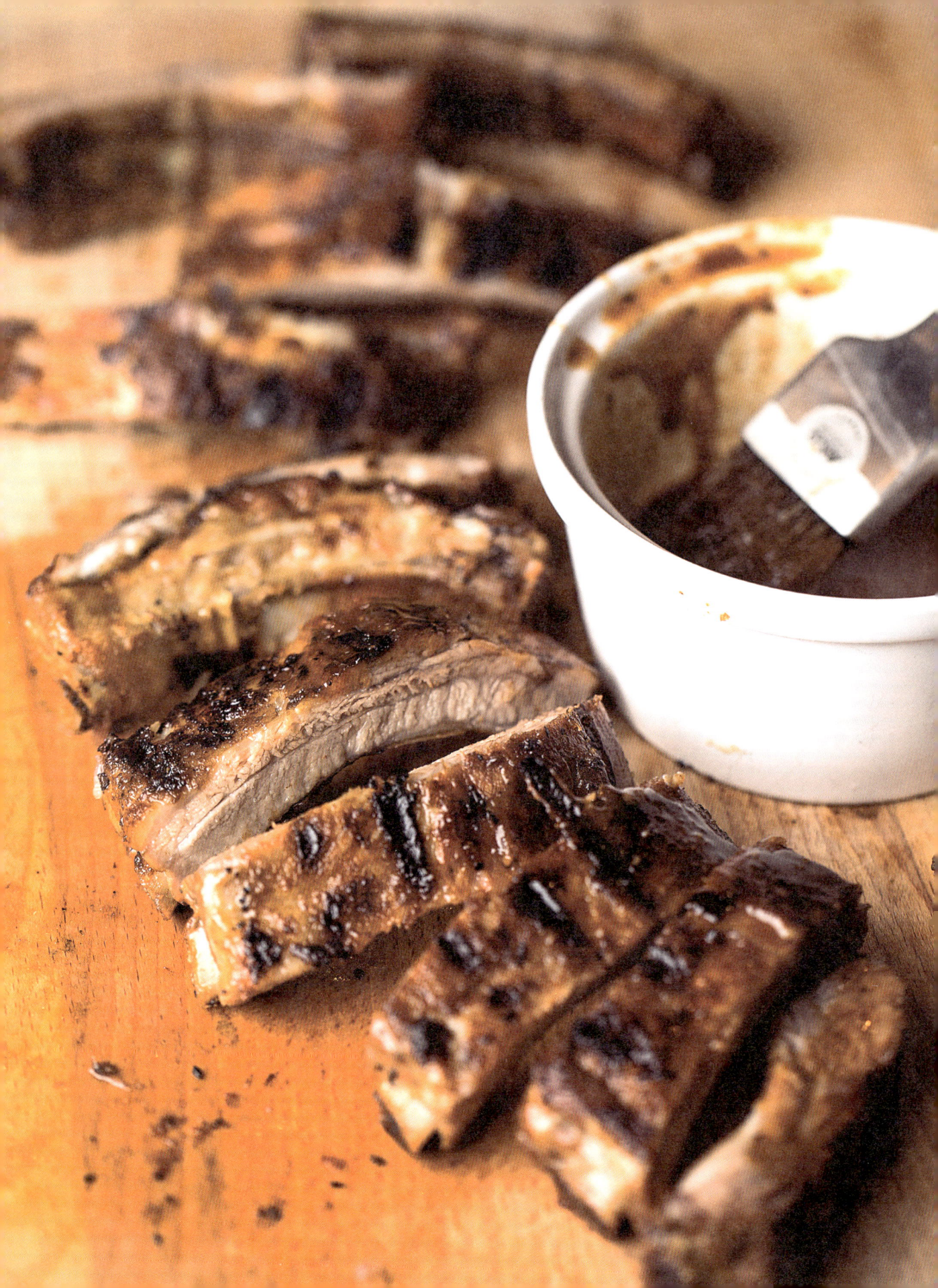

baby back ribs
4 servings
for the barbecue

MAKING THESE RIBS FOR A GROUP OF FRIENDS OR FAMILY AT OUR LAKE HOUSE is so fun and so satisfying. We live in an area with livestock farmers that provide some of the best pork I have ever tasted. You do not need a lot of sauce on these, as the tender baby back is so tasty on its own. Plan on a good half rack per person. They won't go to waste!

1 tablespoon fine sea salt

1 tablespoon dry mustard

1 tablespoon paprika

½ teaspoon cayenne pepper (*more if you like it spicy*)

½ teaspoon freshly ground black pepper

4½ pounds of ribs (*2 large or 3 medium racks*)

1½ cups of your favorite barbecue sauce

MBK'S TIPS

Don't wait until the last minute to make this dish. You need the full 2 hours in the oven to make the ribs good and tender before grilling. If using a convection setting on your oven, lower heat to 325 degrees.

GF
DF

1. Preheat oven to 350°.

2. Combine the first five ingredients in a small bowl.

3. Place each rack of ribs on a double layer of tinfoil and sprinkle rub over ribs. Wrap each rack and divide between 2 baking sheets. Bake ribs until tender, but not falling apart, about 2 hours.

4. Carefully unwrap ribs and save any accumulated juices in a glass measuring cup. Let ribs cool slightly while you heat grill to medium-high temperature. Add prepared barbecue sauce to rib juices and mix well.

5. Return ribs to grill, basting with sauce, turning frequently until charred, lacquered and cooked throughout, 7-10 minutes.

6. Pull from the grill and cut between the bones. Serve with extra sauce if desired.

Enjoy!

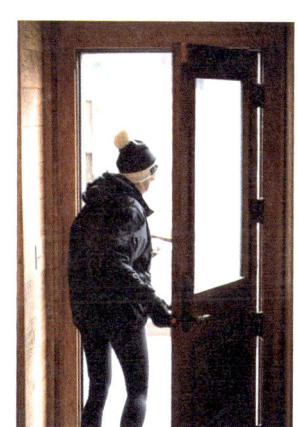

pasta and spinach sauce

6 servings

THIS RECIPE GOES BACK TO MY UNIVERSITY DAYS where I was experimenting with "affordable" dinner options and eating lots of pasta. I always had frozen spinach and canned tomatoes, whereas now I prefer fresh. I shared this with my family one holiday while returning to my hometown of Cleveland and my sister Ellen was instantly a fan. She continues to make this every year on Christmas Day for her family of five. I love when a recipe sticks with someone and it becomes part of their tradition. When I made this batch for the book, my husband was pleased to taste an old familiar dish.

MBK'S TIPS

I love fresh spinach, because it is always available washed and ready to use. Frozen spinach works well also. Always use San Marzano tomatoes - there is no substitute!

Great dish all on its own, or you can add shrimp for an added protein.

NUTRITION EXTRAS

Can be a simple vegetarian meal by eliminating the cream and parmesan

Loaded with vitamin C and A, along with fiber and folate.

GF*
DF*
V*
*(option)

Ingredients

- 3 tablespoons olive oil
- 2 carrots, diced
- 1 onion, chopped
- 4 garlic cloves, minced
- 2 cans San Marzano tomatoes, diced
- 1 pound fresh spinach
- crushed red pepper to taste
- 1 tablespoon dried oregano
- ½ cup heavy cream
- salt and pepper to taste
- fresh parmesan

Instructions

1. Heat 3 tablespoons oil in a large non-stick pan on medium heat. Saute carrots, onion and garlic until vegetables have softened, approximately 7-10 minutes.

2. Add tomatoes, spinach, red pepper and oregano. Simmer on low for 20 minutes.

3. Add cream, cooking until incorporated and sauce has returned to a boil.

4. Serve warm sauce immediately over pasta of your choice. You can also serve with farro, couscous, Kamut, riced cauliflower or other hearty grains.

5. Top with freshly grated parmesan

Enjoy!

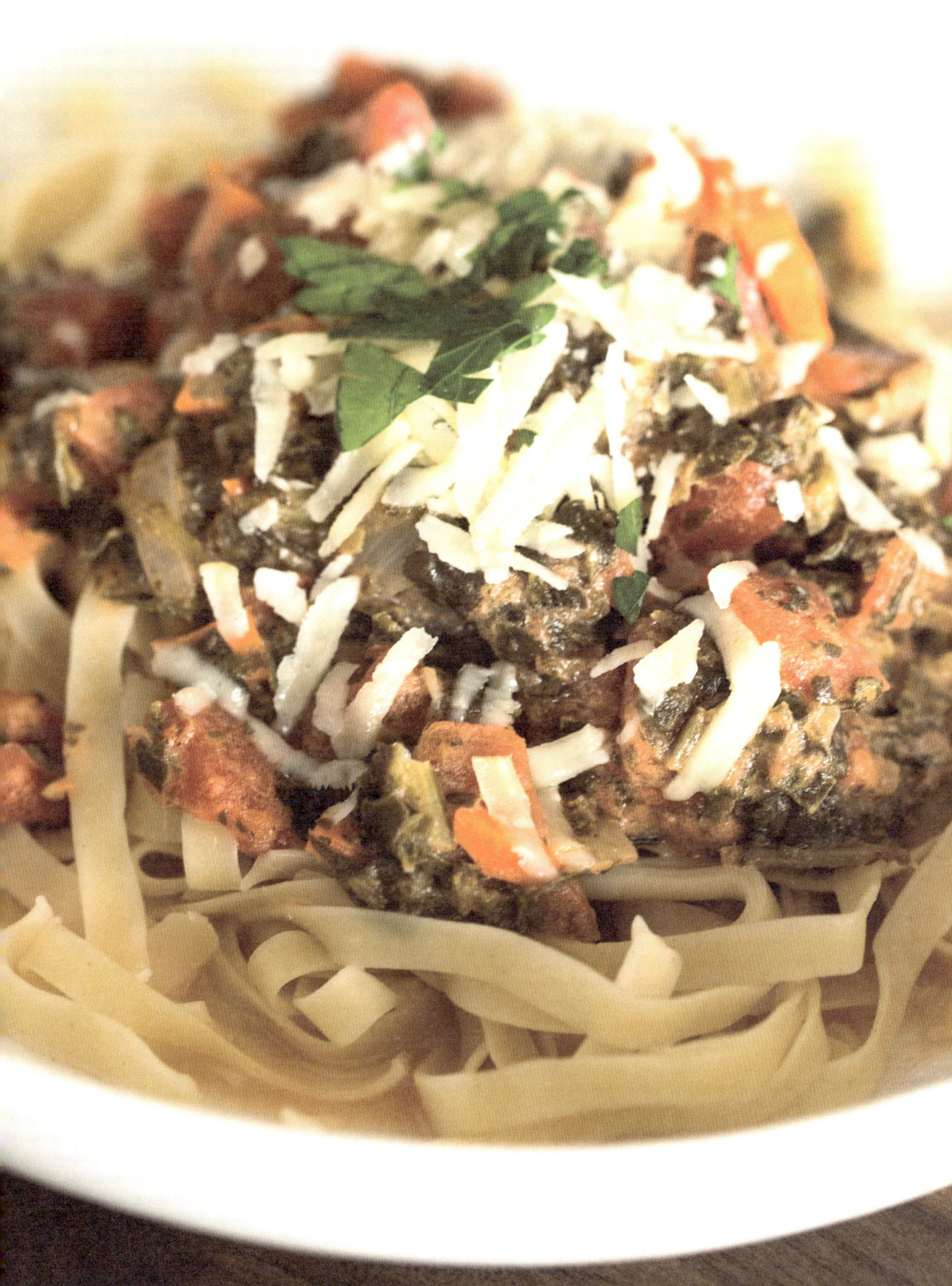

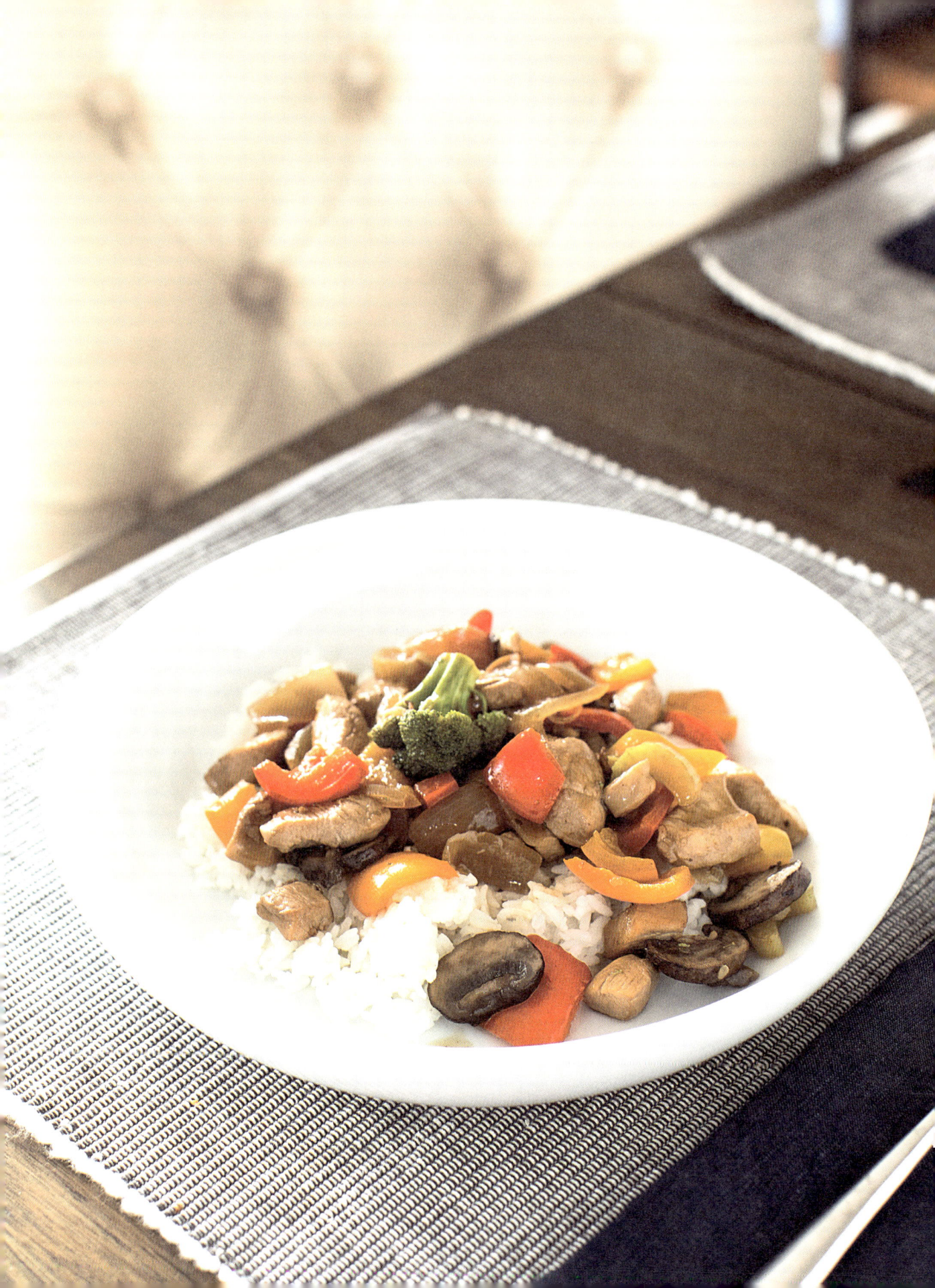

healthy chicken stir-fry
4 servings

THIS STIR-FRY DISH TAKES US BACK TO THE BASICS OF WOK COOKING. I love sharing this recipe with clients because it is quick and healthy and anyone can pull it together. Be sure to buy fresh, organic vegetables, organic chicken and rice. Children love this dish, even ones that are picky eaters. It's a dish that should go into the weekly rotation of weeknight meals for feeding a family. The leftovers are great for lunch the next day.

1 cup organic basmati rice, prepared as directed

¼ cup robust red wine

1-2 tablespoons cornstarch

3 tablespoons avocado oil

1 large sweet onion, cut into 1-inch pieces

2 stalks of celery, cleaned and sliced

1 large carrot, cleaned and sliced

2 chicken breast halves, cut into ¾ inch pieces

1 large red pepper + 1 large yellow bell pepper, cleaned and cut into 1-inch pieces

6 ounces baby bella mushrooms, sliced

½ cup low-sodium soy sauce

¾ cup low-sodium chicken stock

MBK'S TIPS

If you do not have a wok, a large frying pan will do. I like stainless steel, so you can get the oil hot, and cook the vegetables quickly on high heat. I love avocado oil for high temperatures, but organic canola oil will work as well.

1. Prepare all of the vegetables and cook rice according to directions.

2. In a small bowl mix soy sauce, red wine and cornstarch.

3. In a large 14-inch saucepan or wok, heat oil on medium-high heat and add onion, celery, carrot and chicken. Once vegetables have started to cook, about 3 minutes, add peppers, mushrooms and soy sauce mixture.

4. After 5-7 minutes of cooking, add chicken stock and mix thoroughly. Turn off heat. Stir-fry and rice should finish at the same time.

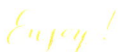

NUTRITION EXTRAS

This dish is a high protein, low in saturated fat, full of fiber-rich vegetables and loaded with antioxidants. You will not go to bed feeling full after this meal. This stif-fry provides a real nice proportion of meat to veggies - the healthiest way to eat a meal.

GF
DF
LS

roast leg of lamb
with crispy potatoes

6-8 servings

THIS LAMB DISH WAS INSPIRED FROM A RECIPE by Ina Garten and has been an Easter tradition in my home for several years. I wish I had discovered this when I used to make Easter dinner for my parents. They both loved lamb and really loved me showing up to their house to take over their kitchen! The fat drippings on the potatoes with the salt, garlic and rosemary make them so scrumptious! Serve this with several green side dishes and you have a holiday feast. It's effortless to prepare and serve.

MBK'S TIPS

If you have tasted duck fat fries, you get the idea.... Yum!

GF
DF

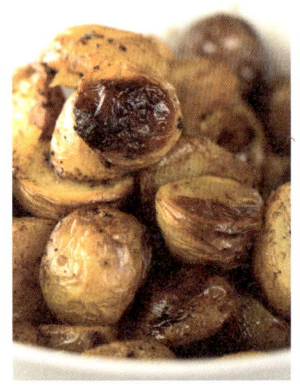

- 4-5 pound leg of lamb
- fresh rosemary
- olive oil
- 6 garlic cloves, crushed
- salt and freshly crushed pepper
- juice from 1 fresh lemon
- 3 pounds Yukon gold potatoes, medium-size, cleaned and cut in half

1. Preheat oven to 425° convection, if available.

2. Combine 3 tablespoons of fresh chopped rosemary with 4 tablespoons of olive oil, crushed garlic and a generous portion of salt and pepper. Rub herb paste over the entire surface of room temperature leg of lamb.

3. In stainless steel roasting pan layer potatoes on the pan's bottom and spray with a light coating of olive oil. Squeeze ½ of fresh lemon over potatoes and sprinkle with sea salt. Set herb-coated lamb, directly on top of potatoes so the rendered fat drips directly onto vegetables. Squeeze the second half of lemon over the lamb and place into the preheated oven.

4. Roast for approximately 1 hour, stirring and turning potatoes once or twice during the cooking process. Test for doneness and remove from oven. Let sit for 15 minutes before serving.

Enjoy!

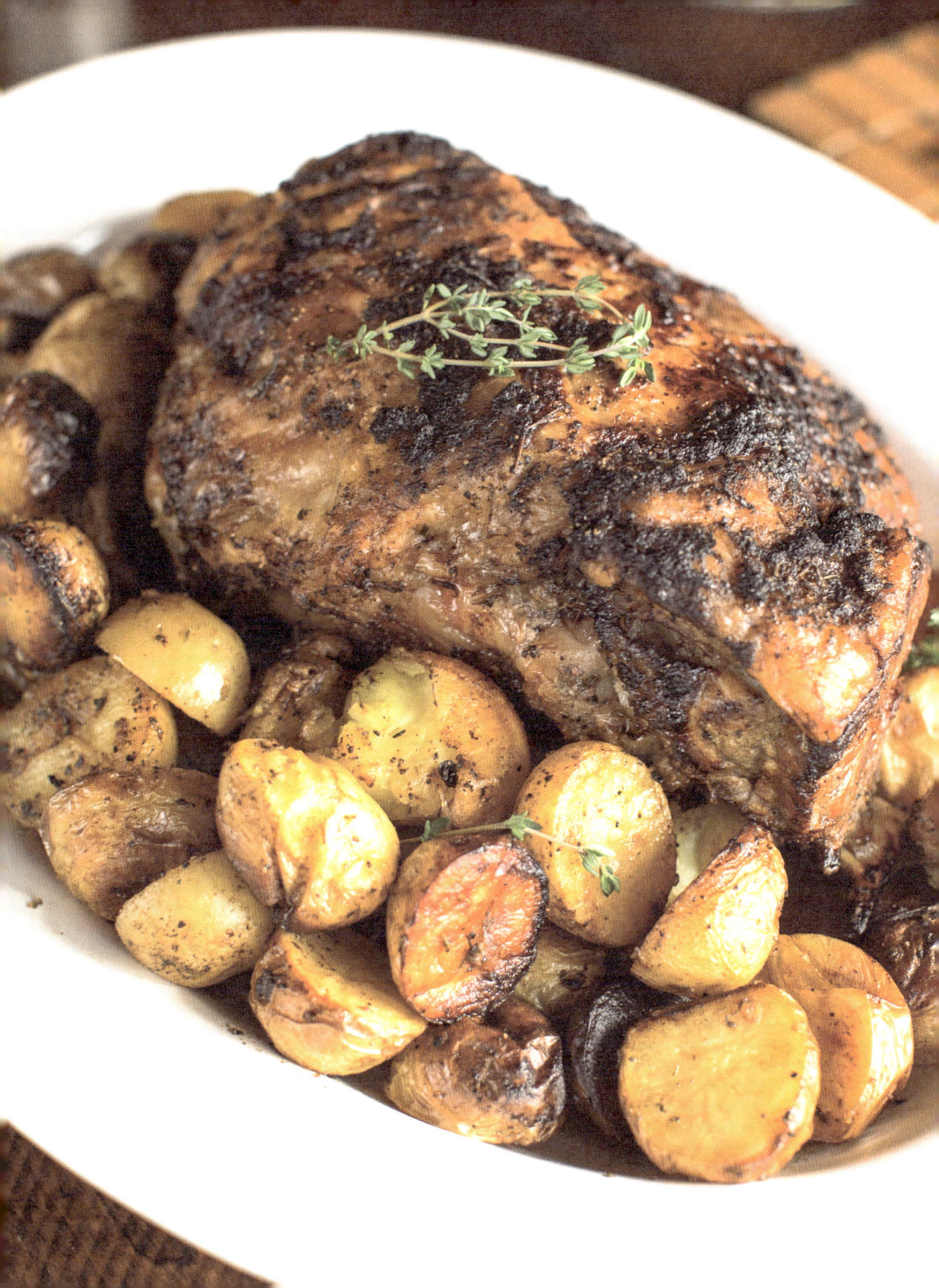

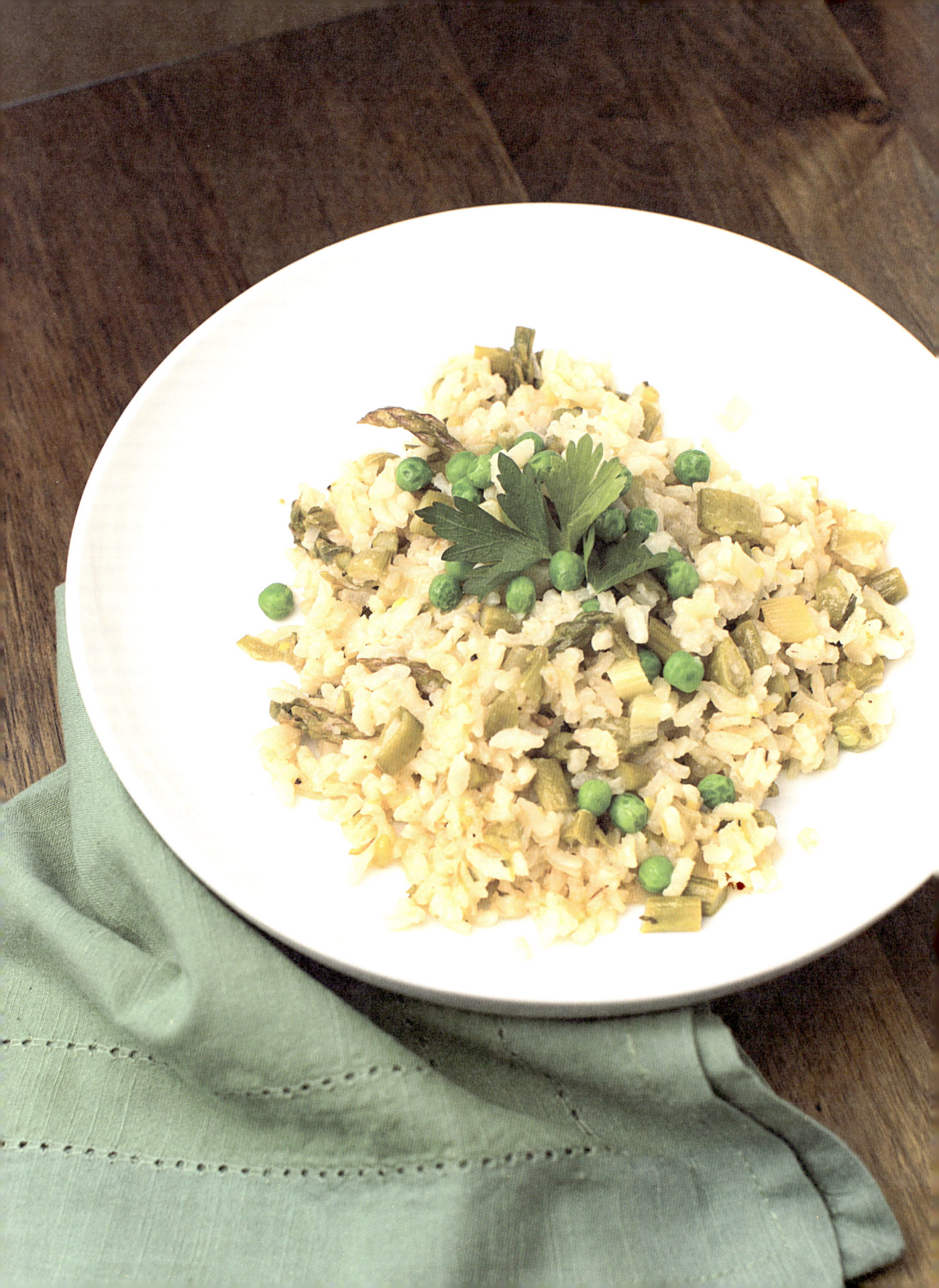

spring green risotto

6-8 servings

PICKING ONLY ONE RISOTTO FOR THE COOKBOOK was very challenging, because every season I come up with a new favorite recipe for this very versatile Italian rice. I decided to go basic, so anyone can learn to make this at home and start experimenting on getting the technique down. Sometimes this recipe is the base for added scallops, shrimp or lobster. In the winter, I use lots of mushrooms and a much heavier stock with leeks and butter. This dish is an excellent version that is wonderful with the first of fresh spring asparagus.

- 3 tablespoons olive oil
- 2 leeks, white part only, cleaned and chopped
- 1 large fennel bulb, cleaned and chopped
- 1½ cups Arborio rice
- ⅔ cup dry white wine
- 4-5 cups chicken stock *(kept simmering on the stove)*
- 1 pound asparagus, trimmed, cut into 1-inch pieces and blanched for 5 minutes *(drain and cool in ice water)*
- 10-ounce package frozen peas, defrosted
- zest from 1 lemon
- zest from 1 lime
- 2 tablespoons fresh lemon juice
- sea salt and fresh pepper to taste
- 2/3 cup parmesan, freshly grated
- 3 tablespoons fresh chives, minced

MBK'S TIPS

Don't plan on leaving the kitchen while making risotto. You need to stir often and add stock slowly throughout the cooking process. Taste rice along the way for preferred texture.

The stock must stay warm to ensure even, continuous and thorough cooking.

GF

1. In large non-stick saucepan heat oil on medium heat. Add leeks and fennel and saute for 5-7 minutes.

2. Add rice and cook for 2 minutes. Add white wine and simmer until the wine is absorbed.

3. Add chicken stock, ½ cup at a time, allowing for the stock to be absorbed. Stir occasionally and continue cooking for 15 minutes

4. Add asparagus, peas, lemon zest, lime zest, lemon juice and fresh peper. Contiue adding stock in increments, for an additional 10 minutes until rice is tender but still firm. At this point the risotto should ready.

5. Right before serving add parmesan, chives and additional salt, if necessary. Serve warm with extra parmesan for topping.

Enjoy!

grilled rosemary lamb chops

IN RECENT YEARS AMERICAN LAMB HAS GOTTEN very popular. It's no longer necessary to purchase lamb from other parts of the world. You can usually find local lamb all year long. This recipe is easy to make and so delicious and works for a quick, weeknight meal or entertaining guests. If you are hungry for lamb, this is a recipe that will please. Just remember to marinate it well in advance.

12 - 1-inch thick loin lamb chops

salt and pepper, to season chops

¼ cup balsamic vinegar

6 tablespoons olive oil

6 garlic cloves, minced

3 tablespoons fresh lemon, juiced

3 tablespoons fresh rosemary, minced

NUTRITION EXTRAS

As most lamb is pasture-raised on a natural diet, it is a great healthy protein choice for dinner.

GF
DF
LS

1. Salt and pepper lamb chops and place in a single layer in a 13x9 inch glass dish.

2. Mix remaining ingredients to create a marinade for chops. Pour over lamb and refrigerate for at least 4 hours and up to 8, turning meat occasionally.

3. Prepare grill on medium-high heat and grill chops to desired doneness, basting often with marinade, about 4 minutes per side.

Enjoy!

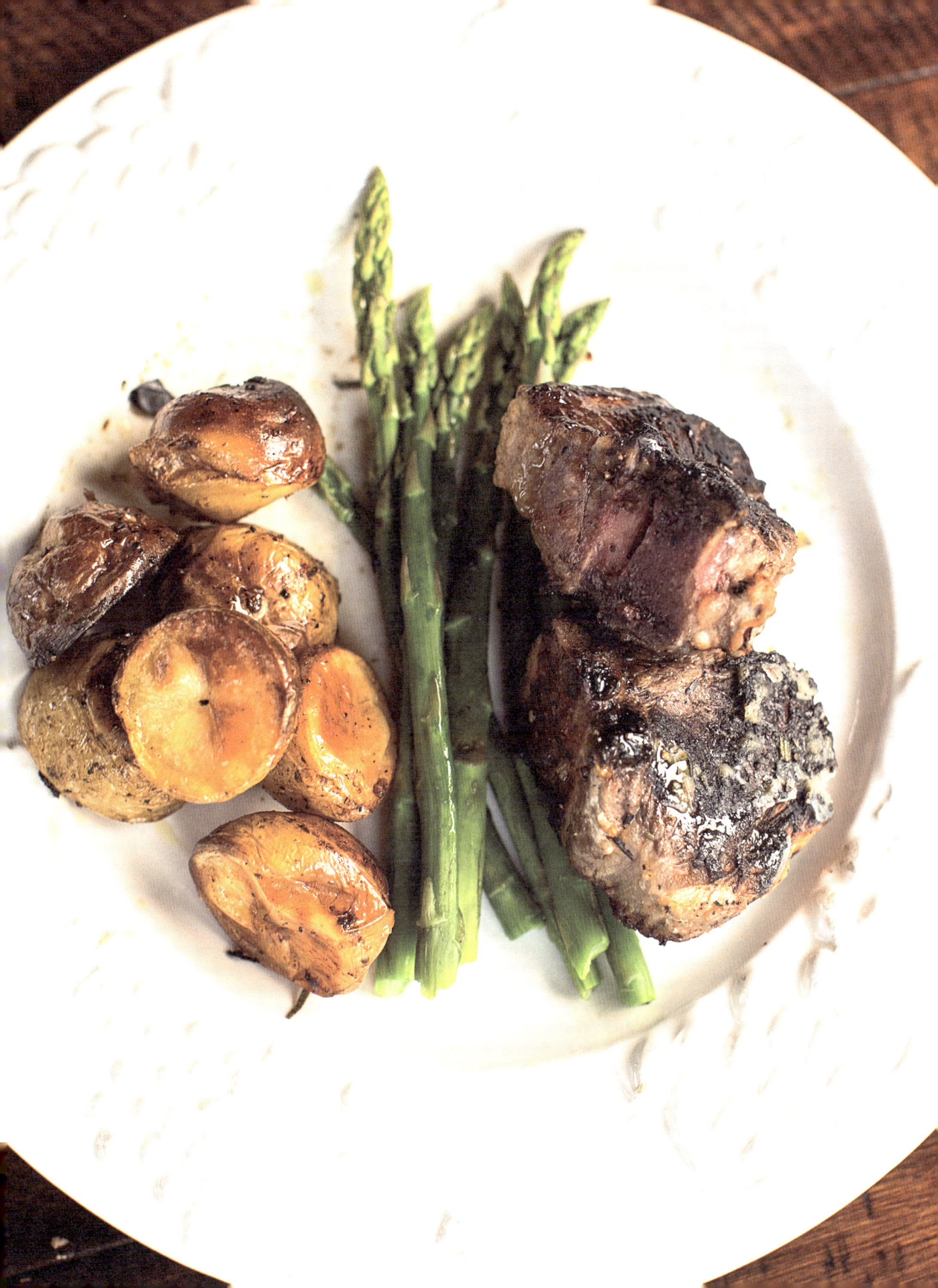

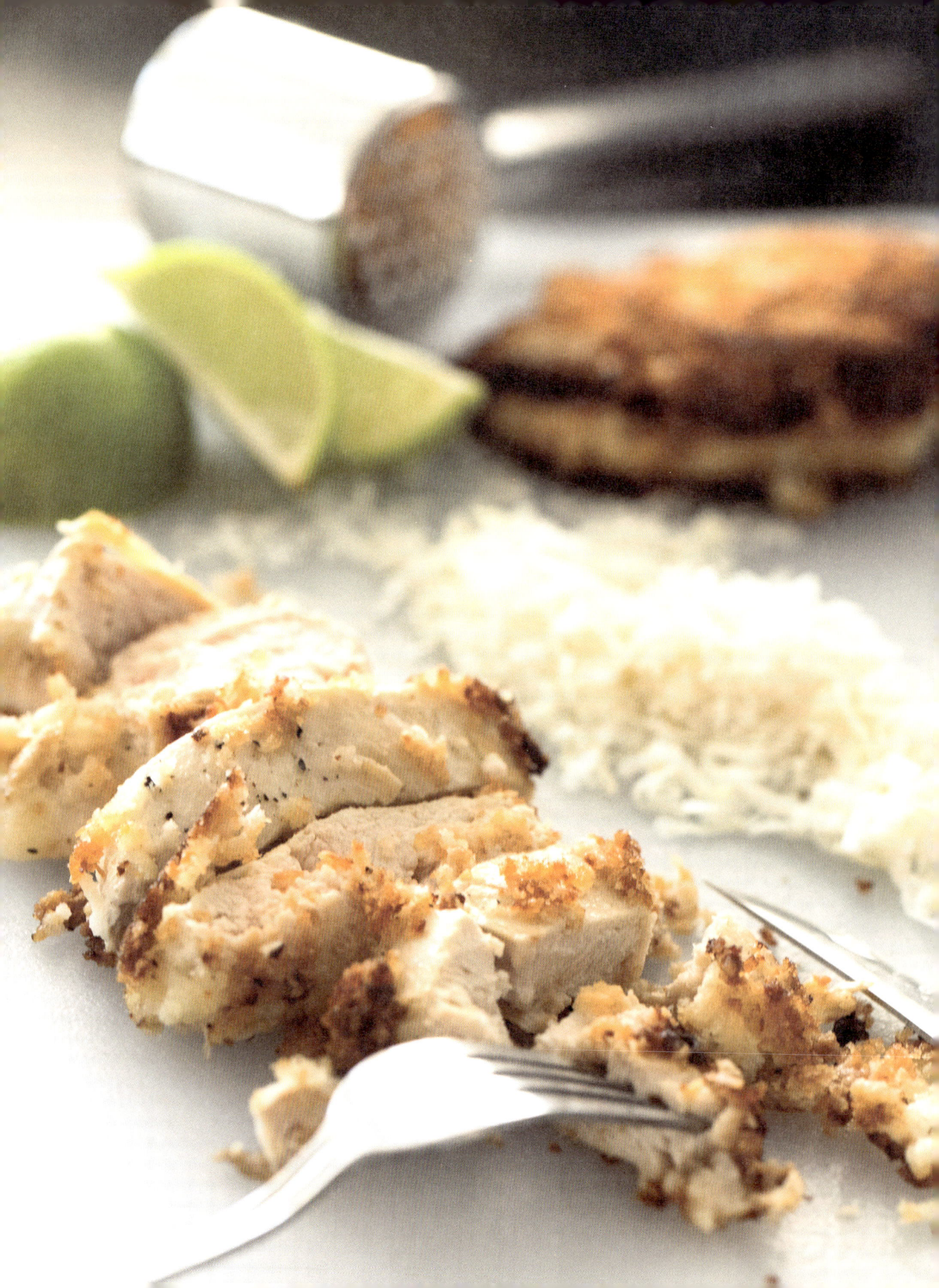

coconut chicken
6 servings

THIS RECIPE IS ADAPTED FROM A DISH CREATED BY Marcus Samuelsson, head chef and proprietor of The Red Rooster in Harlem. I love how easy this dish is to make and how flavorful the coconut panko crust becomes. I will warn you that there is no grey when it comes to coconut, people either love it or hate it, so it's a bit of a gamble to serve when entertaining. I have tried doubling the recipe for a large group, and it got a little messy. Keep this one reserved for an intimate party or family dinner.

6 medium-sized chicken breasts, pounded to tenderize

2 cups buttermilk

½ cup coconut milk

2 garlic cloves, minced

salt and fresh pepper

2 cups panko

3 tablespoons unsweetened, finely shredded coconut

avocado oil for cooking chicken

MBK'S TIPS

If you are trying to stay gluten-free, there are plenty of good options for panko with no gluten as an alternative.

Make sure to get the oil good and hot, because you only want to have to turn the chicken once. Keep the breasts on the smaller side.

1. In a ziplock bag combine chicken, buttermilk, coconut milk and garlic. Refrigerate for 2-4 hours.

2. Drain chicken and season with salt and pepper.

3. In a shallow bowl combine panko, coconut and additional ½ teaspoon salt and pepper.

4. Dip cutlets in panko, coating both sides of meat and place back in the refrigerator for 10 minutes.

5. In a large skillet heat ⅓ cup of oil, on medium-high heat. Once the pan is hot, cook chicken, turning once, approximately 6 minutes per side. Moderate the heat so the chicken does not burn.

6. Drain on paper towels and rest the meat for 10 minutes before serving.

Enjoy!

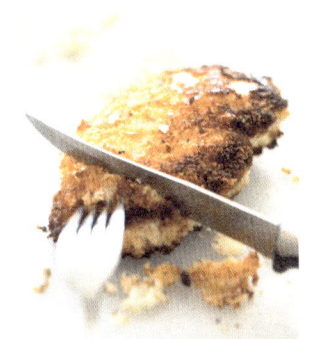

fresh tomato sauce

NEVER IS THE QUALITY OF THE PRODUCTS IN YOUR PANTRY more critical than those that go into your fresh tomato sauce. San Marzano tomatoes are the best and sometimes very pricey, but well worth it. Shop around and stock up when you see them on sale. Fresh basil is always available thankfully, and adds a subtle sweetness to the sauce. Very different than dried basil. I use this sauce for many dishes, including my homemade pizza, as it freezes beautifully. I almost always have some already prepared in the refrigerator or freezer.

MBK'S TIPS

In my opinion, the handheld blender is at the top of the appliance chain. This handy tool saves you from having to use the Vitamix or Cuisinart to puree your sauce.

I would only keep this sauce in the refrigerator for a week, before needing to freeze the leftovers.

NUTRITION EXTRAS

This sauce is a good source of vitamin A and vitamin C as well as potassium.

GF
DF
V

- ⅓ cup olive oil
- 1 large sweet onion, chopped
- 4 garlic cloves
- 3 - 28-ounce cans San Marzano tomatoes
- 1 - 15-ounce can good quality tomato sauce
- 1 - 28-ounce can tomato puree
- 4 cups of water
- ½ bottle of red wine
- 1 cup fresh basil, chopped
- 2 tablespoons dried basil
- 2+ tablespoons dried oregano
- 2 teaspoons crushed red pepper
- 2 tablespoons dark brown sugar
- 2 bay leaves

1. In a large stockpot over medium-low heat, heat oil and saute onion and garlic until translucent, approximately 7 minutes.

2. Add all remaining ingredients except bay leaves. Cook on a low boil for 30 minutes.

3. Puree sauce with a handheld mixer.

4. Add bay leaves and continue to cook. At this point, you can add meatballs and Italian sausage, if desired. Continue to cook on low for 1-2 hours.

Enjoy!

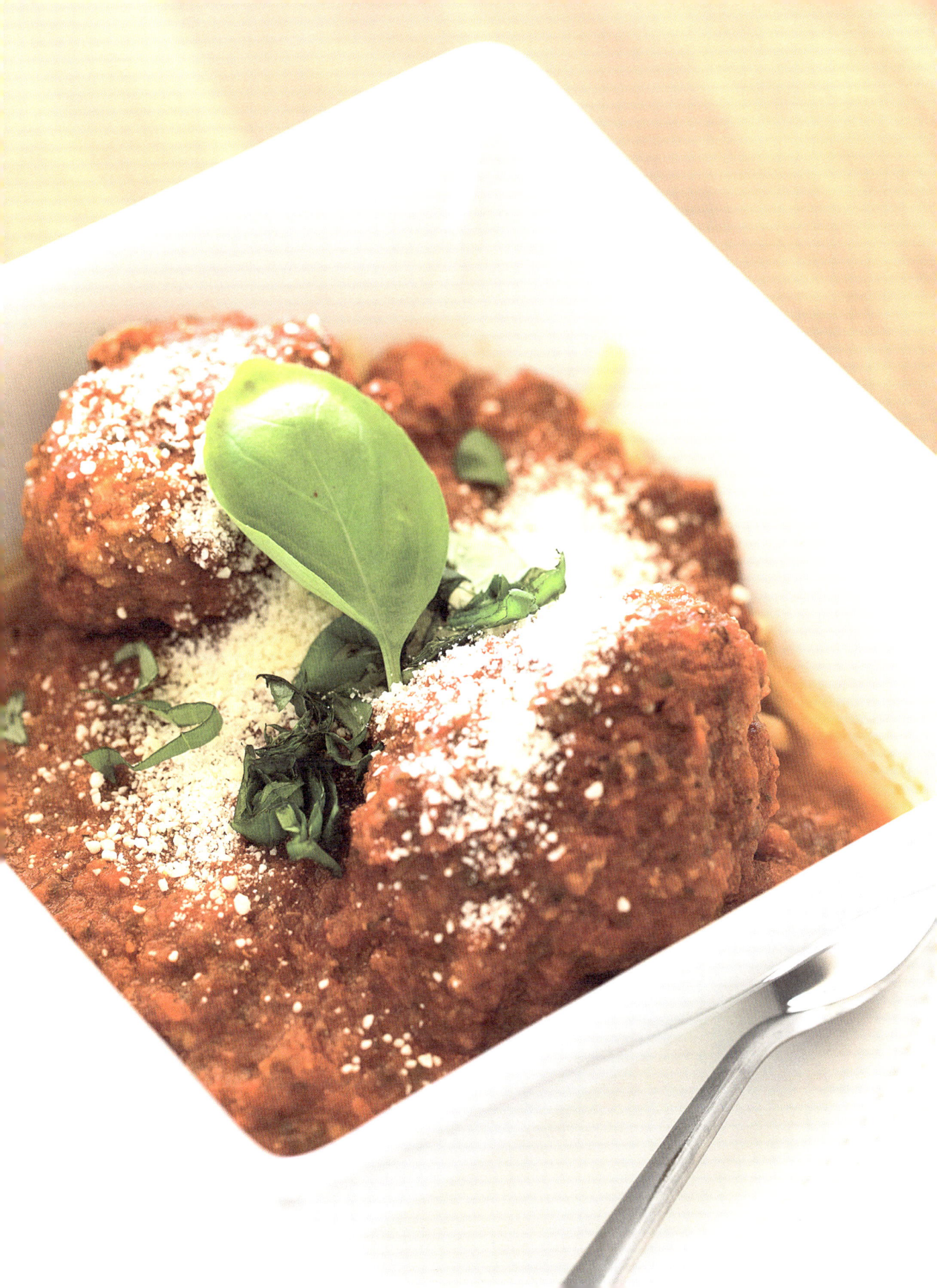

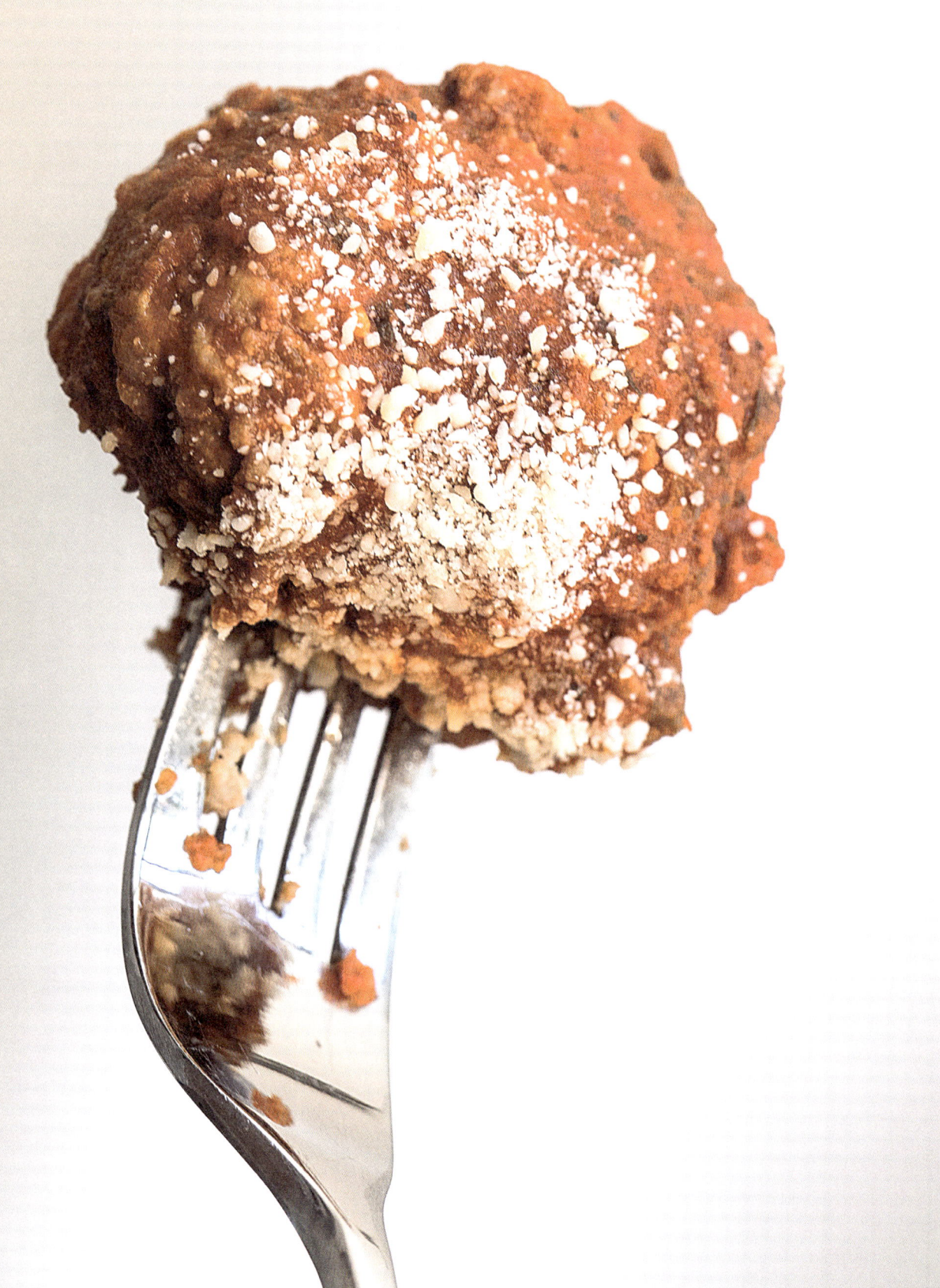

meatballs!

THERE IS NOTHING COMPLICATED ABOUT MY MEATBALLS and people always seem to want the recipe. Credit goes to the quality of my ingredients and the homemade sauce that they are swimming in. My nephew Connor always requested this dish when he came for dinner. The secret is out and it's not a big one!

- 1 pound lean ground beef
- 1 pound ground pork
- 2 medium eggs
- 1 cup Italian style breadcrumbs
- ½ cup parmesan cheese, finely grated
- 1 tablespoon + 1 teaspoon oregano
- 2 teaspoons pepper
- 1 teaspoon salt

1. Gently mix all ingredients by hand in a large glass mixing bowl.
2. Form small, even meatballs and drop directly into the already prepared tomato sauce.
3. Cook for a good hour on a low simmer.

Enjoy!

MBK'S TIPS

I prefer freshly grated parmesan, which most of the stores now offer in the cheese department. You're going to need lots of cheese for the dish, so stock up.

The old school thought is to brown the meatballs before putting into the sauce. I never thought it necessary. Who needs an extra dirty pan?

crab cakes
4 servings

IF YOU LIVE IN MARYLAND AND YOU ENJOY COOKING chances are you have a crab cake recipe. I have tried many variations, always using jumbo lump Maryland crab and I think I have nailed the perfect version with this recipe. I never tire of making crab cakes and often prepare these for my husband Jeff, as he loves this delicious traditional Maryland seafood dish.

MBK'S TIPS

If you are doubling this recipe, it's perfectly ok to buy lump crabmeat to mix with the jumbo lump, to save a few dollars on the total cost. It will still be a very rich, loaded crab cake that has very little filler.

You can use plain bread crumbs, plain panko or ground up saltine crackers - they all work.

NUTRITION EXTRAS

Can be gluten-free, simply purchase GF Panko

DF
LS

- 1 pound fresh jumbo lump Maryland blue crab, drained and clean
- ⅓ cup organic mayonnaise
- ½ cup fine cracker crumbs or panko
- 1 teaspoon dry mustard
- 1 teaspoon old bay
- ⅛ teaspoon cayenne pepper
- 2 teaspoon fresh lemon juice
- 1 tablespoon fresh parsley, chopped
- ¼ teaspoon fine sea salt
- ¼ teaspoon white pepper
- 1 egg, beaten
- avocado oil
- lemon wedges for serving

1. Mix mayonnaise, cracker crumbs, dry mustard, old bay, cayenne, lemon juice, parsley, salt and pepper.

2. Gently fold in 1 pound of drained, clean crab meat.

3. Carefully fold in beaten egg.

4. Mold mixture into six medium or four large crab cakes. Set on wax paper to refrigerate for 15 minutes *(or until needed)*.

5. In large saute pan heat 3 tablespoons avocado oil on medium-high heat. Cook crab cakes, approximately 4 minutes per side or until cooked throughout. Serve with lemon.

Enjoy!

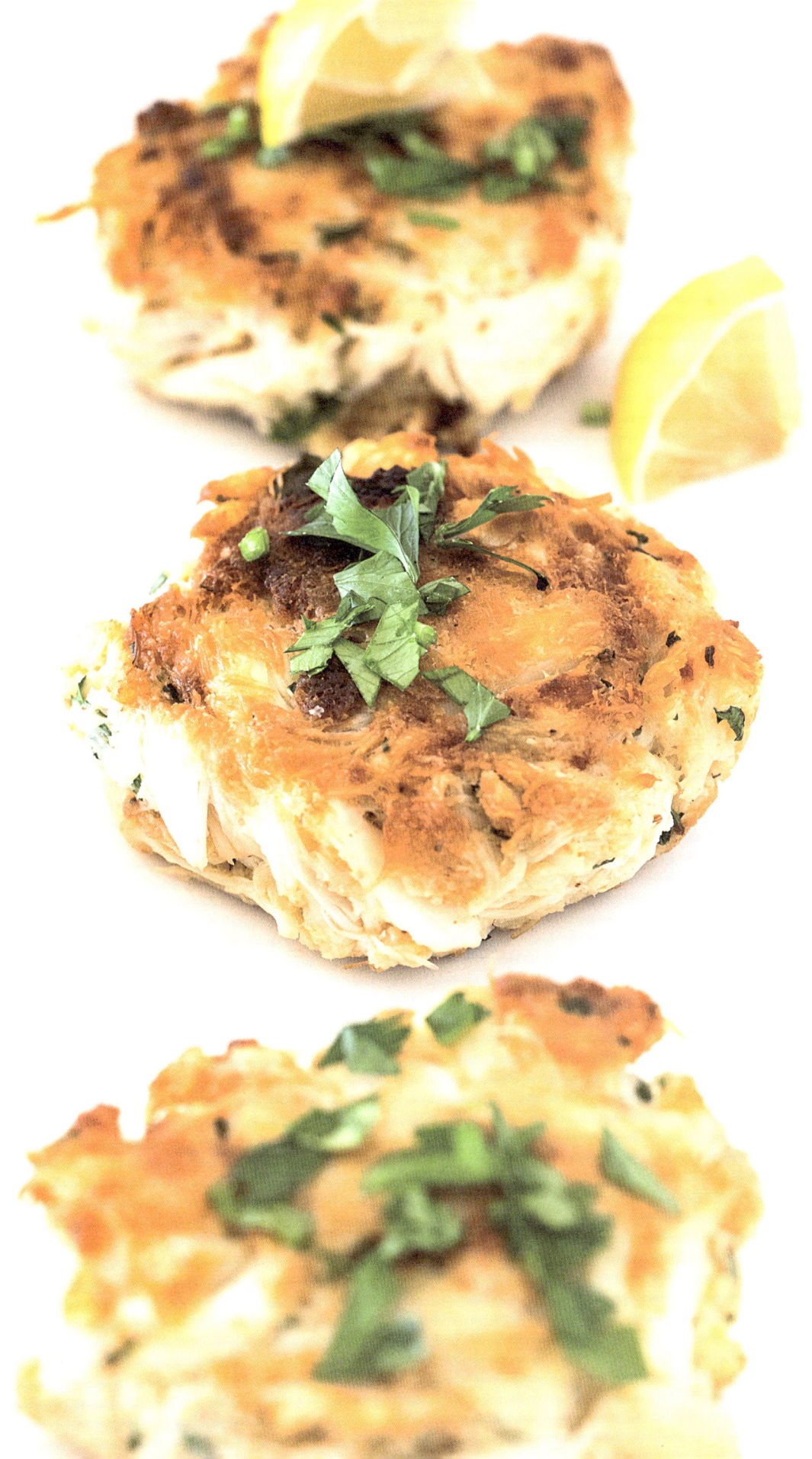

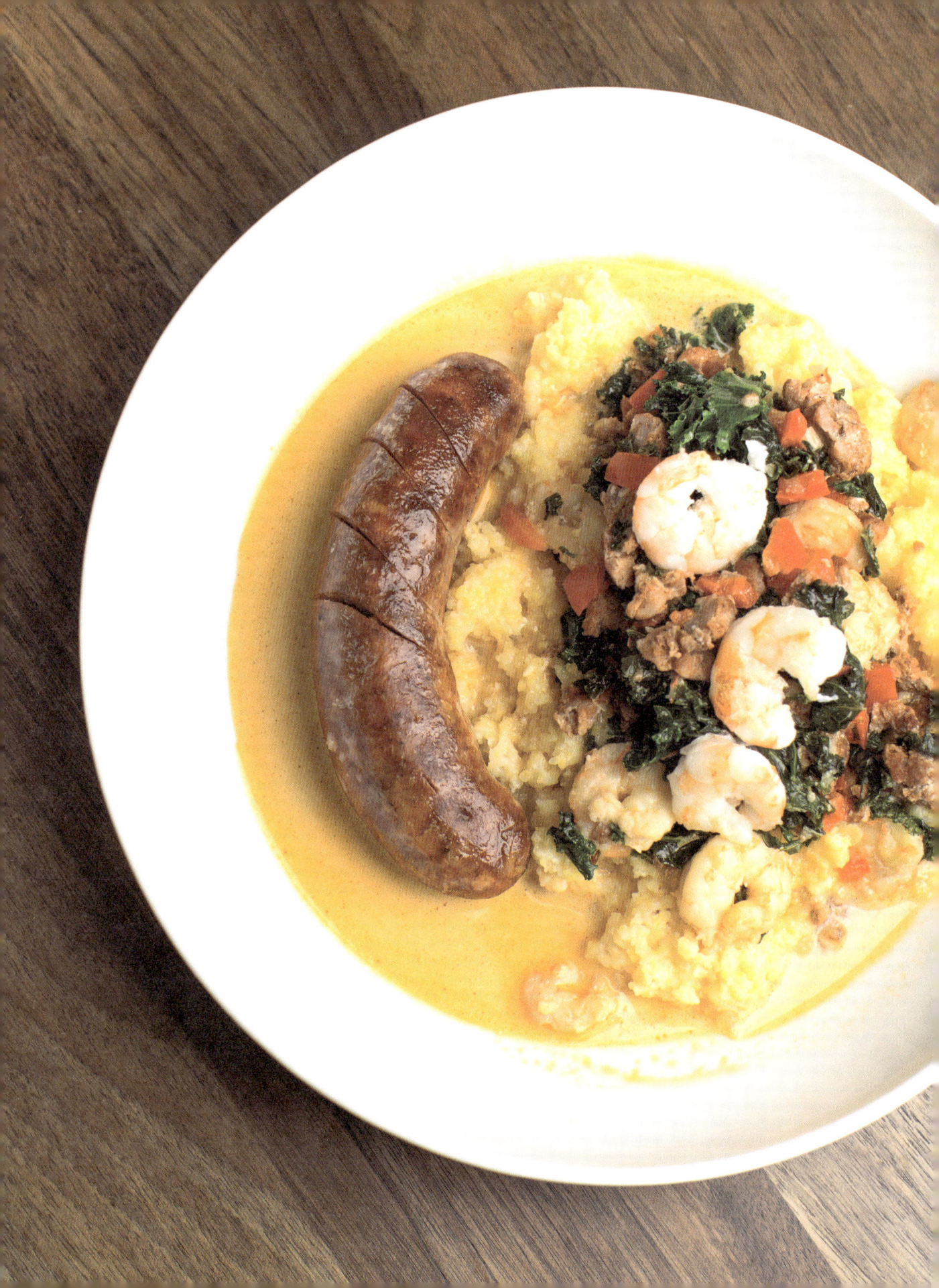

shrimp and grits
with chorizo & kale

4 servings

THIS RECIPE IS MY TAKE ON A VERY VERSATILE dish that I have seen prepared in so many ways. I have tasted other creamier or cheesier versions and thought it was unnecessary to make this such a heavy dish. I lightened the sauce with stock, added some fresh greens and quickly turned this classic into my healthy version of shrimp and grits.

1 cup cooked grits, prepared as directed

olive oil

2 large chorizo sausage links, casing removed

1 medium shallot, diced

1 red pepper, diced

1 bunch of swiss chard, stems removed and sliced thinly *(approximately 2 cups)*

1 cup chicken or vegetable stock

½ cup heavy cream

1 pound shrimp, cleaned and deveined

salt and pepper to taste

fresh parsley

1. Prepare grits according to directions. Keep warm.
2. Heat 2 tablespoons of oil in a large skillet. Add chorizo and cook until brown and cooked through, breaking up meat as it cooks. Drain fat and remove meat from the pan.
3. Add 2 tablespoons of oil to the pan and saute shallots, red pepper and swiss chard and cook until tender.
4. Add stock and meat. Turn heat to medium and create a low boil for 2-3 minutes.
5. Add cream and shrimp while the sauce is simmering and cook until the sauce thickens, an additional 2-3 minutes. Adjust seasoning, adding more salt and pepper, if necessary.
6. Serve over warm grits. Top with fresh parsley.

Enjoy!

MBK'S TIPS

Any dark, leafy green will work, but my favorite is chard. It's a little softer than most kales and not as bitter.

GF

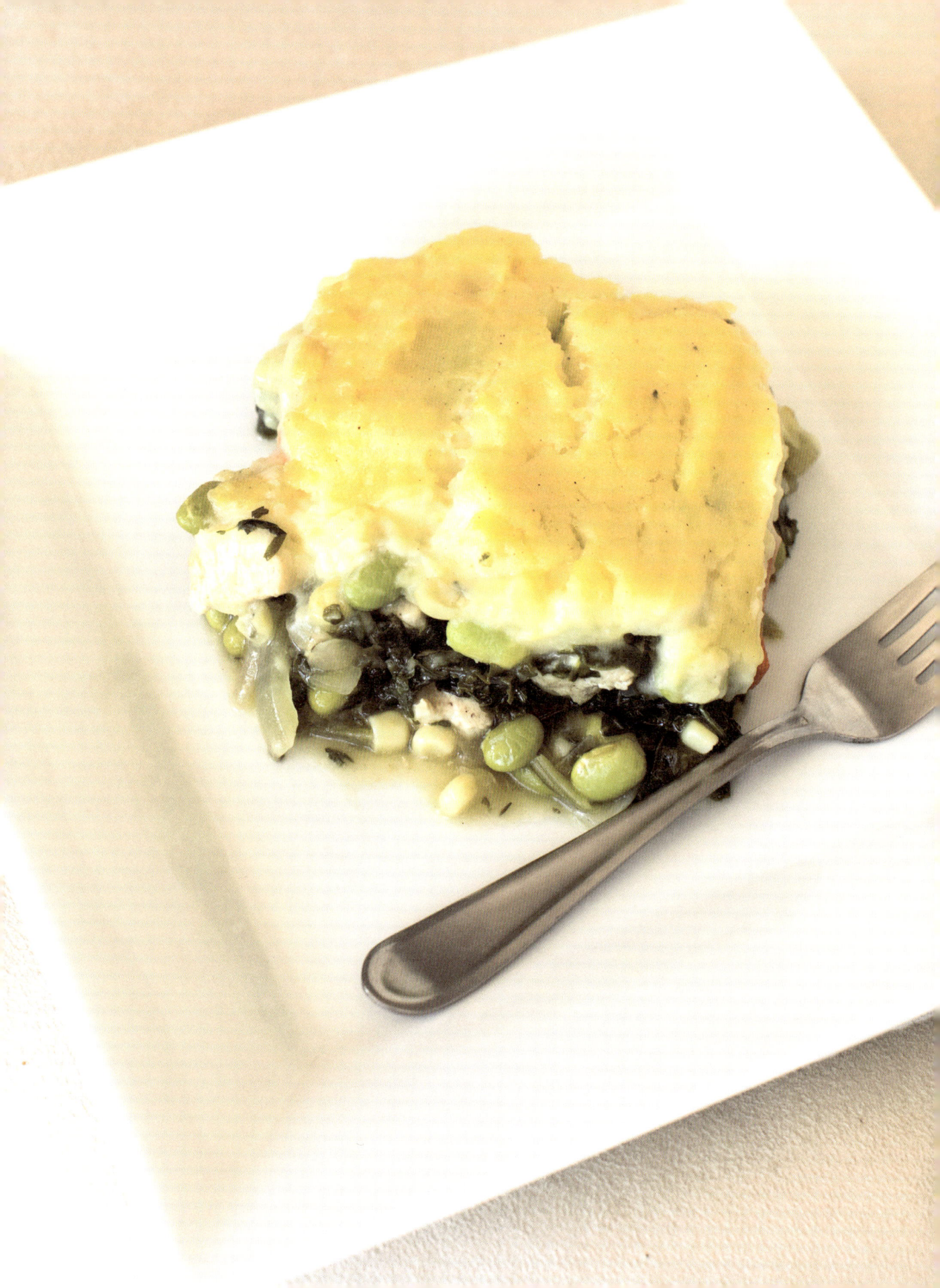

post-thanksgiving
shepherd's pie

6 servings

I ONLY MAKE THIS DISH ONCE A YEAR AND I ENJOY it so much I always wonder why I don't make it more often. It's a great dish to make with Thanksgiving leftovers and a great way to clean out the refrigerator. You can add any additional vegetables you might have because everything goes well under the blanket of mashed potatoes!

3 tablespoons olive oil

2 medium onions, chopped

3 carrots, chopped

4 celery stalks, chopped

2 cups frozen peas, thawed

2 cups left over turkey breast, chopped

2½ cups chicken stock, (hopefully some leftover gravy can be part of this portion)

2 tablespoons corn starch

2 teaspoons dried thyme

salt and pepper to taste

4 cups leftover mashed potatoes

1. Preheat oven to 375°.

2. In a large saucepan heat oil on medium heat. Saute onions and carrots until vegetables soften, approximately 10 minutes.

3. Add celery, peas, turkey and stock. Bring mixture to boil and add corn starch that has been diluted with equal parts water. Simmer for 10 minutes, adding thyme, salt and pepper to taste.

4. Pour mixture into a large 8x12 glass baking dish and spread mashed potatoes evenly over the top.

5. Bake uncovered for 30 minutes or until potatoes are starting to brown and mixture is boiling. Pull from oven and let rest 15 minutes before serving.

Enjoy!

MBK'S TIPS

My basic recipe here includes 4 vegetables, Adding additional greens makes it that much more nutrient-rich.

The picture here includes spinach and edamame, to show a variation on the dish.

NUTRITION EXTRAS

The edamame gives this dish a protein boost in addition to the protein from the turkey. It's loaded with enough vegetables, that it stands on its own as a complete meal.

GF

roasted chicken
with vegetables

EVERY HOUSE NEEDS A RECIPE TO FEED A FAMILY, and this one is my eldest son Blake's favorite meal. I have cooked and re-cooked this recipe hundreds of times. Over the years, I've been able to get the seasoning and cooking time down just right. This dish is a tried and true perfect Sunday dinner with wholesome deliciousness.

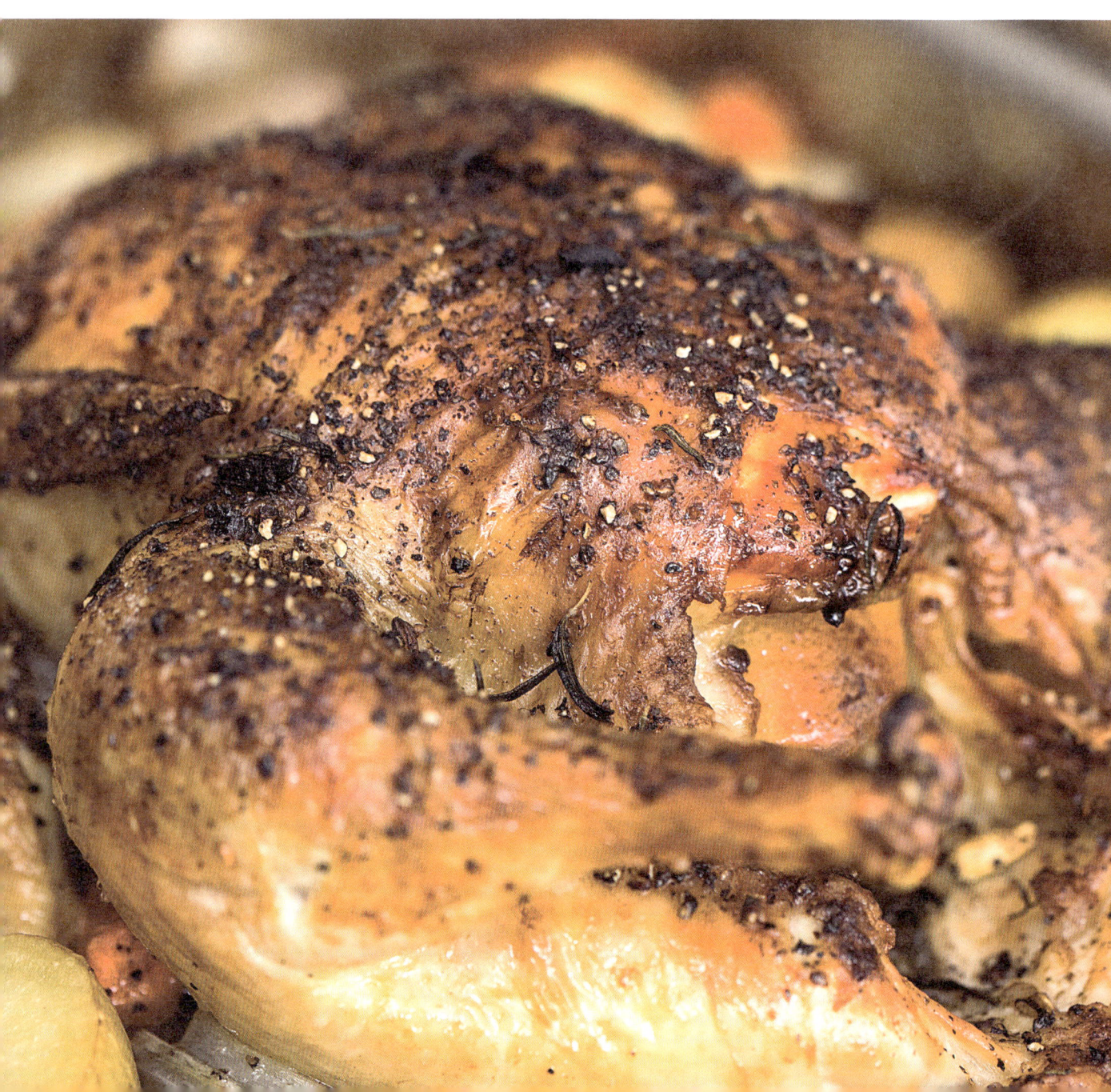

4-5 pound organic roasting chicken

1 lemon

olive oil

course sea salt and fresh ground pepper

1 tablespoon dried rosemary or 2 tablespoons fresh rosemary, chopped fine

cooking spray

1½ pounds Yukon gold potatoes and sweet potatoes, cut into uniform size portions

1½ pounds large carrots, cut into similar size portions

2 large sweet onions, quartered

2 cups chicken stock or white wine

MBK'S TIPS

Mix and match any choice of vegetables to roast under the bird. I love fennel, sweet onions and roasted sweet potatoes, along with good ole Yukon gold. Make sure vegetables are only one layer deep. You don't want to crowd the vegetables and you want to ensure an even cook.

1. Preheat oven to 425° convection.

2. Squeeze juice from lemon all over the bird, then rub olive oil to coat the chicken.

3. Generously cover the chicken with salt, pepper and rosemary. Insert the lemon halves into the cavity of the bird.

4. Spray a large roasting pan, fitted with a rack with olive oil and cook the chicken, approximately 30 minutes.

5. Remove from oven, add a layer of vegetables to the bottom of the pan and spray lightly with olive oil. Add 1½ cups chicken stock or wine and stir to coat before going back into the oven.

6. Toss vegetables every 20 minutes, adding more stock if necessary during the cooking process. Continue cooking for 1 hour or until chicken is done and vegetables are browned and caramelized.

7. Remove from oven and allow the chicken to rest for 15 minutes before serving. Top vegetables with pan drippings and serve alongside chicken.

Enjoy!

NUTRITION EXTRAS

After making this you will have great leftovers for lunches the following week. Chicken is something I always have in my house, as it yields very high amounts of protein per gram of calories and fat.

As always, shop local and buy organic.

GF
DF

eggplant parmesan
4-6 servings

I CRAVE THIS DISH ALL YEAR ROUND, and luckily, access to eggplant is usually available. I like to buy organic eggplant on a smaller scale because it holds up better when browning. Besides, the fruit tends to be firmer. The general rule of thumb is, the larger, more mature the eggplant, the mealier the produce becomes. When my children were little, it took some convincing that this dish could be as delicious as chicken. Thankfully, now they all love this dish, as much as I do. It's a great meatless dinner option.

MBK'S TIPS

Keep it on the light side, by serving on top of roasted spaghetti squash, instead of heavy pasta. Make sure the breadcrumbs are very fine, so the coating does not get too heavy.

NUTRITION EXTRAS

Loads of fiber from both the eggplant and the spaghetti squash. This dinner is low-carb and has plenty of protein for one meal.

- 2 medium eggplants
- 2 eggs, blended
- 1½ cups fine breadcrumbs, seasoned with 1 teaspoon oregano + 1 tablespoon grated parmesan
- ⅓ cup avocado oil
- 6 ounces of fresh mozzarella, finely sliced
- fresh parmesan, grated
- fresh tomato sauce *(see recipe)*

1. Preheat oven to 375°. Have tomato sauce readily available at room temperature or slightly warmed.

2. Peel and cut the eggplant into even size rounds, ½ inch slices.

3. Dip eggplant first into the egg mixture, then breadcrumbs and set aside.

4. Heat oil on medium-high heat *(use large skillet good for browning foods)*. When the oil is slightly smoking, place eggplant evenly on the surface of the hot pan. Brown for approximately 3-5 minutes per side. Drain on paper towels.

5. In a large rectangular pan cover the bottom of the pan with a thin layer of sauce and place eggplant evenly on top.

6. Cover with mozzarella and additional sauce, approximately 3 cups. Top with grated parmesan *(optional)* and bake for 40 minutes.

Enjoy!

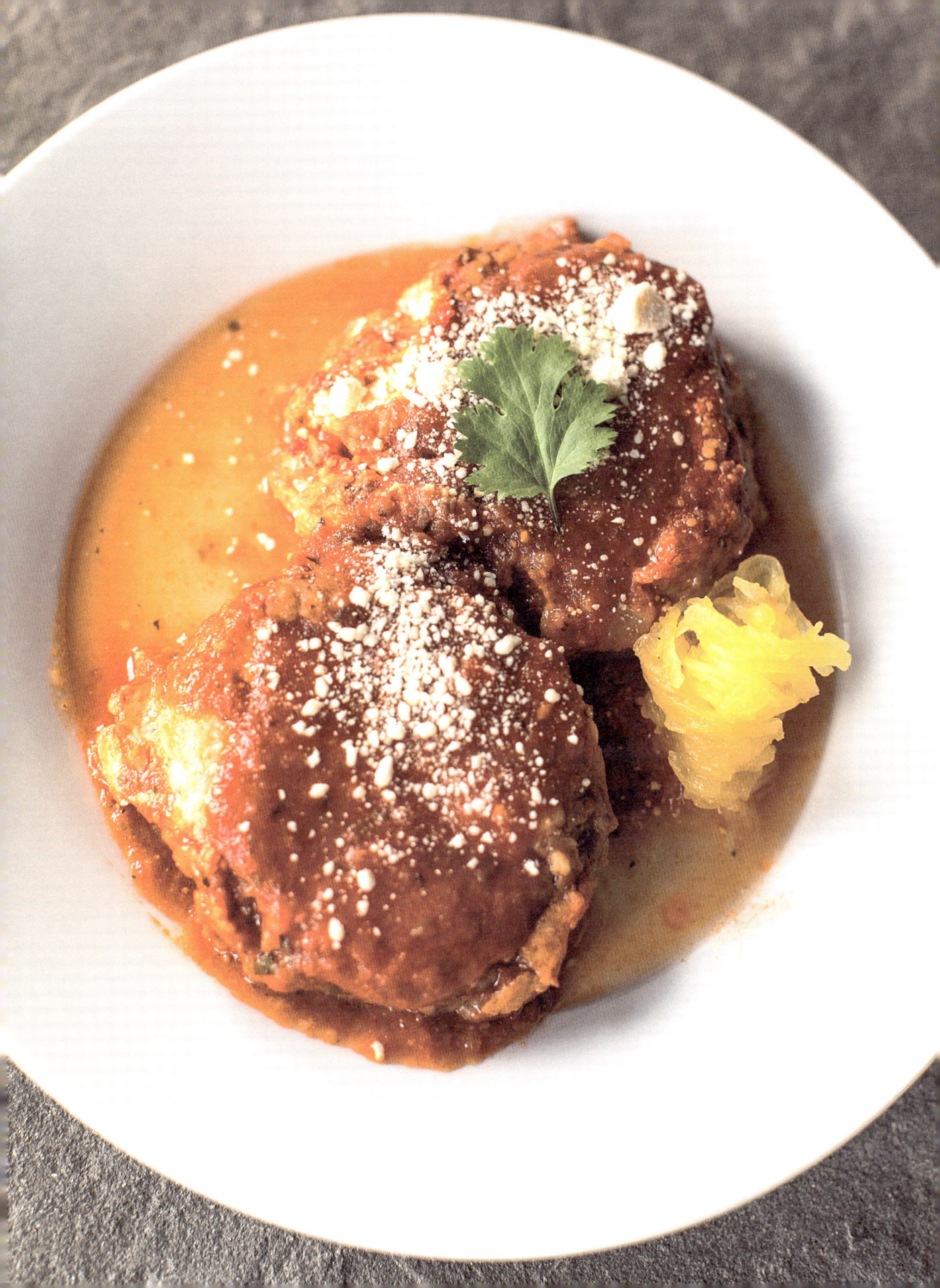

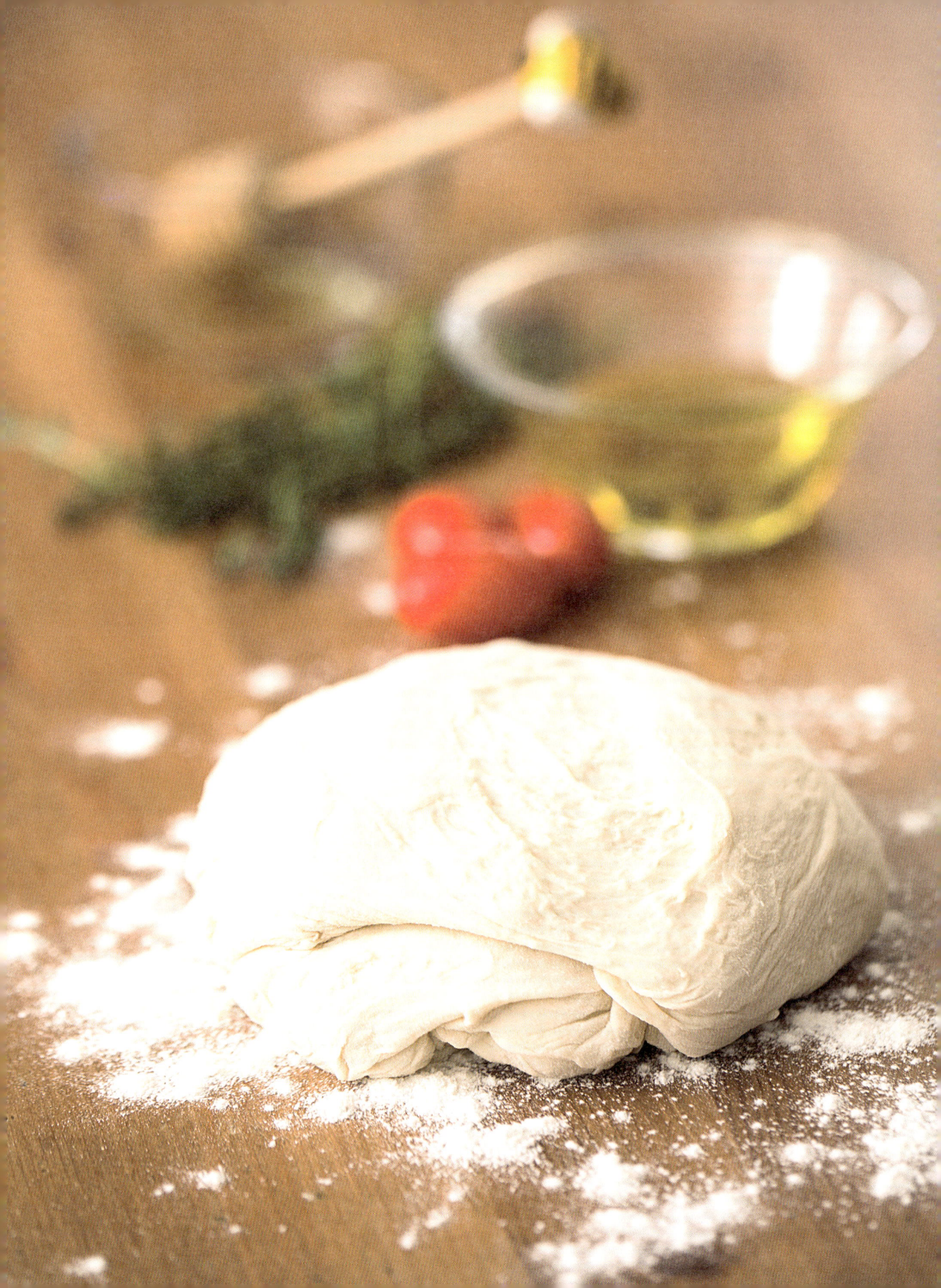

fresh pizza dough

Making this recipe at home makes this dough so much fresher and tastier than store bought. It's well worth the effort! I have attempted gluten-free flour and cauliflower pizza crusts, with little success. Fresh, artisanal, organic flour, that has been left to rise for plenty of time, rolls out to a beautiful, thin, tasty, crispy crust. Nothing compares!

- 1 teaspoon honey
- 1 teaspoon active dry yeast
- 2¼ cups flour + more if needed
- extra-virgin olive oil
- 1 teaspoon salt
- 2 tablespoons cornmeal

1. Add the honey and yeast to 1 cup of warm water. Stir to dissolve. Let the mixture sit for 3 minutes to make sure the yeast is alive. It should foam and start to bubble.

2. Place the flour and salt in a stand-up mixer fitted with a dough hook. Add the yeast mixture and mix on low speed until the mixture starts to come together.

3. Turn the speed up to medium and mix for 8 minutes. The dough should remain soft and sticky as it starts to pull away from the sides of the bowl. Add 1 extra tablespoon of flour, if needed.

4. Coat your hands in a bit of olive oil and form the dough into a ball. Place dough in a bowl that has been coated with olive oil. Cover with a towel and rest the dough in a warm place until it doubles in size, about 1 hour.

5. Knockdown the dough and cut into four equal pieces, if making smaller pizzas or reform into a ball, if making one large pizza. Rest the dough for an additional hour.

6. Sprinkle cornmeal on pizza pan sprayed with olive oil. Roll dough out on a floured surface to the desired size.

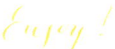

MBK'S TIPS

Always check dates on the yeast package. Out of date yeast will not be active and will cause your dough to not rise. Active yeast should bubble when you mix with the warm water.

DF
V

fresh pizza with the works

4 servings

I WANT TO SAY, THIS IS MY SON WARREN'S FAVORITE MEAL, but I think my other three children would fight for that spot. Everyone loves homemade pizza! There is no comparison to most of the pizzas that are available to purchase. What I love most is the homemade crust that you can roll out to as thin as you like. I have had many pizza parties over the years. This pizza has been enjoyed after evening tennis games with friends, crowds at our lake house, and children's birthday parties. Everyone gets involved in creating their pie. It requires two ovens if you are feeding a lot of people. It can serve as such a fun themed party. Guests have every reason to hang in the kitchen when making this recipe!

MBK'S TIPS

Prepare all the toppings long before anyone gets their hands on the dough. If everything has been organized in advance, the assembly should be super simple.

After spraying the pan with olive oil, sprinkle with cornmeal. It adds texture and taste to the bottom of the crust.

You want the dough good and cooked before removing from the oven. Don't be afraid to see your toppings start to brown.

Ingredients

- fresh pizza dough (*see recipe on the previous page*)
- olive oil spray
- 2 tablespoons cornmeal
- flour for rolling out the dough
- ½ cup tomato sauce
- ¾ cup baby bella mushrooms, sliced
- 1 fresh tomato, sliced thin
- 4 baby bell peppers, in all colors, seeded and sliced thinly
- 1 small sweet onion, sliced thinly
- nitrate-free pepperoni or salami to taste, thinly sliced (*approximately 1/2 stick or 2 large links of Italian sausage*)
- 8 ounces of fresh mozzarella
- dried oregan
- dried crushed hot red pepper flakes
- grated parmesan
- fresh basil

Instructions

1. Preheat oven to 500° for at least 30 minutes before baking.
2. Spray round or rectangle pizza baking sheet with olive oil, then spread the cornmeal evenly, dusting the bottom of the pan.
3. Roll out dough on a floured surface to desired size. Transfer to prepared pan and spread out evenly.
4. Top with tomato sauce, then cut vegetables, sliced meat and cheese.
5. Sprinkle 2 teaspoons of dried oregano, along with 1 teaspoon crushed red pepper, then ¼ cup grated parmesan. Bake for 10-14 minutes, until the desired doneness. Top with fresh basil and let rest 5 minutes before cutting into slices.

Enjoy!

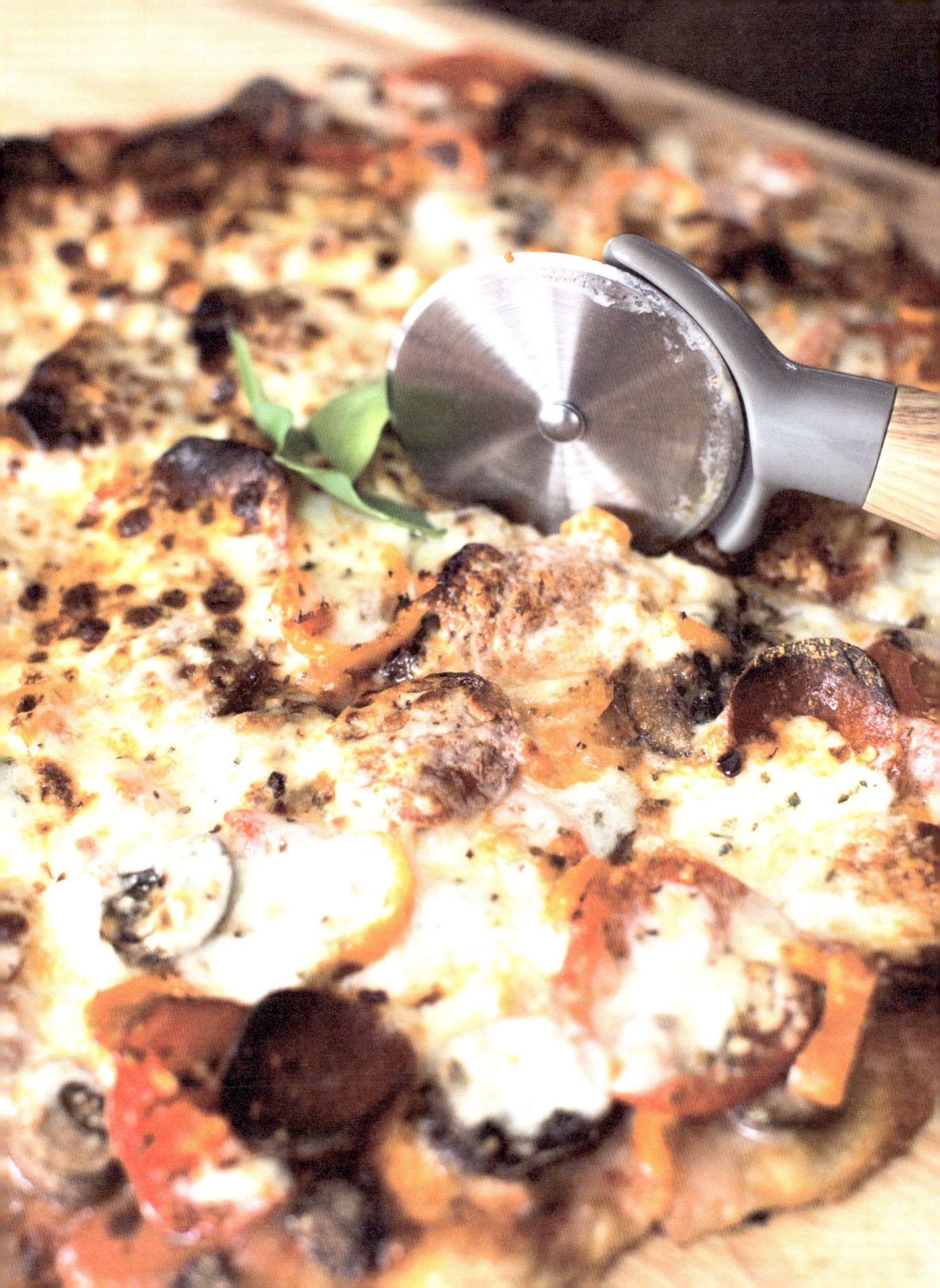

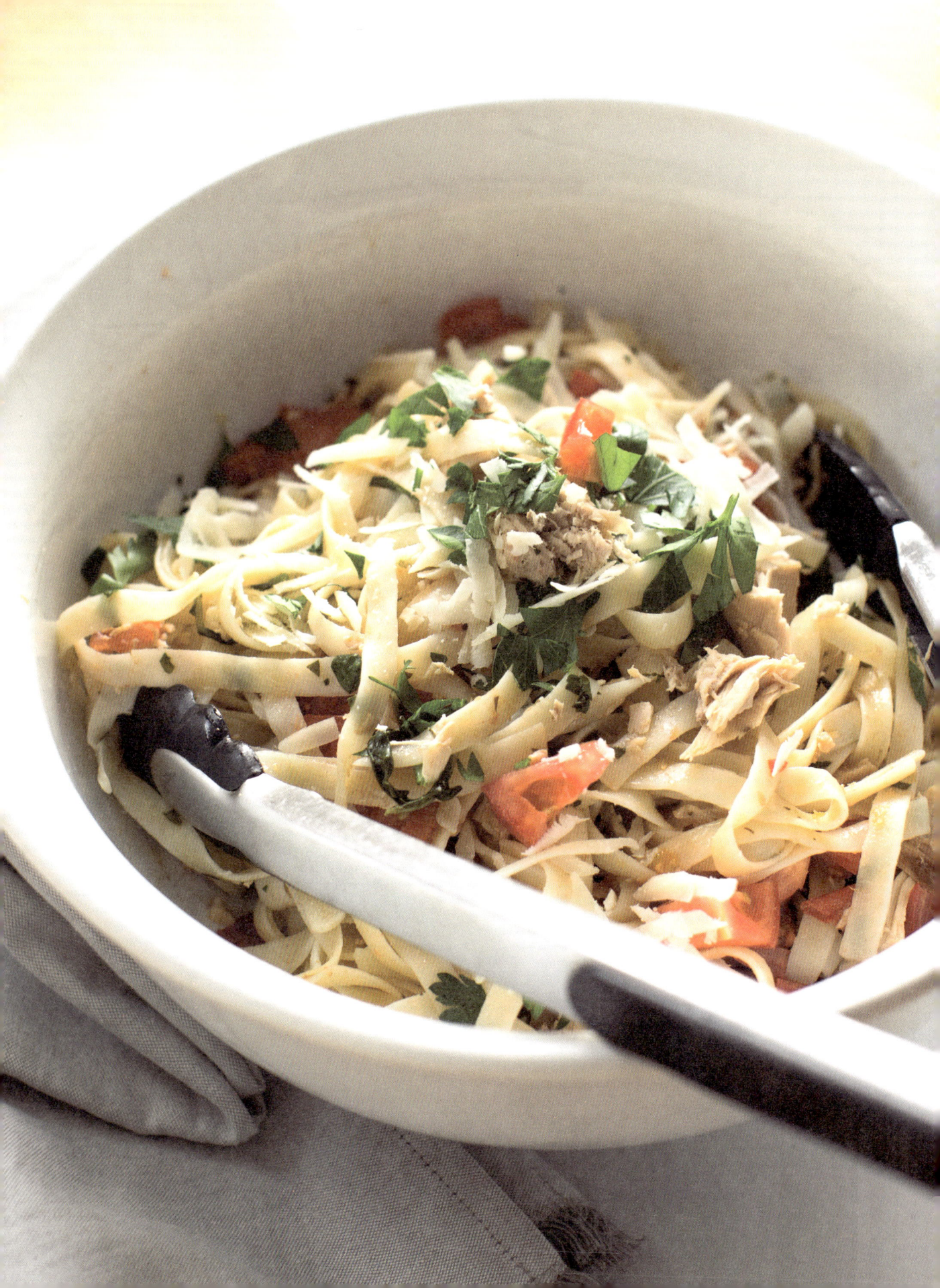

pasta with kale & tuna
4 servings

THIS DISH COULD BE A LIGHT SUMMER LUNCH OR DINNER. It takes very little time to prepare and it's so simple and delicious. I love that it requires nothing fancier than canned tuna. A budget meal that anyone can afford to pull together.

- 8 ounces whole-grain pasta
- 3 tablespoons olive oil
- 4 garlic cloves, finely chopped
- 1 bunch of kale, finely chopped
- ½ cup tomatoes, chopped (fresh or canned)
- ¼ cup parsley, chopped
- 1 can of good quality wild-caught tuna
- lemon juice to taste (one half to one full lemon juiced
- fresh parmesan, grated to taste

MBK'S TIPS

Purchase sustainably caught tuna. It's a personal preference if you like tuna packed in oil or water, but I generally prefer water with light salt added.

1. Cook pasta according to directions.
2. In a saute pan heat oil over medium heat and cook garlic until fragrant, 1-2 minutes. Be careful not to scorch.
3. Add kale and saute until wilted.
4. Add tomatoes.
5. Return pasta to pan with garlic and kale. Add parsley, tuna, and lemon.
6. Warm to taste and top with fresh parmesan.

Enjoy!

NUTRITION EXTRAS

Canned tuna is an excellent protein that is high in omega 3 fatty acids. Kale is rich in Vitamin A, C and K, along with folate, a vitamin that is good for brain development.

chicken piccata
4 servings

THIS LIGHT AND REFRESHING DINNER IS SO EASY to make and hits the spot when you don't want a heavy meal, but want something warm and savory. I usually serve with two greens that pair well with the lemon and wine sauce. Maybe baby broccoli and sautéed spinach? I love lots of mushrooms with every bite, so I tend to use a full container. It's the perfect light meal to reset our bodies after a weekend of heavy dinners.

2 boneless skinless chicken breasts, halved

flour for dredging chicken

olive oil for browning chicken

2 tablespoons unsalted butter, divided

2 whole garlic cloves

sea salt and fresh ground

½ cup white wine

juice of 1 lemon

1 cup chicken stock

2 cups baby bella mushrooms, sliced

¼ cup fresh parsley

NUTRITION EXTRAS

This is a great meal that is high in protein and fiber-rich vegetables. Mushrooms are medicinal, and are known to reduce the length of illness.

1. Pound chicken breast halves between 2 pieces of parchment paper to tenderize. Prepare a shallow dish with flour for dredging chicken.

2. In a saute skillet large enough to hold chicken comfortably, heat 2 tablespoons of oil + 1 tablespoon butter over medium heat. Add garlic and cook just long enough to flavor the oil, approximately 2 minutes. Remove garlic and discard. Turn heat to medium high for browning the chicken.

3. Season chicken with salt and pepper and dredge in flour. Place in hot pan and brown thoroughly on both sides, approximately 4 minutes per side.

4. Remove chicken and add white wine and lemon. Reduce sauce for 2 minutes, whisking any brown bits into sauce.

5. Add stock, remaining butter and mushrooms. Return chicken to pan, reduce heat to a low boil and cook for approximately 15 minutes.

6. Top with fresh parsley, 2 minutes before removing from heat.

Enjoy!

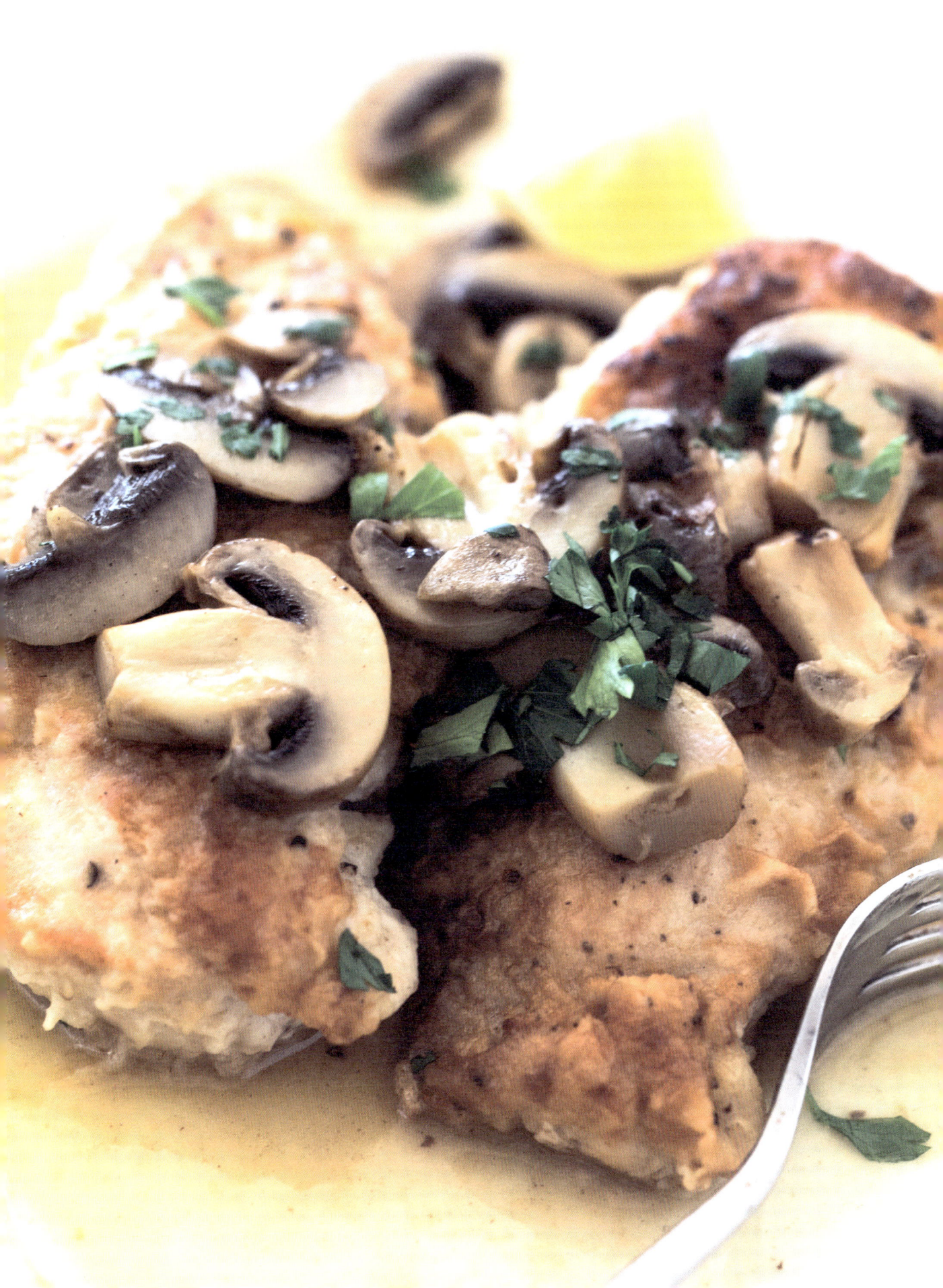

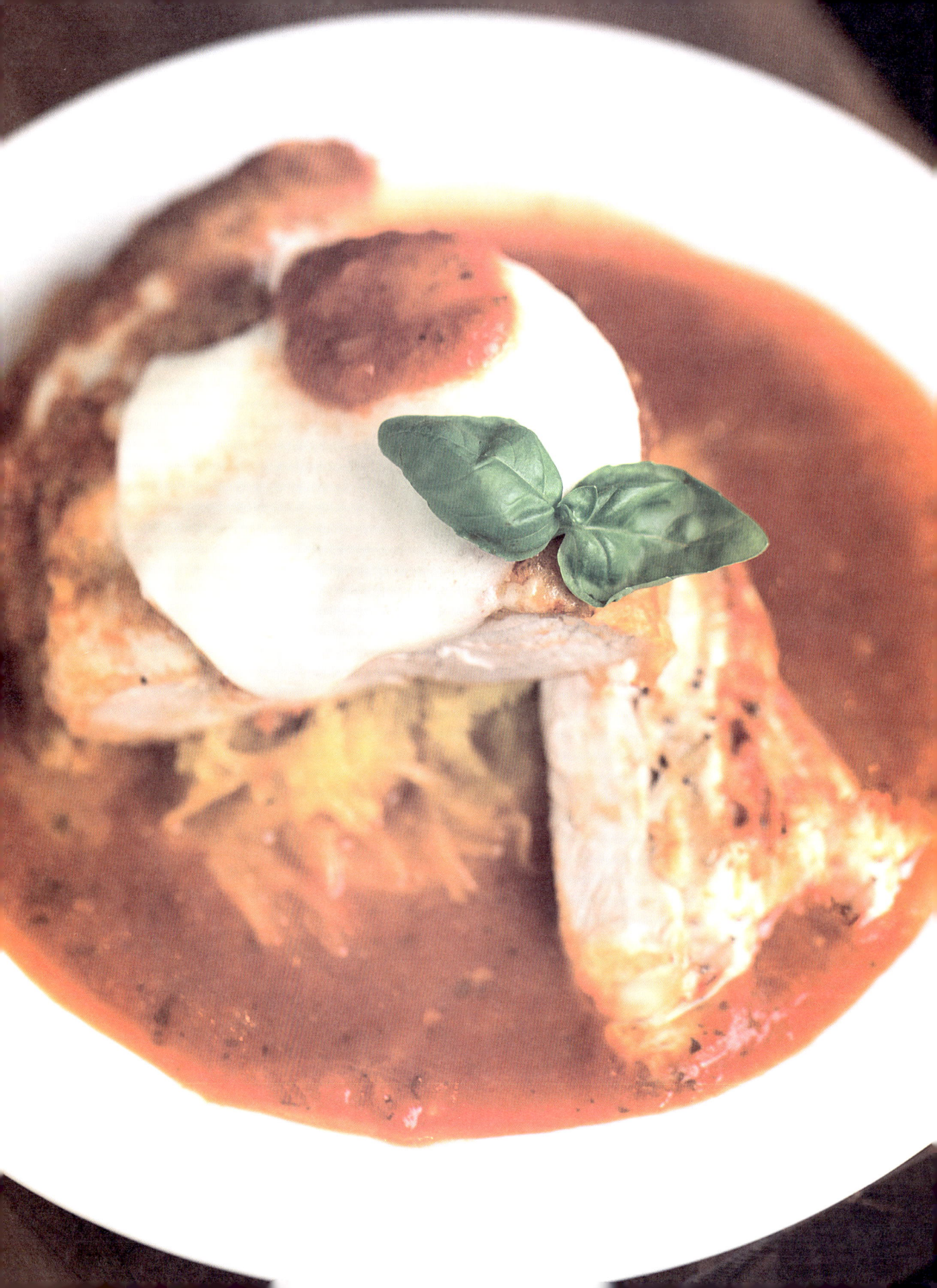

chicken parmesan
4-6 servings

THIS MEAL IS BY FAR MY DAUGHTER BRITTANY'S favorite family dinner. She loves when I make a fresh sauce, and chicken parmesan for Sunday get-togethers with our ever-expanding families. Our grandchildren love this dish as well! I usually have fresh Italian pasta, but pasta alternatives work well also. This dish hits the spot on a cold winter night and leftovers for lunches throughout the week are much appreciated.

5 boneless skinless chicken breast or cutlets, room temperature

sea salt and fresh ground pepper

Italian style bread crumbs *(approximately 1 cup)*

5 tablespoons olive oil, for browning chicken

5 ounces mozzarella cheese, thinly sliced

prepared homemade tomato sauce *(see recipe)*

parmesan cheese

1. Preheat oven to 350° and let chicken settle to room temperature.
2. Pound chicken, so meat becomes tenderized. Season lightly with salt and pepper.
3. Dip chicken into breadcrumbs, evenly coating both sides.
4. In a stainless pan heat oil on medium-high heat. Add chicken to pan and brown equally for 5-7 minutes per side.
5. Remove and blot chicken on paper towels to remove any excess oil. Place in glass pyrex pan and coat with sliced mozzarella. Be generous with the cheese.
6. Cover with homemade tomato sauce and sprinkle with fresh parmesan. Place in oven and bake for 40 minutes.
7. Let chicken rest for 10 minutes before serving. Serve with a side of pasta!

Enjoy!

MBK'S TIPS

This is a lighter version of the classic dish that typically calls for the chicken to be dipped into egg before breading. This is just as satisfying and not as heavy!

You can use chicken thighs if you prefer, be sure to trim off the fat before breading.

CHAPTER 6

sides

twice-baked potatoes with a sweet twist 166

southwest sweet corn succotash 169

sour cream mashed potatoes 170

scalloped potatoes with goat cheese and herbs de provence 173

roasted vegetables 175

roasted brussels sprouts with lemon 176

roasted beets 179

parmesan potatoes 180

oven-roasted fresh corn with summer squash and avocado 183

fresh roasted asparagus 184

charred onions and sauteed greens 187

carrot yam puree 188

broccoli cheddar quinoa muffins 191

I LOVE COOKING LOTS OF VEGETABLES and having leftovers the next day to add to a breakfast egg dish or lunch salad. I double the recipe, whenever roasting fresh vegetables for this reason alone. These sides are just some of my favorites and classic dishes that I still make often, whether for dinner for two or a family gathering. Root vegetables, tubers, healthy greens, it does not matter - they are all rich in phytonutrients and fill my pantry and refrigerator. My husband and I love them all, so mixing it up depends on what's on my mind for dinner. I often say, "I never met a potato I did not like" and it's true. This can also be said of roasted vegetables. To me, comfort food means a good portion of mashed potatoes!

twice-baked potatoes
with a sweet twist

6 servings

EVERYONE LOVES A TWICE-BAKED POTATO and this recipe takes tradition up a notch. I discovered this by accident once when I did not have enough regular potatoes for the family and I needed to stretch the recipe. I enjoyed it so much that I now only make this version. It adds a little creamy sweetness to the overall flavor. If your sweet potato skin doesn't hold up to filling with the mixture, discard and overstuff the russet potato skins. It should divide easily into six large portions.

MBK'S TIPS

Check potatoes after 1 hour. Depending on the size of the vegetables, they could be ready in less than 90 minutes.

NUTRITION EXTRAS

Both sweet and regular potatoes are highly nutritious. Potatoes provide more potassium, but sweet potatoes offer more vitamin A. They are comparable in calorie, carb and protein content.

GF

- 3 large russet potatoes
- 1 large sweet potato
- ½ cup sour cream
- 3 tablespoons unsalted butter
- 1 cup shredded extra-sharp cheddar cheese
- 4 strips bacon, chopped and pan-fried until crisp
- ¼ cup chives
- sea salt and fresh pepper

1. Heat oven to 425°.
2. Pierce holes in whole potatoes and bake in preheated oven for 90 minutes. Remove and allow potatoes to cool. Lower oven temperature to 325°.
3. Cut all four potatoes down the middle. Scoop out insides and put direcly into a mixing bowl fitted with a whip attachment.
4. Add all remaining ingredients and mix just until thoroughly combined.
5. Place potato shells on a baking sheet lined with parchment and fill skins evenly with potato mixture.
6. Place back in the oven, and cook for approximately 35 minutes or until completely thoroughly heated.

Enjoy!

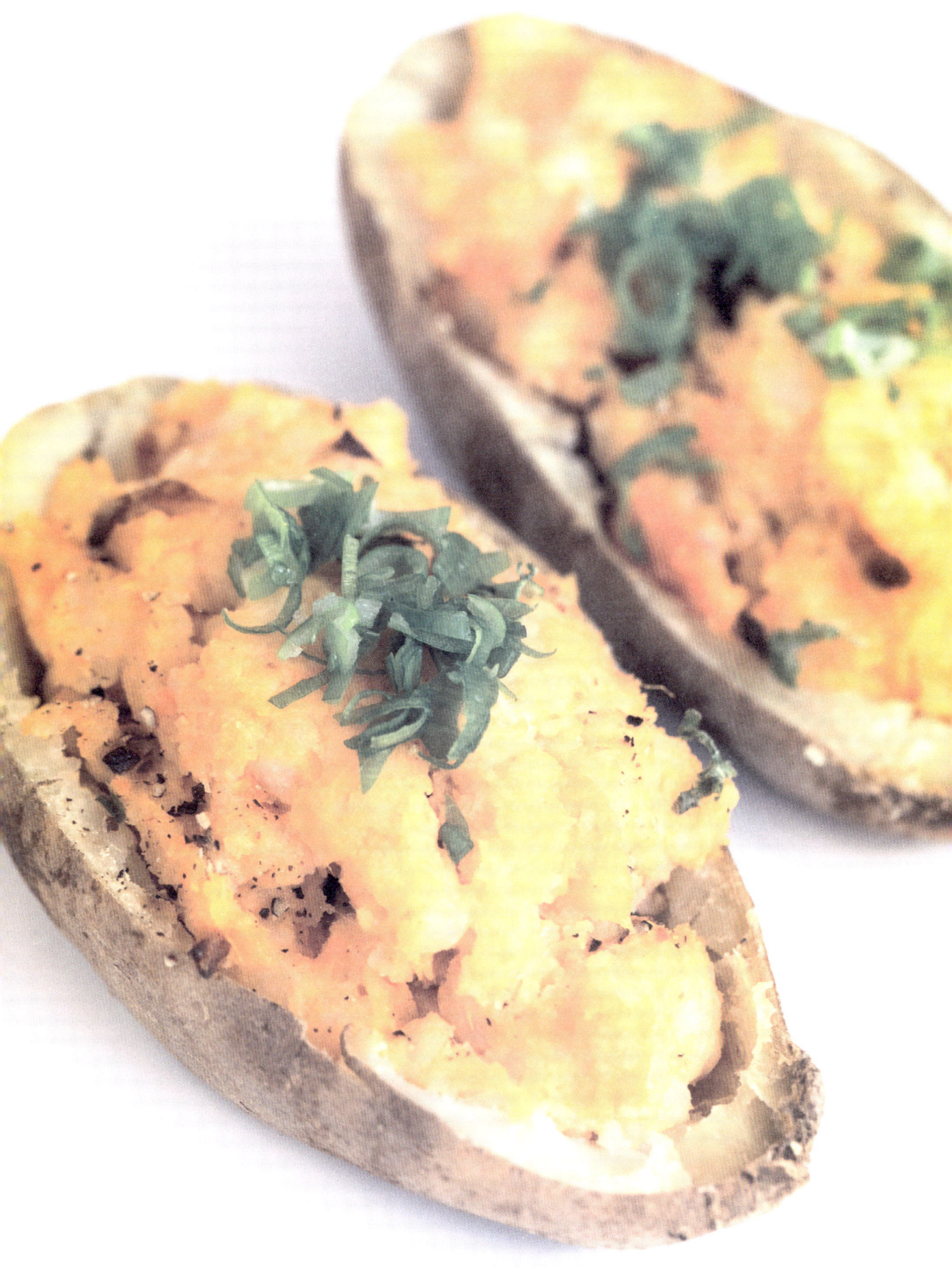

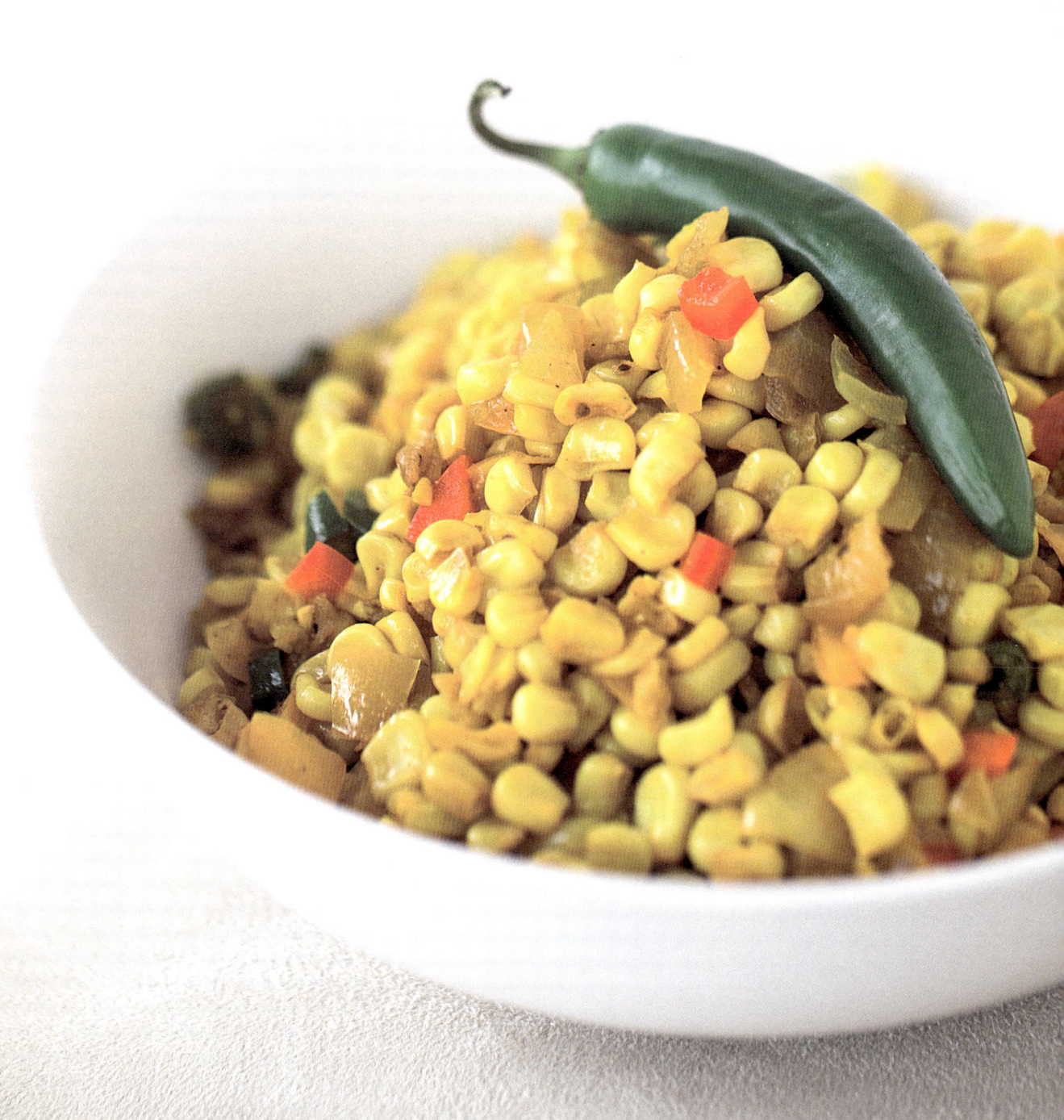

southwest sweet corn succotash

6-8 servings

I STARTED MAKING MY VERSION OF SUCCOTASH 20 YEARS AGO, and pulled this name *(succotash)* from a dish my siblings and I did not particularly care for while growing up. Back then it was lima beans and frozen vegetables and was never a welcome sight on the dinner table. This recipe was such a hit that my sister Connie and her husband Pat put it on the menu of one of their restaurants in the Canadian Rockies. I am sure they incorporated the vegetables available in their climate. This version stems from the fresh Maryland corn and peppers, in which we wait half the summer to arrive. I like a little heat, so I spice mine up a bit, but you can use mild peppers and forego the jalapeños.

- 4-6 tablespoons olive oil
- 1 large Vidalia or other sweet onion
- 2 jalapeno peppers, deseeded and diced
- 1 red pepper, chopped
- 5 fresh ears of sweet corn, shucked and cut from the cob
- 1 tablespoon cumin
- 1 teaspoon cayenne pepper
- 1 teaspoon turmeric
- sea salt and fresh pepper
- ½ cup fresh cilantro, chopped

MBK'S TIPS

Get to know your farmers and make sure your corn is non-GMO and organic. Corn is abundant in late July and all of August. Even better, it's cheap, delicious and good for you. I guarantee you will be making this more than once!

GF
DF
V

1. Heat oil in a large nonstick pan over medium heat. Saute onion and peppers until soft, approximately 5 minutes.

2. Add corn and seasoning and continue to cook until corn is cooked completeky and starting to brown. Stir often, so the corn does not stick to the bottom of the pan.

3. Adjust seasonings to taste and add cilantro before serving.

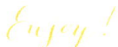

sour cream mashed potatoes
6 servings

MASHED POTATOES ARE ALWAYS WELCOME, not just at Thanksgiving. Sometimes it's that simple recipe that requires a blueprint. This recipe is my essential go-to when potatoes are calling. The sour cream adds a richness that is full of flavor.

MBK'S TIPS

It's a personal preference if you peel your potatoes before or after you boil them. I like to peel before cooking, for skinless, clean mashed potatoes.

You can use a mixer to mash the potatoes, but be careful not to turn it on high or over-mix, as the dish will be ruined. The potatoes will release starch and become gummy.

Don't be afraid of extra salt. Potatoes call for more than your average vegetable.

GF

3 pounds Yukon gold potatoes, peeled and cut into equal quarters

¾ stick unsalted butter

¾ cup sour cream

¾ cup whole milk

generous amount of sea salt and white pepper

1. Place potatoes in a large pot with enough cold water to cover. Bring to a boil and add 2 teaspoons of salt to the water. Cook potatoes on a low boil for 20 - 25 minutes, or until potatoes are tender.

2. Drain potatoes and return to pot or a clean mixing bowl.

3. Add all remaining ingredients. Season with salt and pepper to taste and mash with a handheld masher until well incorporated. Don't over-mix.

4. Taste and adjust seasoning if necessary.

Enjoy!

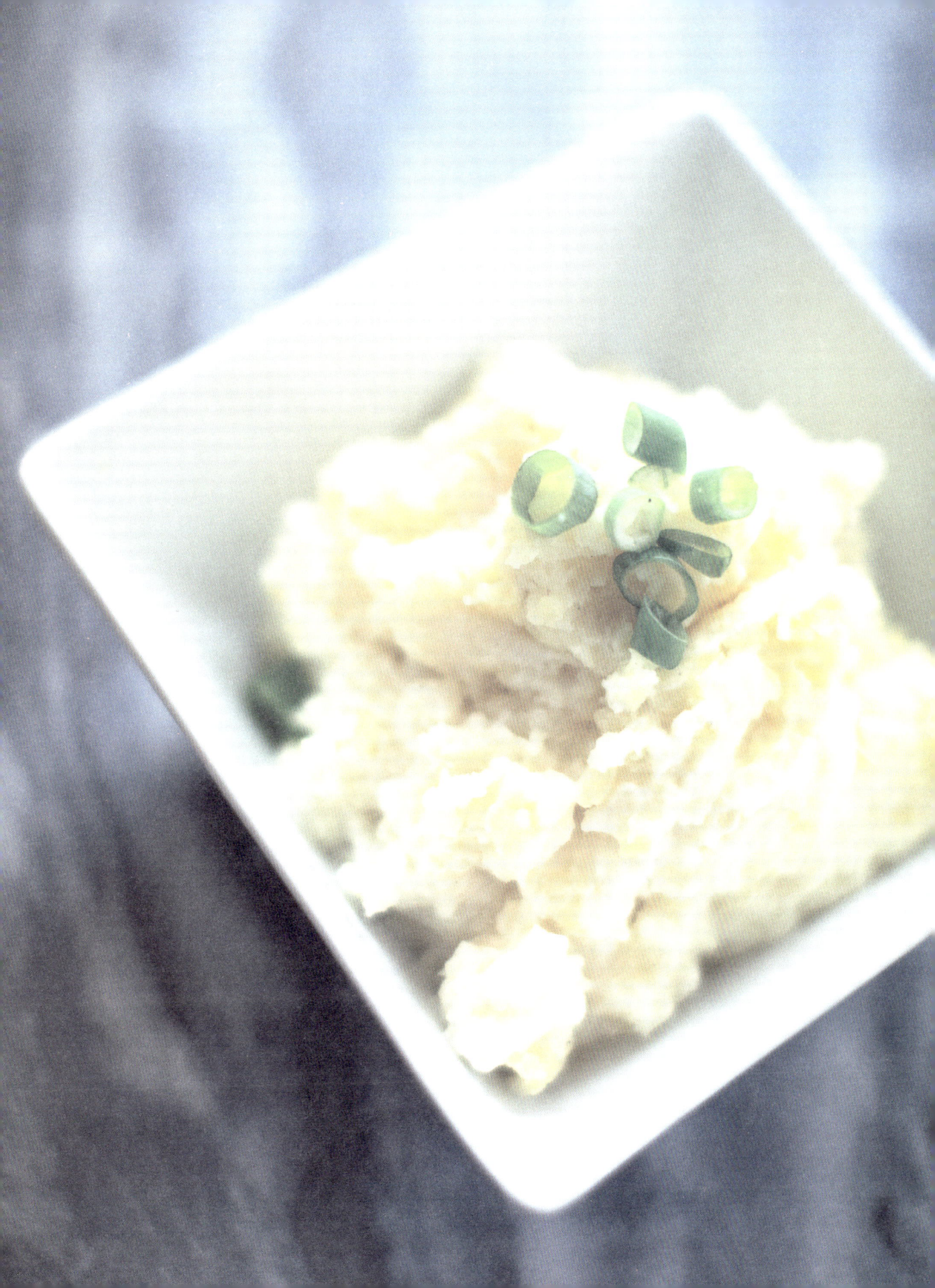

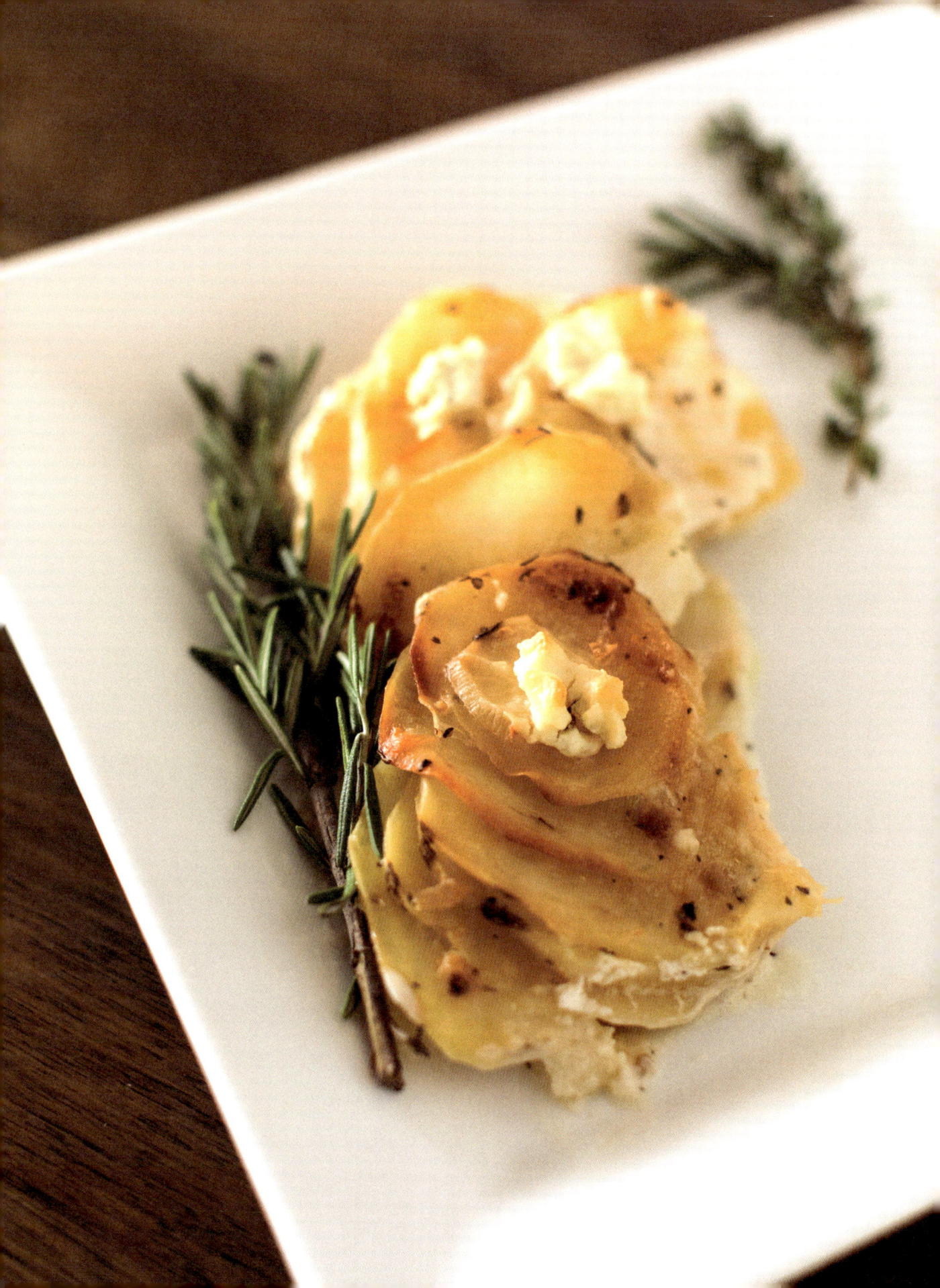

scalloped potatoes
with goat cheese & herbs de provence

6-8 servings

I MAKE THESE POTATOES EVERY CHRISTMAS and that makes my daughter Brittany very happy. The house smells so aromatic. Between the shallots and the herb de provence, you are salivating by the time they are finished. They are a fantastic side to the standing rib roast that I also make only on Christmas. I am not sure why I wait all year for this, but I do!

- 1½ cups heavy cream
- 1½ cups chicken stock
- 1 cup dry white wine
- ½ cup shallots, minced
- 3 garlic cloves
- 4 teaspoons herbs de provence
- 1/2 tsp sea salt
- 1 tsp fresh ground pepper
- 1 - 10-ounce log soft goat cheese, divided
- 4 pounds of russet potatoes, peeled, thinly sliced
- olive oil

1. Preheat oven to 400°.
2. Coat a 13x9x2 inch glass baking dish with olive oil.
3. Mix first eight ingredients in large, deep rimmed saute pan. Bring to simmer over medium heat and add half of the goat cheese. Whisk until smooth. Chill the remaining cheese.
4. Add potatoes to the pot and bring back to a simmer. Transfer potato mixture to the glass baking dish, cover with foil and bake for 15 minutes.
5. Uncover and bake for an additional 50 minutes.
6. Remove from oven and dot remaining cheese evenly across the surface of the dish.
7. Place back in the oven and cook for an additional 10 minutes or until cheese softens. Remove and let sit for 15 minutes before serving.

Enjoy!

MBK'S TIPS

Pull out the mandolin or the Cuisinart for these. It will save you lots of time, and the dish will come together more quickly.

GF

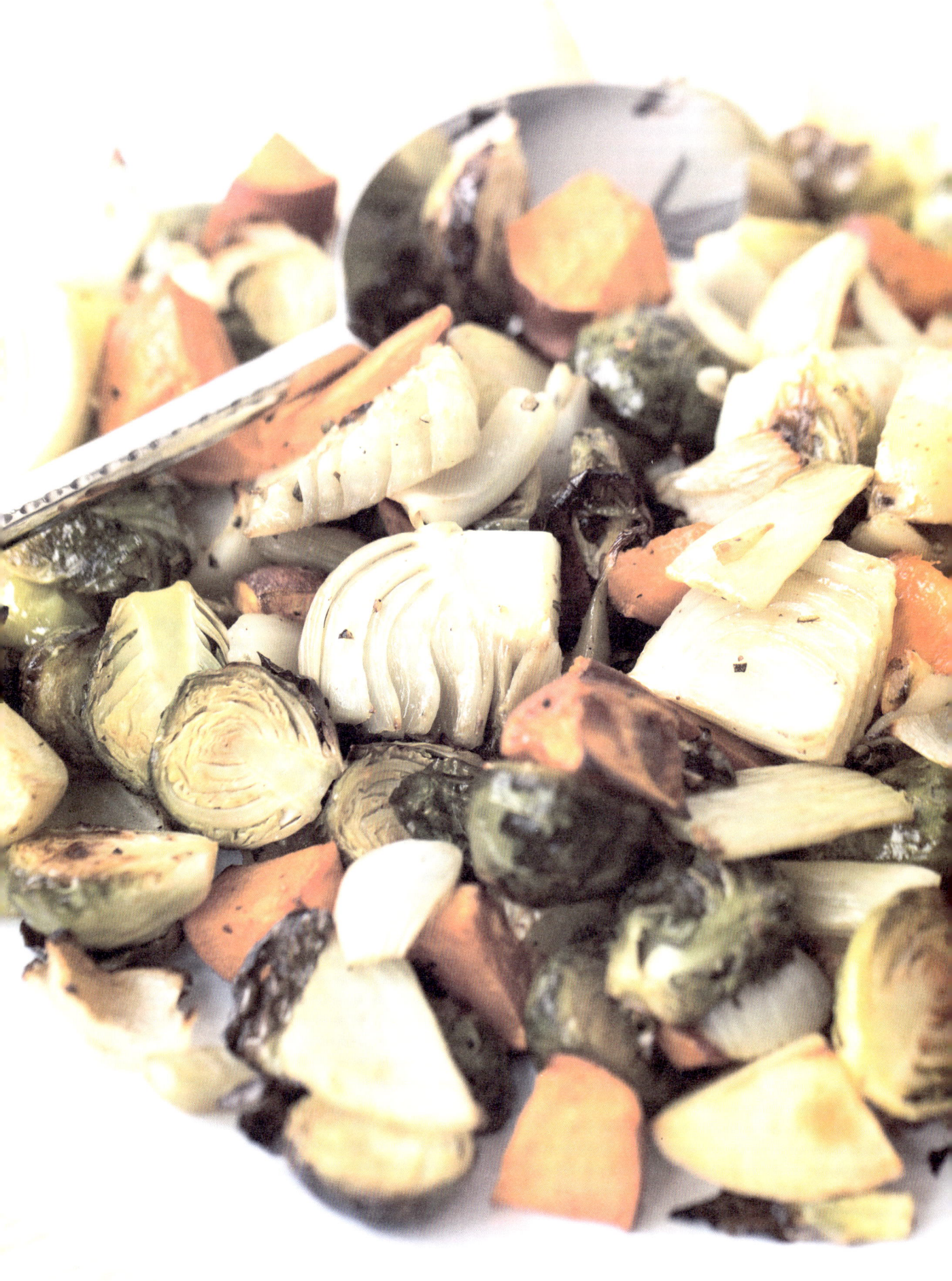

roasted vegetables
6 servings

I MAKE ROOT VEGETABLES EVERY WEEK IN THE WINTER MONTHS. The leftovers are great to throw into hearty salads or snack on when you need a quick bite of something satisfying and starchy. They also go well with eggs for breakfast, as they are so versatile. This combination of vegetables is one of many that can be roasted together at the same time, as the timing to cook is similar. Sometimes I will choose three types of potatoes. Other times I throw fennel in the mix along with some freshly grated parmesan cheese, but I always include an onion. It all depends on what's in the pantry.

- 2 medium sweet potatoes
- 2 large sweet onions
- 1 pound brussels sprouts, cleaned, trimmed and halved
- olive oil
- salt and pepper to taste

1. Preheat oven to 425° convection.
2. Cut sweet potatoes and onions into even size pieces, approximately the same size as the halved brussels sprouts.
3. Mix all vegetables thoroughly, coating with olive oil and fresh salt and pepper. Spread onto a single layer on a rimmed cookie sheet that has been sprayed with olive oil or lined with parchment paper.
4. Bake for 15 minutes. Stir the mixture to ensure browning on all sides, baking for another 15 minutes or desired doneness.

Enjoy!

MBK'S TIPS

Keep parchment paper on hand to make clean up a breeze.

NUTRITION EXTRAS

Root vegetables are rich in vitamin A, vitamin C, fiber, magnesium and several antioxidants. These are a welcomed carb in all healthy eating plans.

GF
DF
V
LS

roasted brussel sprouts
6 servings

with lemon & breadcrumbs

BREADCRUMBS GIVE THESE BRUSSEL SPROUTS a touch of added texture that makes an already tasty vegetable that much more attractive. The trend to dress up these little cabbages has been on the restaurant circuit for some time now, with everything from bacon to sriracha. I like to keep them simple and roast them with very minimal added flavor.

MBK'S TIPS

You can use parchment paper instead of spraying a pan with olive oil. Makes for an easy cleanup.

NUTRITION EXTRAS

This dish is loaded with dietary fiber and lots of vitamin C and some vitamin A. Rich in potassium as well.

2½ pounds brussels sprouts, trimmed and halved

2 garlic cloves, minced

3 tablespoons olive oil

sea salt and black pepper

½ stick unsalted butter

⅓ cup fresh bread crumbs

3 tablespoons lemon juice, squeezed from 1 fresh lemon

1. Heat oven to 425°.
2. Toss sprouts, garlic, olive oil, salt, and pepper together. Layer evenly on a baking sheet sprayed with olive oil.
3. Roast, turning once, approximately 20 minutes *(convection if possible)*.
4. Brown breadcrumbs with ½ stick butter in a frying pan on medium heat. Do not burn.
5. Toss brussels sprouts in a large serving bowl with breadcrumbs and lemon.

Enjoy!

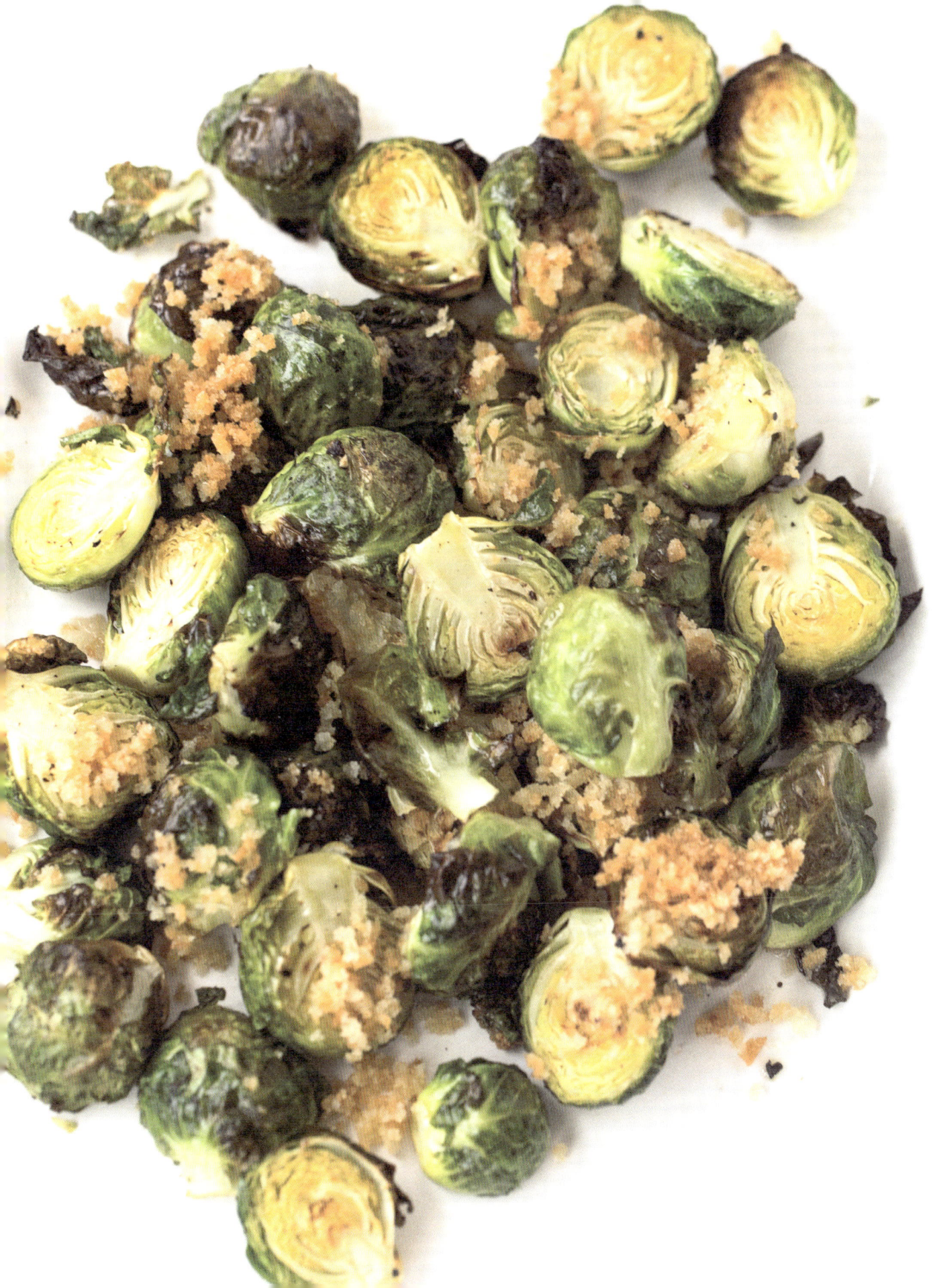

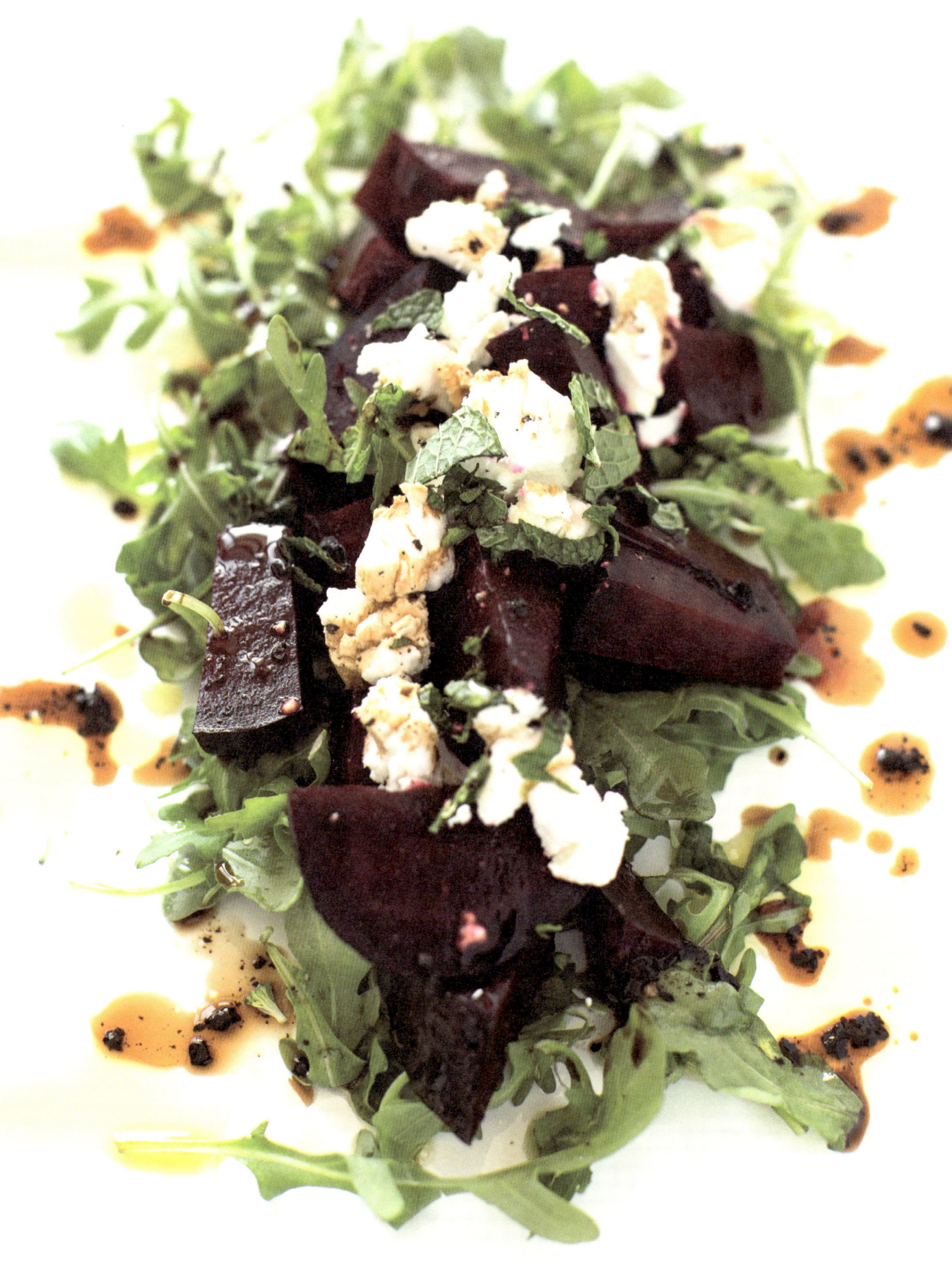

roasted beets

ROASTING BEETS IS SO EASY and having these sweet, root vegetables ready to eat in the refrigerator, should be a staple in every house that loves beets as much as we do. They are available year-round, inexpensive and they add so much flavor to salads of all types. Pictured here are my beets with arugula, goat cheese and fresh mint and topped with my homemade balsamic dressing. Yum! Such a refreshing salad any time of the year.

1 pound fresh beets, stems removed and cleaned

1 tablespoon olive oil

sea salt and pepper to taste

1. Preheat oven to 425°.

2. Place beets in the center of a large sheet of heavy-duty aluminum foil. Drizzle with olive oil, salt and pepper. Wrap to seal beets completely.

3. Place in the center of oven and bake, approximately 45 minutes to 1 hour, depending on size of beets.

4. Cool beets and peel the outer skin. Slice to desired thickness.

Enjoy!

MBK'S TIPS

Add these to a quinoa salad, for an addition of texture. These can keep in the refrigerator, once roasted, for well over a week. Keep the beets covered and slice as needed.

GF
DF
V

parmesan potatoes
6 servings

THIS SIMPLE DISH HAS BEEN PASSED AROUND and served on more tables than any of my recipes. Most of my sisters make these in their homes. Even picky eaters love this recipe! It's delicious accompanied with grilled salmon and a large, mixed green salad. This is my go-to summer dinner for a crowd and it can be pulled together quickly.

MBK'S TIPS

I like Yukon gold, but russet potatoes work just as well. Don't skimp on the cheese. The potatoes can take a lot of salty parmesan for flavoring. Rotate once and flip halfway through the cooking process.

GF

6-8 medium-size yellow skin potatoes, cleaned and diced evenly into medium-size pieces.

1 cup parmesan cheese, finely grated

¼ cup olive oil

salt and pepper to taste

1. Preheat oven to 400°.

2. Combine all ingredients and spread evenly onto a nonstick baking sheet or parchment paper-lined baking sheet.

3. Roast until potatoes are golden brown and starting to crisp, approximately 30 minutes.

Enjoy!

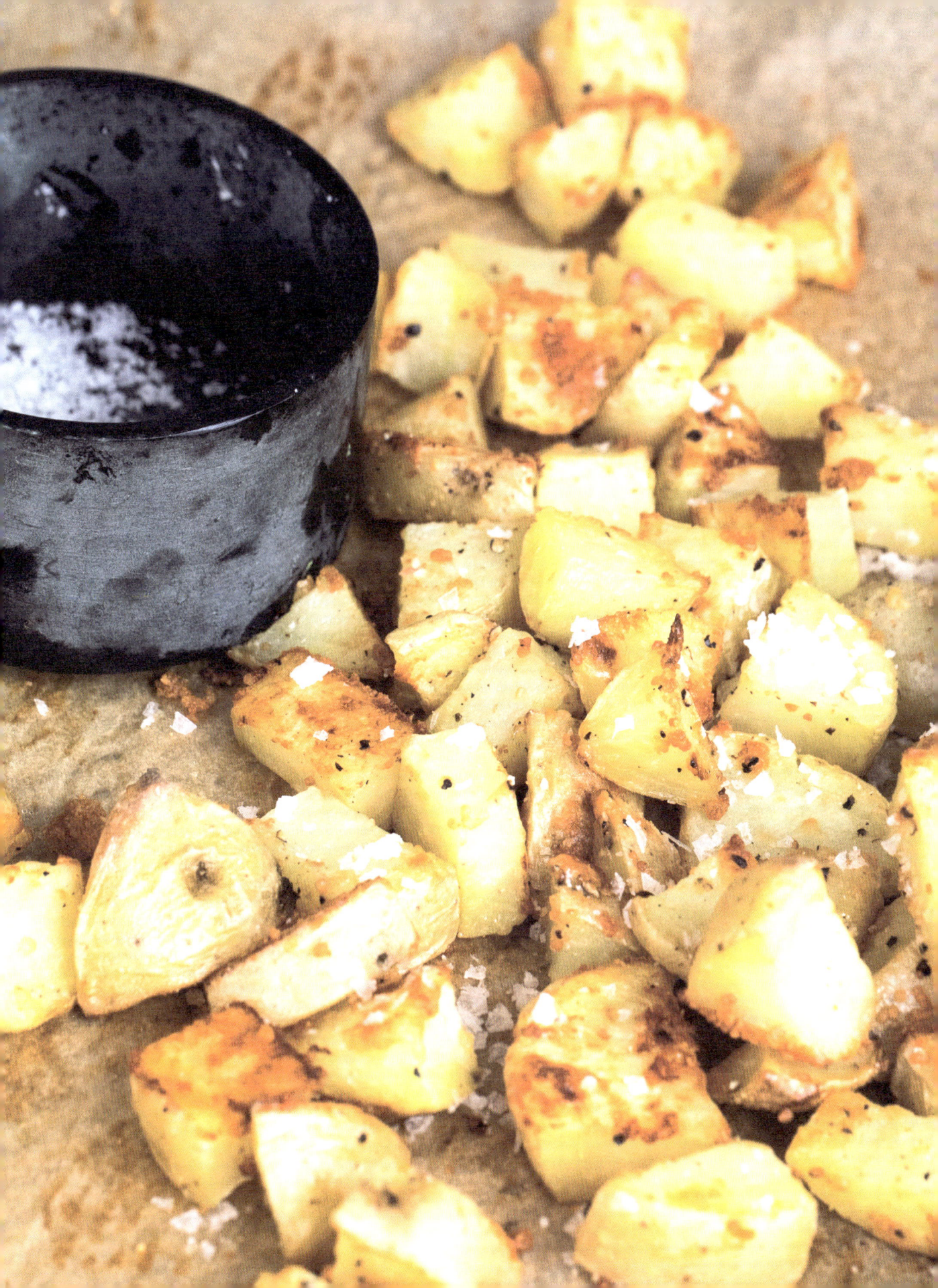

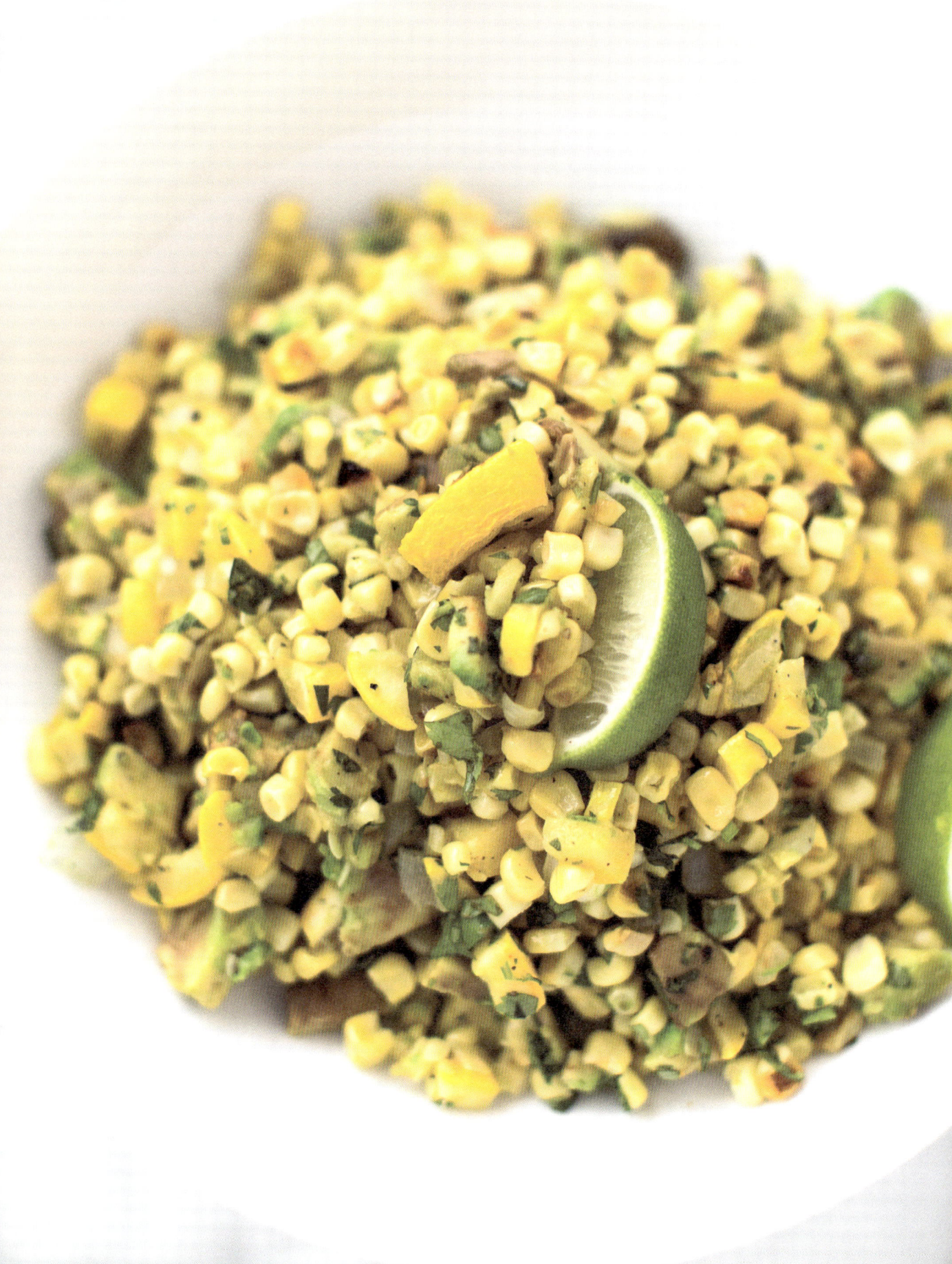

oven-roasted fresh corn
with summer squash & avocado

8 servings

I CAME UPON A RENDITION OF THIS RECIPE YEARS AGO when looking for ways to make corn off the cob for a crowd. Not everyone loves to eat corn on the cob and it can be quite messy if you are trying for a more formal dinner setting. In late August, summer corn and summer squash are in such abundance, that having a mix of recipes on hand is helpful for variety. This dish is full of texture with the creamy avocado mixed in and it's loaded with southwestern flavors from the added spice and lime. This dish pairs well with any grilled meat or ribs.

- 6 ears fresh corn, cut off the cob
- 1 medium yellow squash, seeded and chopped
- 1 sweet onion, chopped
- 3 tablespoons olive oil
- salt and fresh ground pepper
- 2 avocados, diced
- 1 large lime, juiced
- ½ teaspoon cayenne pepper
- ¼ cup chopped fresh, cilantro

MBK'S TIPS

You can use raw avocado if you don't like the idea of cooking the fruit. It's delicious either way, but the roasting adds a deeper flavor.

Use leftovers to combine in any salad to provide a more abundant flavor and texture.

1. Place oven rack six inches from broiler in the oven. Preheat oven to the broiler setting.
2. Line a long, sturdy baking sheet with heavy aluminum foil.
3. In a large mixing bowl add cut corn, squash, onion, 2 tablespoons olive oil and fresh salt and pepper to taste and stir until combined.
4. Spread evenly onto prepared pan and place under a preheated broiler for 6 minutes, stirring once to evenly roast.
5. Remove from oven. Add avocado evenly on top of the mixture and place it back under the broiler for an additional 2 minutes.
6. Remove and place back into the serving bowl. Add lime juice, cayenne, and an extra tablespoon of olive oil. Taste and add additional salt and pepper if needed.
7. Add fresh cilantro before serving. Serve it warm or at room temperature.

Enjoy!

NUTRITION EXTRAS

This is a fiber-rich dish, which also includes healthy fats from the olive oil and avocado.

GF
DF
V

fresh roasted asparagus
6-8 servings

YOU COULD STOP AT OLIVE OIL WITH SALT AND PEPPER, but sometimes the added balsamic and parmesan *(or one or the other)* dresses it up a bit. It sure looks pretty on a buffet table with the fresh cheese for added flavor. When asparagus is in season it's amazingly delicious and almost always a crowd-pleaser. I don't know many people who don't love eating this green.

MBK'S TIPS

Cooking time will vary depending on the thickness of the asparagus. Check after about 7 minutes to see how crisp your vegetables remain. Take it out when you feel it's finished cooking, just don't let it get too mushy.

2 pounds asparagus, trimmed and semi-peeled

extra virgin olive oil

sea salt and fresh ground pepper

3 tablespoons balsamic vinegar

¼ cup parmesan, shaved

NUTRITION EXTRAS

Asparagus is considered a prebiotic, due to its high fiber content. Also high in folate and vitamins A,C,E and K. Winner winner!

GF

1. Preheat oven to 400°.

2. Arrange asparagus spears in a single layer on a large rimmed baking sheet. Spray or drizzle with extra virgin olive oil. Roll spears to ensure a light coat. Season moderately with salt and pepper.

3. Roast in pre-heated oven for approximately 12 minutes, turning once during the cooking process.

4. Transfer to serving platter and drizzle vinegar onto spears. Top with shaved parmesan, using a vegetable peeler, before serving.

Enjoy!

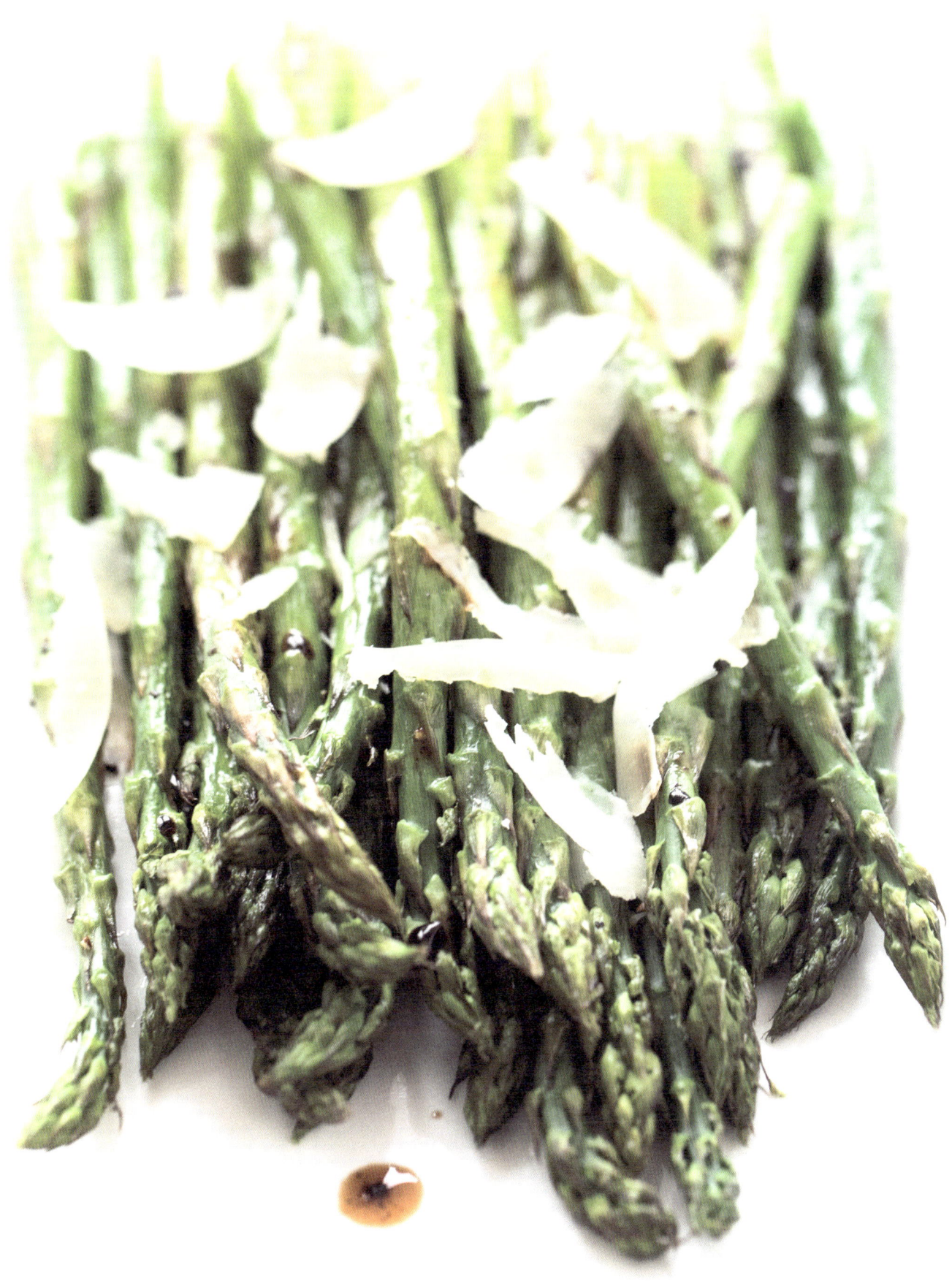

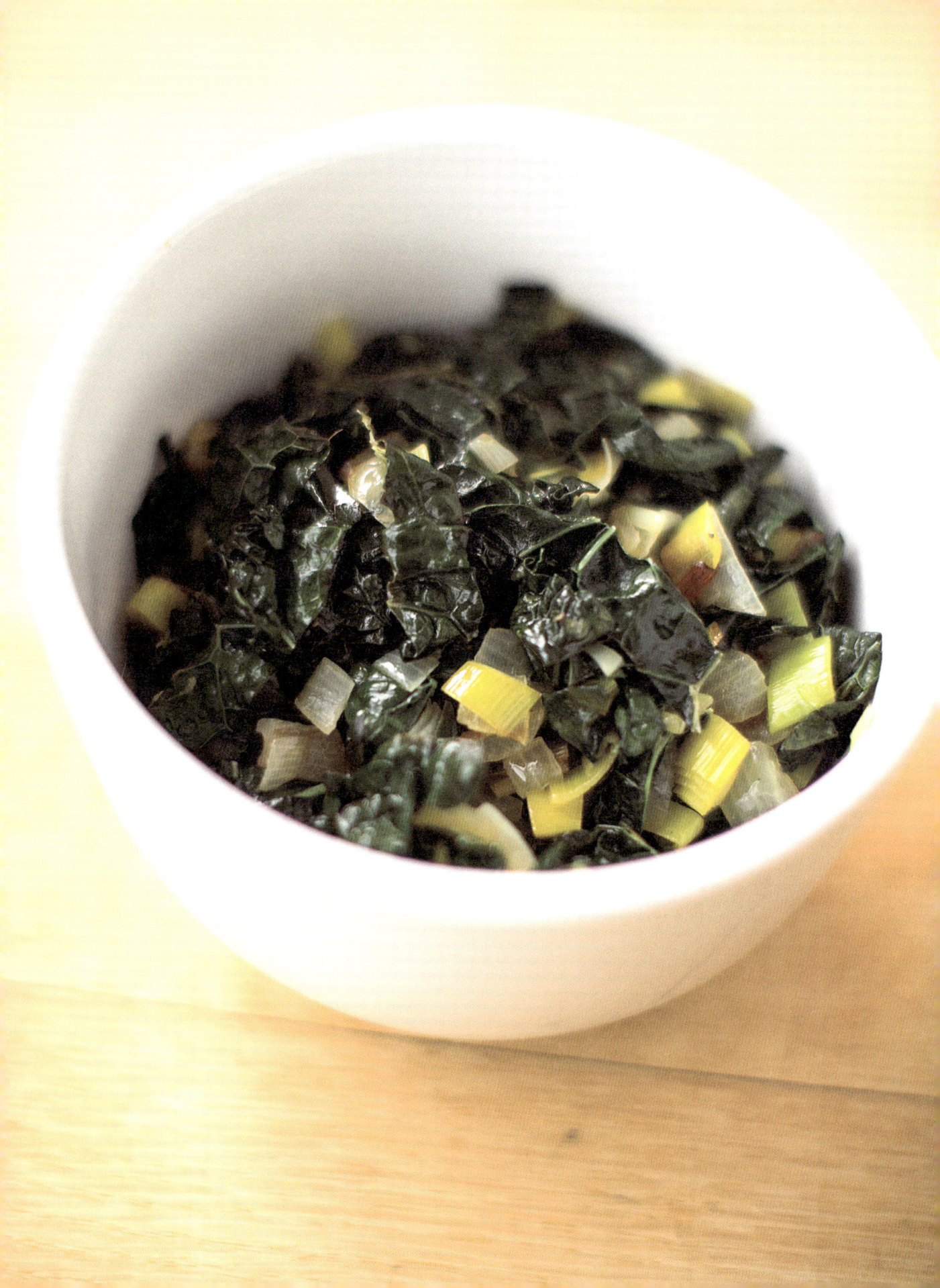

charred onions and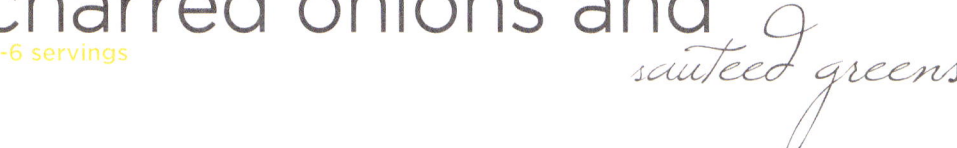

4-6 servings

I LOVE COOKED GREENS AND ONIONS FOR A SIDE DISH once in a while instead of a salad. These are so full of nutrients and flavor that they can accompany any protein you are serving. You do not have to slow cook greens for an extended amount of time, as once thought. I prefer swiss chard, but any other dark green leafy vegetable works.

3 tablespoons olive oil

1 large sweet onion, cut into large chunks

1 medium leek, white and light green parts, cleaned and sliced into rounds

8 cups clean, stemmed, greens of any choice (*kale, spinach, mustard greens*)

salt and fresh pepper to taste

 lemon, juiced

1. Heat oil in a large non-stick frying pan on medium heat. Saute onion and leek for about 10 minutes or until starting to brown on the bottom.

2. Add greens, salt and pepper to taste and continue to saute, approximately 7 minutes.

3. Remove from heat and squeeze ½ lemon over vegetable mixture. Serve immediately.

Enjoy!

NUTRITION EXTRAS

The list of nutrients is long. Greens are full of fiber, iron, magnesium, potassium and calcium. They also contain lots of Vitamins A, C, E and K and many of the B vitamins. There is a reason these go to the top of the charts when it comes to nutrition and why I try to eat them daily, whether cooked or raw.

GF
DF
V

carrot yam puree

6 servings

CARROT YAM PUREE IS A NICE SIDE DISH AT THANKSGIVING and a sweet change from mashed potatoes. This dish also goes well with roasted pork. It's all prepared in one pan, which makes it a quick and easy side that brings loads of flavor to your meal.

¼ cup olive oil

1 large sweet onion, diced

2 garlic cloves, minced

2 pounds carrots, peeled and sliced

2 pounds sweet potatoes, peeled and cut into ¾ inch pieces

4½ cups low sodium chicken broth

fresh salt and ground pepper

MBK'S TIPS

Start in a deep pan, so there is plenty of room to mix the dish. Add extra liquid in small increments, as you do not want the dish to get too watery - 1/4 cup of reserved liquid at a time.

GF
DF
V *(substitute vegetable stock for chicken stock)*

1. Heat oil in a large deep saucepan on medium heat. You need a pan large enough for all the above ingredients.

2. Add onion and cook until tender, approximately 5 minutes.

3. Add garlic and cook for an additional minute.

4. Add carrots, sweet potatoes, salt, and pepper and continue to cook for 5 minutes or until softened.

5. Add broth and bring to a low boil. Reduce heat and simmer until vegetables are tender, approximately 25 minutes.

6. Using a soup ladle, remove 2 cups of the liquid and reserve.

7. Using an emersion blender, puree the mixture until slightly chunky, adding reserved liquid as needed, ¼ cup at a time. If required, adjust seasoning with additional salt and pepper to taste.

8. Serve immediately or keep on low heat until needed.

Enjoy!

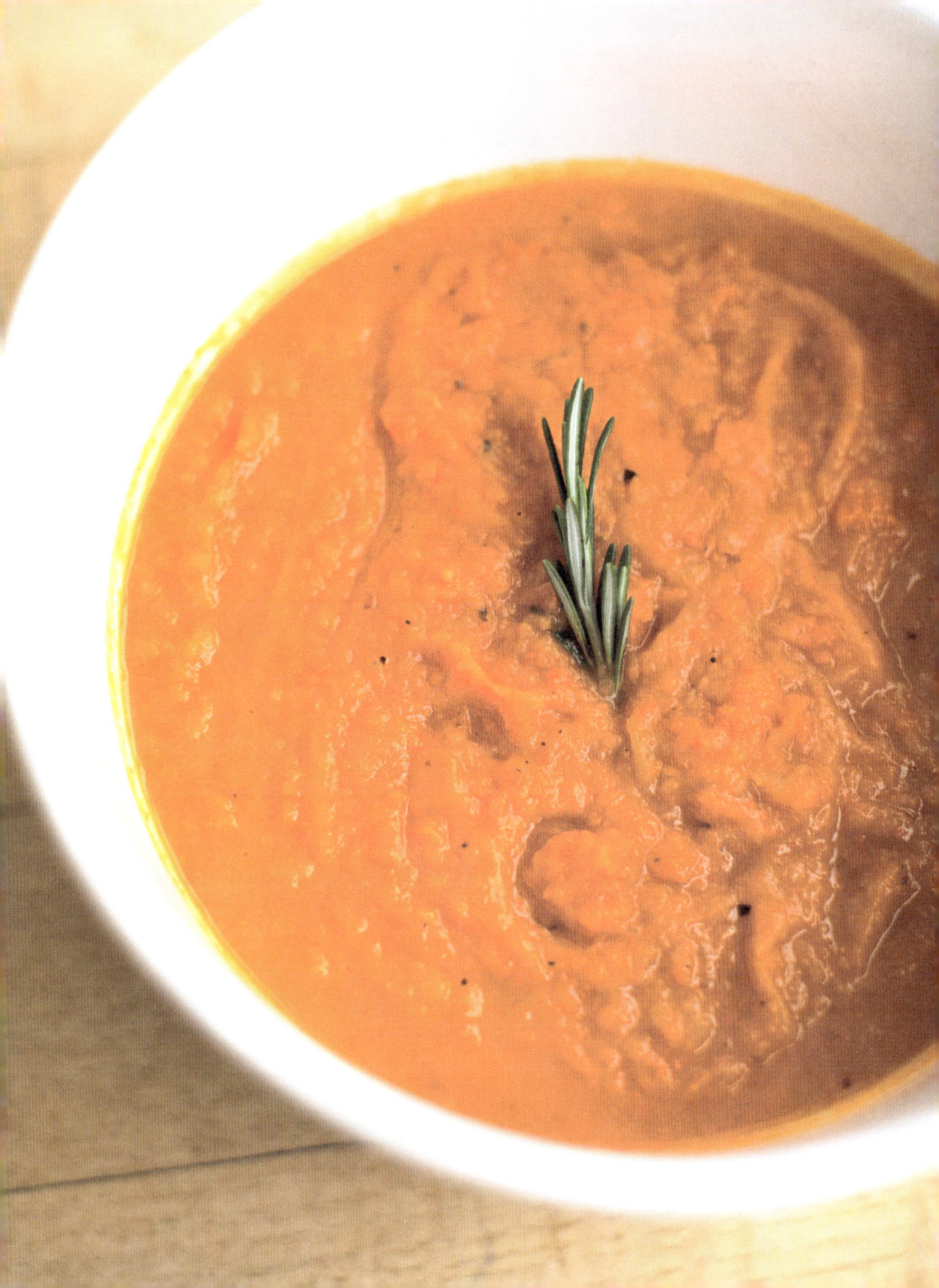

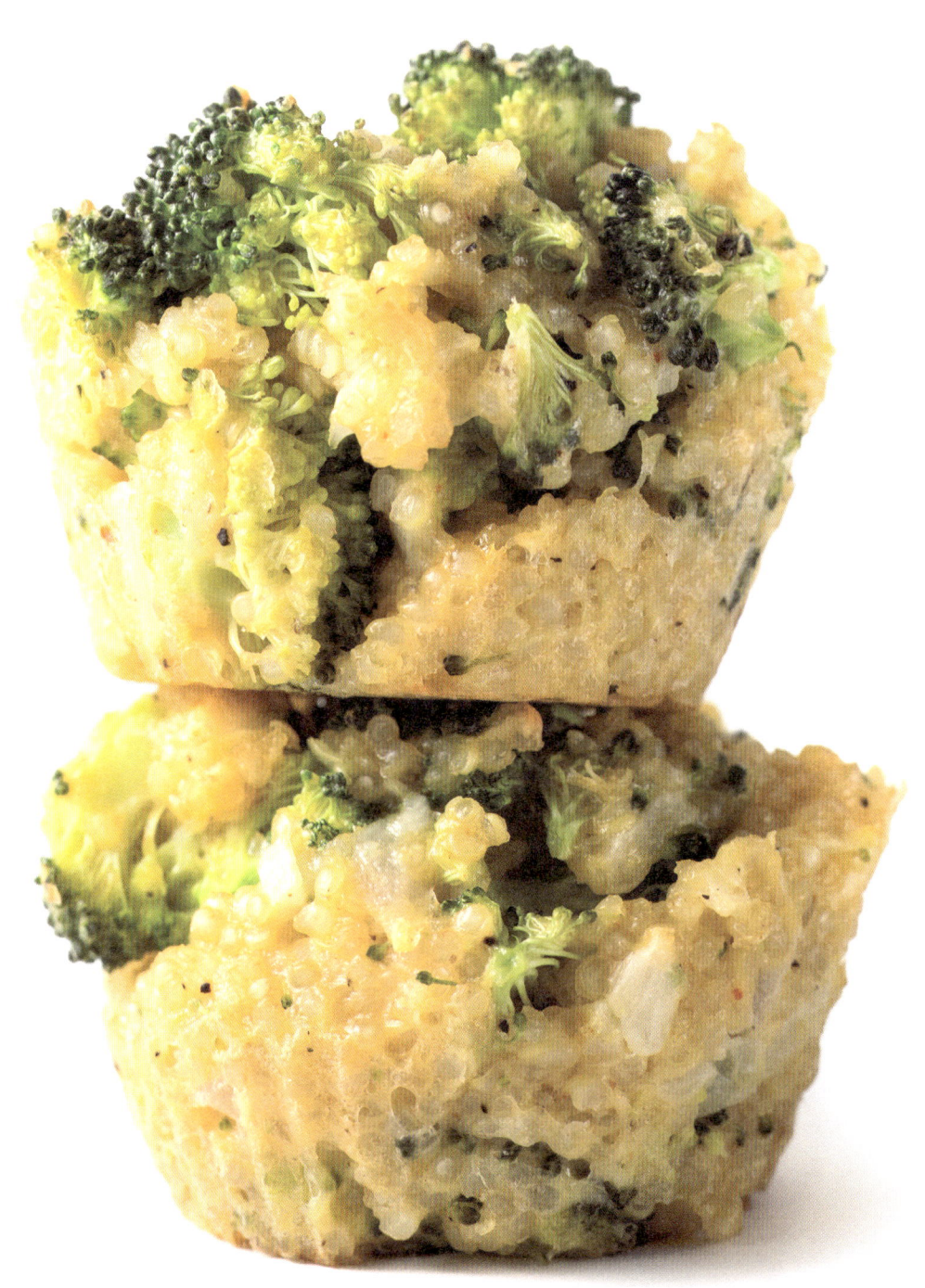

broccoli cheddar quinoa muffins
24 muffins

IF YOU ARE LOOKING FOR A SIDE DISH TO FILL KIDS with healthy carbs - look no further. It's impossible to eat just one of these. These gluten-free muffins are that good and can be made for lunch or dinner for a nice change. I love broccoli in all shapes and sizes, raw or cooked. These are just one more way to enjoy this healthy vegetable.

¾ cups quinoa, rinsed, cooked according to directions

2 eggs, lightly beaten

2 cups broccoli florets, finely diced

1 cup sweet onion, finely diced

1 clove garlic, minced

1½ cups cheddar cheese, shredded

½ teaspoon paprika

crushed red pepper to taste

1. Preheat oven to 350°.
2. In a large bowl, combine cooked quinoa, eggs, broccoli, onion, garlic, cheese and paprika.
3. Spray the inside of 2 muffin tins with non-stick olive oil spray.
4. Put a quarter cup of mixture into each muffin cup. Bake for 15 to 20 minutes or until edges turn golden brown.
5. Remove from oven, let cool 5 minutes before removing from pans.

Enjoy!

MBK'S TIPS

Dice your vegetables, uniform in size, to help the dish stick together when done. Press mixture into muffin cups, so the egg will bind with the ingredients while cooking.

GF

CHAPTER 7
muffins & biscuits

carrot cake banana muffins 194

whole wheat banana muffins 197

corn muffins 198

blueberry scones 201

blueberry muffins 202

herb biscuits 205

NOTHING CAN TOP A WARM, FRESH MUFFIN or biscuit coming out of the oven. Some of these recipes are a great companion to a soup or gumbo, others are breakfast delights that have been circulating my morning repertoire for decades.

When making these recipes, I always make extra to freeze and have on hand when needed. They are great to add an additional touch to complete a meal or when I need a little something special with my morning coffee.

A healthy carb in the A.M., that can give me a quick burst of energy, is sometimes just what's needed!

carrot cake banana muffins

12 muffins

THESE ARE MY VERSION OF A MORNING GLORY MUFFIN and should probably be in the breakfast chapter. They are loaded with healthy fat and protein. I have played with the portions of this treat over the years and finally have the right amount of wet to dry ingredients. You can substitute almond flour, if you prefer to make this gluten-free. It is a very moist muffin with both the banana and the coconut oil. I love waking up and having these already made waiting for me to share with my morning coffee. Whether freshly baked or recently frozen - it's great to keep a batch around.

MBK TIPS

You can keep most of these ingredients in your pantry for months at a time. You just need eggs and carrots on hand and you are good to go. Peel and freeze old bananas and pull out an hour before baking. Ripe, frozen bananas work best for baking.

GF*
DF
* (option)

½ cup whole wheat flour

½ cup unbleached all-purpose flour

1 teaspoon ground cinnamon

1 teaspoon baking powder

½ teaspoon salt

¾ cup coconut sugar or organic brown fine cane sugar

½ cup coconut oil, warmed to liquid

2 large eggs, room temperature

1½ cups carrots, coarsely grated

⅔ cup walnuts, chopped

⅔ cup raisins

1 ripe banana, mashed

1. Position rack in the center of the oven and preheat to 350°. Line a muffin pan with 12 paper muffin cups.

2. Sift flours, cinnamon, baking powder, baking soda and salt together in a medium bowl.

3. In the bowl of a heavy-duty mixer fitted with the whisk attachment, combine sugar, oil and eggs. Beat on medium-high speed until mixture has thickened slightly, approximately 2 minutes.

4. Add the dry ingredients, mix it by hand and then add carrots, walnuts, raisins and banana until well combined. Do not overmix. Using a large spoon, distribute evenly in prepared muffin cups.

5. Bake, until the center, comes out clean, 20-25 minutes. Cool completely.

Enjoy!

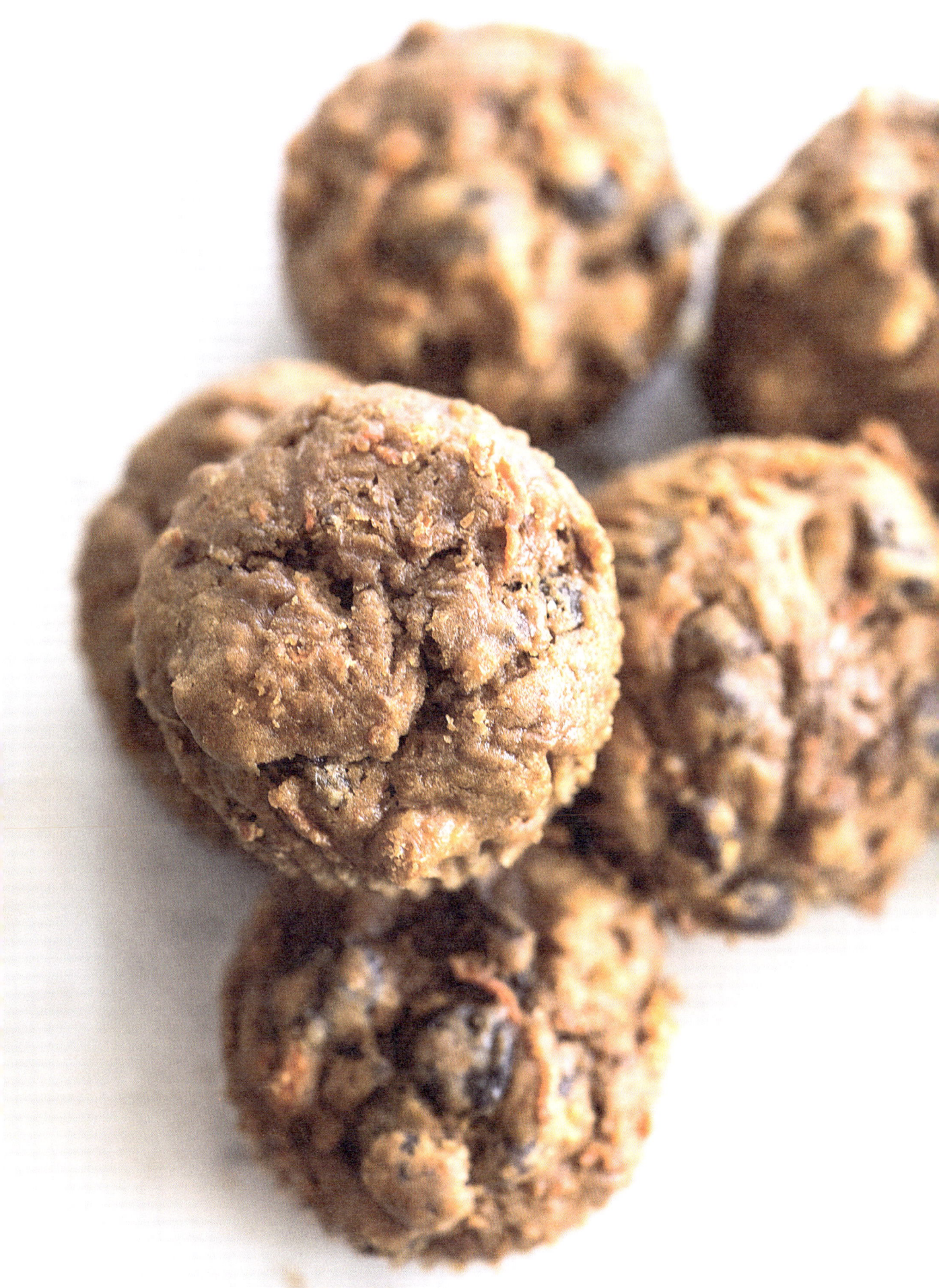

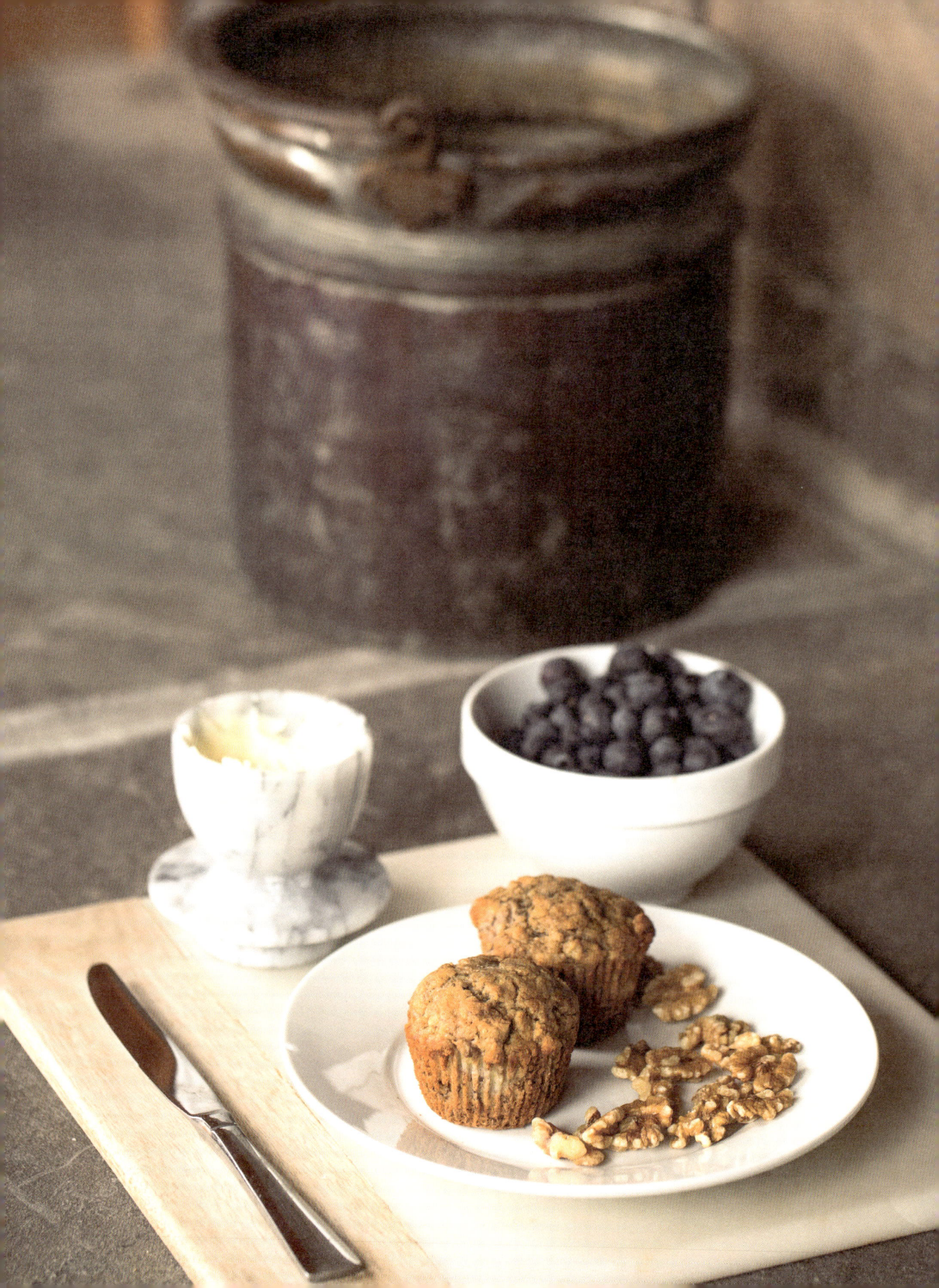

whole wheat banana muffins
12 muffins

MY BANANA NUT MUFFIN RECIPE HERE HAS BEEN IN circulation in my family for many years. My sister Julie, who is the only classically trained chef in the family, always requested this recipe for her son Jack. It's not complicated and it turns out perfect every time. I never tire of banana bread or a good banana muffin, especially one that is not too sweet.

- 3 medium ripe bananas
- ¼ cup buttermilk
- ½ cup unsalted butter
- ½ cup organic brown sugar *(can substitute coconut sugar)*
- 1 egg
- 1 cup organic whole wheat flour
- ½ cup unbleached white flour
- 1 teaspoon baking soda
- ¾ teaspoon salt
- 1 cup walnuts

1. Position rack in the center of the oven and preheat to 350°. Line a muffin pan with 12 paper muffin cups.
2. Mash bananas in a bowl and mix with buttermilk. Set aside.
3. In a mixing bowl, cream butter and sugar until light and fluffy. Add egg and mix well.
4. Sift dry ingredients together. Mix alternatively with creamed butter and banana mixture.
5. Stir in nuts, making sure not to over-mix.
6. Using a large spoon, distribute evenly in prepared muffin cups. Bake for 25 minutes.

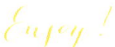

MBK'S TIPS

Always keep old peeled bananas in the freezer and ready for use. Be sure to mash the bananas and buttermilk well, so the flavor of the bananas are evenly dispersed.

corn muffins
12 muffins

EVERYONE NEEDS A CORN MUFFIN RECIPE that they can pull together quickly to accompany a good meal. I like to serve these with my gumbo and other hearty stews and soups. These muffins are also delicious alongside scrambled eggs or a frittata. They are not too sweet, with only 1/3 cup of sugar per 12 muffins, so they compliment many savory foods.

1 cup cornmeal	2 eggs
1 cup unbleached all-purpose flour	¾ cup whole milk or buttermilk
1 tablespoon baking powder	1 stick unsalted butter, melted and cooled to room temperature
½ teaspoon salt	
⅓ cup fine white sugar	

1. Preheat oven to 350°.
2. Mix all dry ingredients in a bowl.
3. In a separate bowl, combine eggs and milk, mix until well combined.
4. Slowly add egg mixture and melted butter to dry ingredients. Mix just until incorporated. Do not over mix.
5. Using a large spoon, distribute evenly in prepared muffin cups. Bake in the center of the heated oven for 20-25 minutes, until tops have started to brown and fork prick comes out clean.
6. Let cool slightly and enjoy with additional fresh butter if desired.

Enjoy!

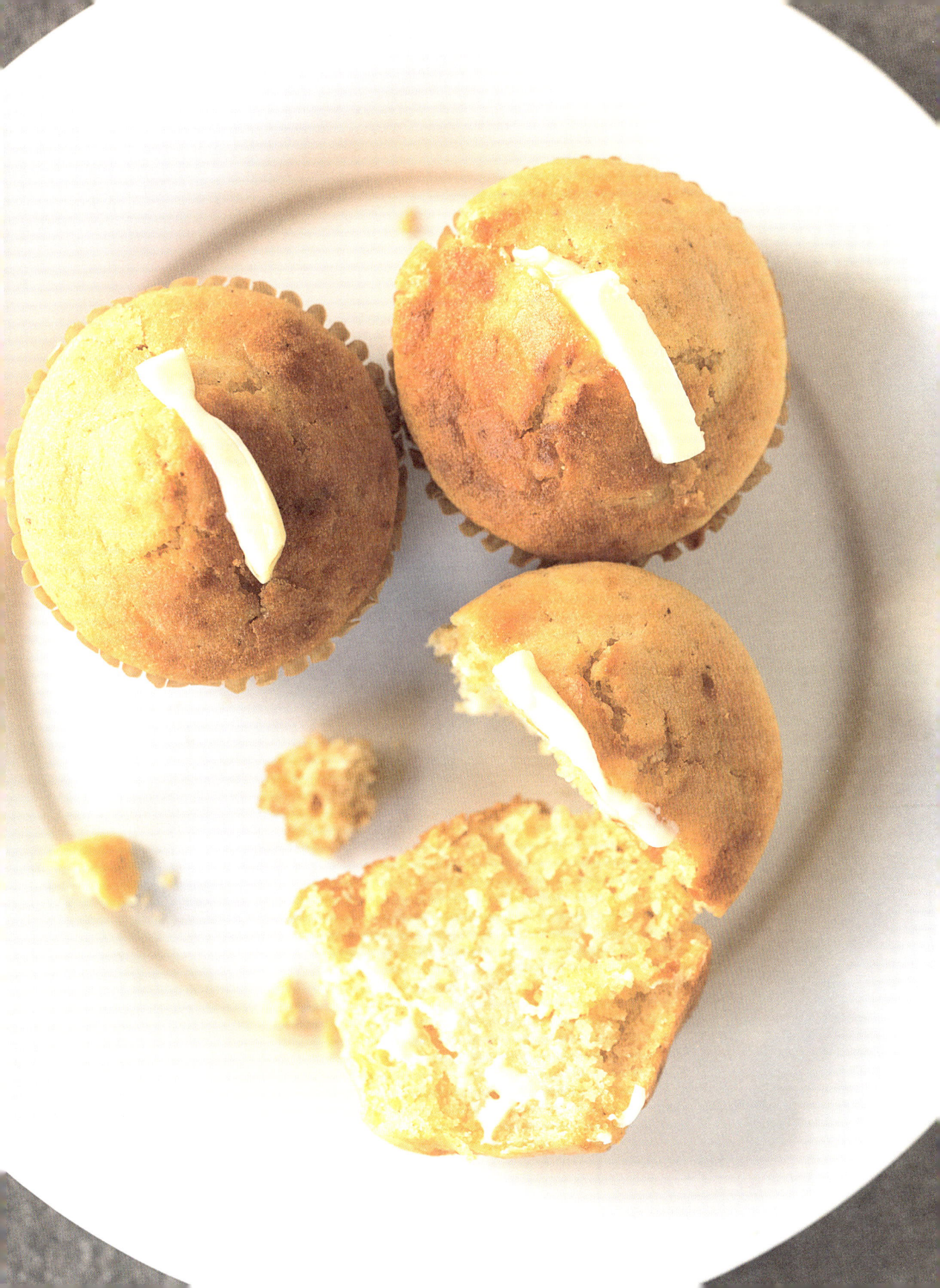

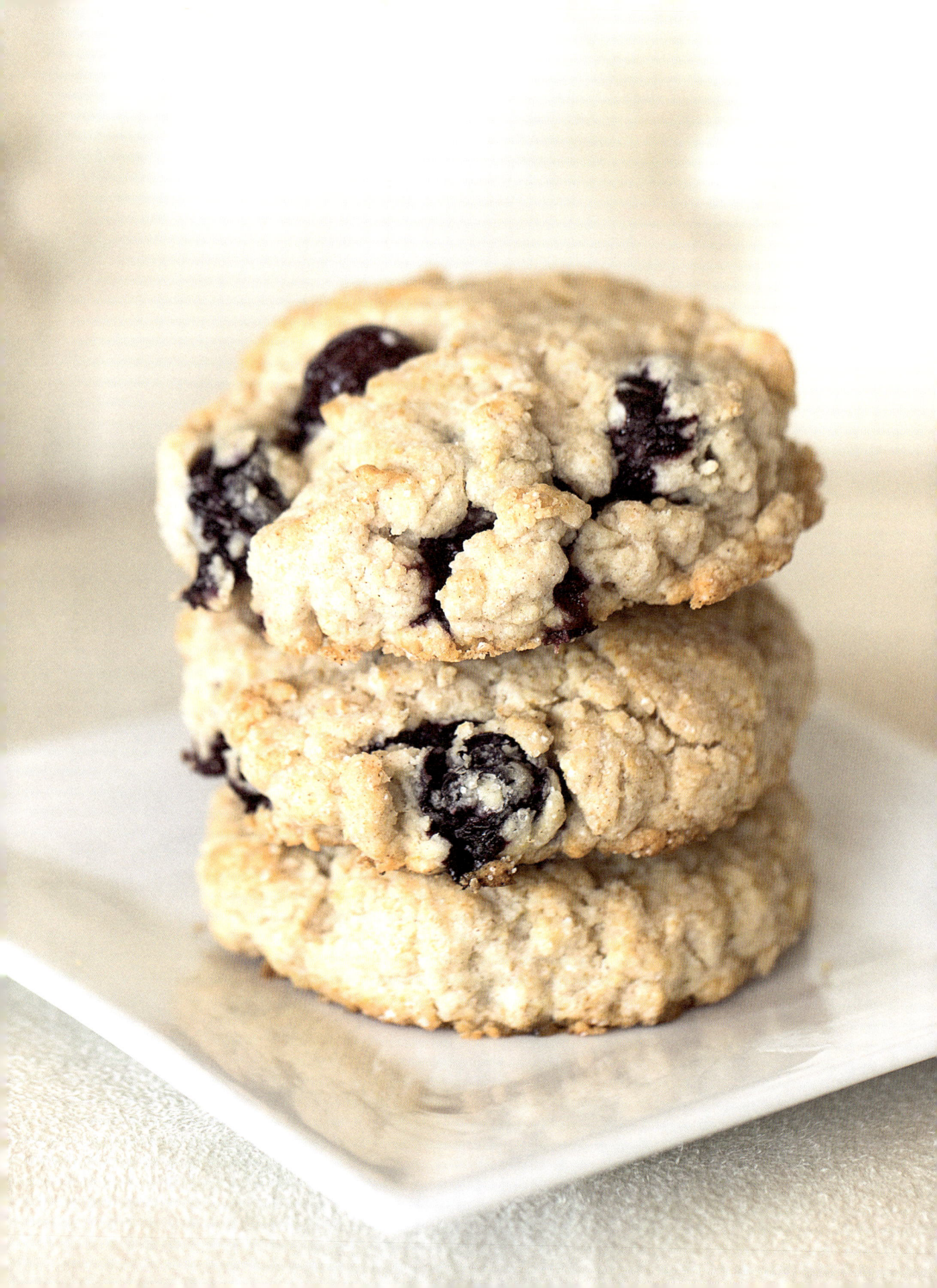

blueberry scones

10 scones

BLUEBERRY SCONES ARE A LITTLE MORE CHALLENGING than muffins and take some practice to master, but so worth the effort. I continually make these treats in the summertime when the berries are dirt cheap and fresh. It requires some counter space and is a little messy, but the flaky treats piping hot out of the oven are worth the heavy clean up.

- 2 cups flour
- ⅓ cup sugar
- 2½ teaspoons baking powder
- ½ teaspoon salt
- ½ teaspoon cinnamon
- ½ cup cold unsalted butter
- 1 egg
- ½ cup heavy cream
- 1 teaspoon vanilla
- 1 heaping cup fresh summer blueberries

1. Preheat oven to 400°.
2. Pulse flour, sugar, baking powder, salt and cinnamon with cut up cold butter in food processor.
3. Add egg, cream and vanilla. Mix gently with several additional pulses.
4. Fold in fresh blueberries *(I use my hands to press berries into dough)*.
5. Turn dough onto floured surface and with floured hands, form an even rectangle.
6. Cut scones into desired shapes and place on baking sheet.
7. Brush tops with additional heavy cream.
8. Bake for 12 to 15 minutes or desired doneness. Broil for 1 minute, at end of baking to make tops golden brown.

Enjoy!

MBK'S TIPS

Watch carefully when you brown the tops, these will burn in seconds if left too long.

I use a cookie cutter sprayed with coconut oil to make uniform round shapes. Free-hand triangles also work just fine!

NUTRITION EXTRAS

Blueberries are one of my favorite fruits for many reasons. Not just high in Vitamin C and fiber, they are also the king of anti-oxidants that protect your cells from free radicals.

blueberry muffins

12 muffins

THIS BASIC MUFFIN RECIPE HAS WITHSTOOD THE TEST of time. Originally adapted from a collection of Williams and Sonoma cookbooks, in which very little has been changed in 30 years. It's hard to reinvent the wheel. I make these often in the summer at our Lake House. Fresh blueberries are in abundance at this time and grazing guests are always looking for a snack. I don't know of many children who turn down a fresh blueberry muffin topped with butter.

---

2 cups organic unbleached flour

1 teaspoon cinnamon *(an option is 1 teaspoon vanilla + ¼ teaspoon almond extract, instead of cinnamon)*

¼ teaspoon salt

2 teaspoons baking powder

½ cup unsalted butter, room temperature

⅔ cup sugar

2 eggs, room temperature

1 cup whole organic milk, room temperature

2 cups blueberries

MBK'S TIPS

I keep a bag of Maine tiny frozen blueberries in the freezer at all times, for when fresh blueberries are not at their peak. Keep frozen until use or your batter will turn purple *(like mine did in the photo)*, as they start to melt and release their juice. Either way, they will taste great! Best when right out of the oven.

1. Preheat oven to 375°. Line muffin pan with 12 paper liners.

2. Mix flour, cinnamon, salt and baking powder together, set aside.

3. Cream butter and sugar for 2 minutes until well combined. Slowly add eggs, mix thoroughly.

4. While the mixer is on low, add dry ingredients, then milk and mix only until well incorporated. Do not over mix.

5. Fold in blueberries gently by hand. Using a large spoon, distribute evenly in prepared muffin cups.

6. Bake for 20-22 minutes testing with a toothpick to ensure the center is dry.

7. For golden muffins, brush tops with melted butter and broil for 1 minute at the end of baking.

Enjoy!

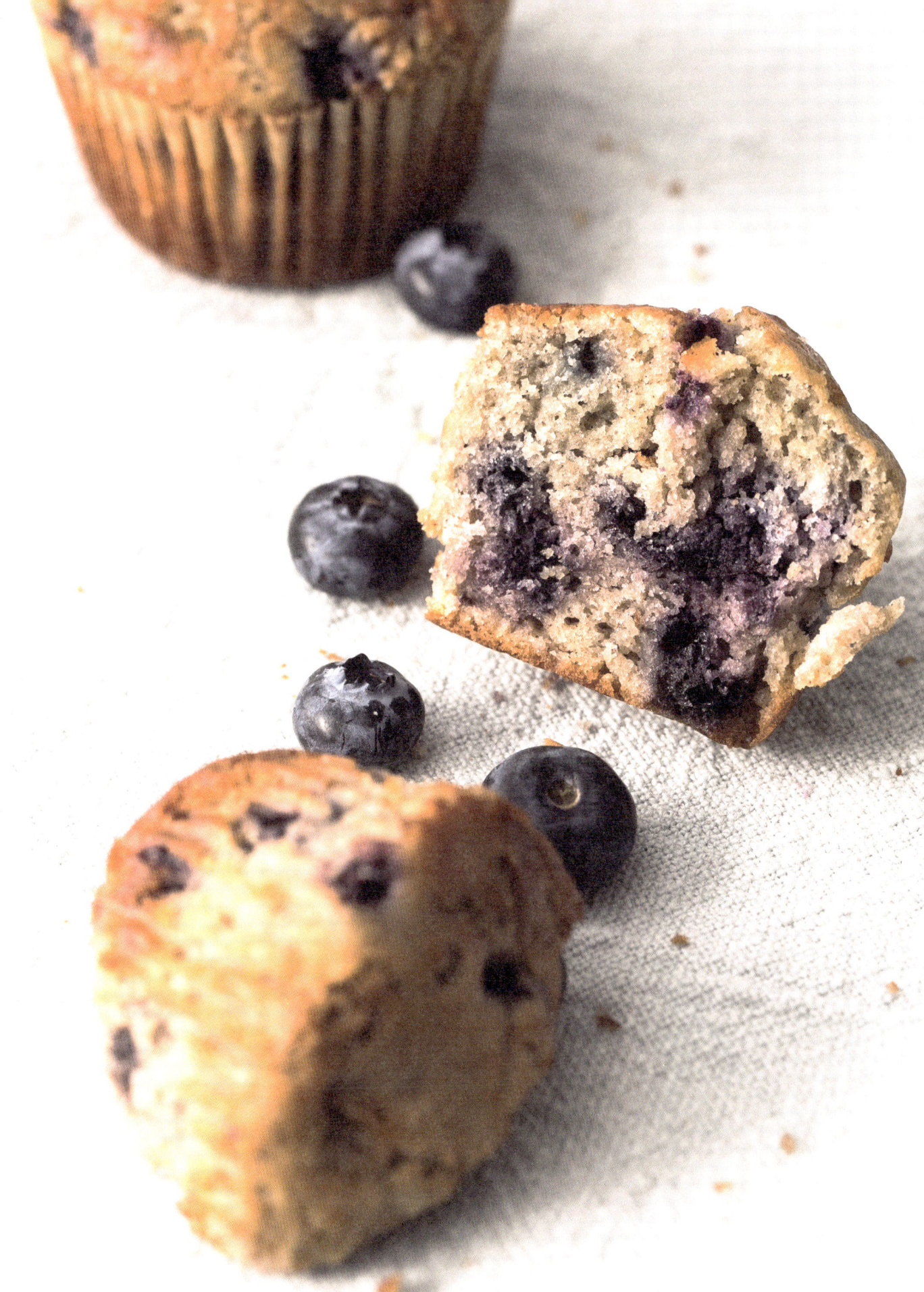

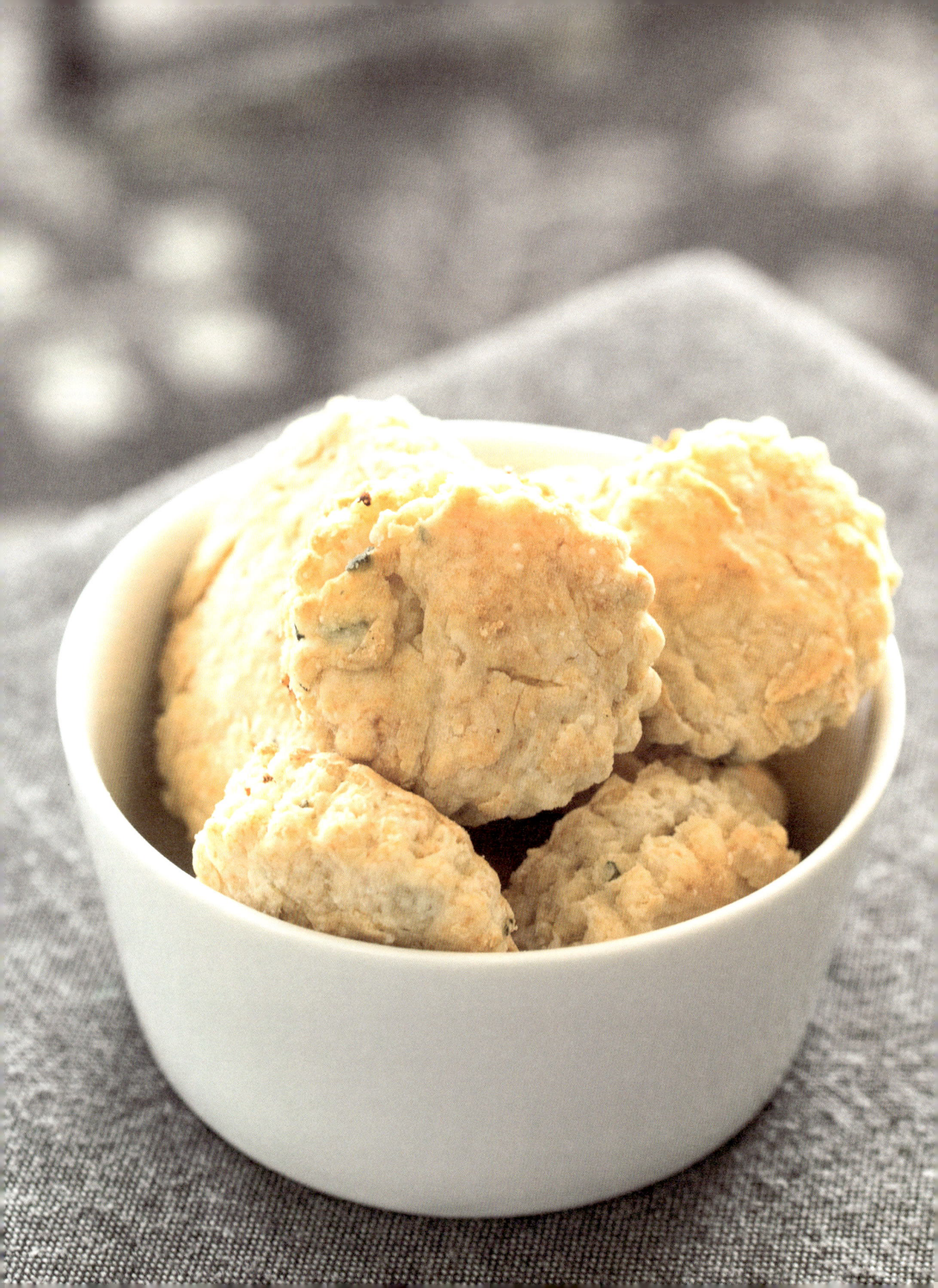

herb biscuits
12 biscuits

THIS MAKES A LARGE NUMBER OF BISCUITS, so cut the recipe in half if you don't need this much dough, as you want to eat these right out of the oven. They tend to go stale quickly unless frozen, so try to time them to be finished when dinner is ready. Unfortunately, reheating is not the same as hot from the oven. They have no sugar and are very savory, so these biscuits pair well with several types of meat, fish and stews.

4 cups unbleached all-purpose flour

2 tablespoons baking powder

1½ tablespoons fresh or dried herb of choice *(thyme, sage, or rosemary)*

2 teaspoons kosher salt

1 teaspoon baking soda

2½ sticks cold unsalted butter, cut into ½ inch pieces

1½ cup buttermilk

1. Pre-heat oven to 400°.
2. In a large mixing bowl combine flour, baking powder, herbs, salt, and baking soda.
3. Add butter using a pastry blender. Cut it in just until crumbly.
4. Add buttermilk and stir until moist. Do not over mix.
5. Transfer dough to a lightly floured surface and knead just enough to bring the dough together. Gently shape into two even 1 inch thick disks.
6. Using a biscuit cutter cut dough into 12 even biscuits and place on two baking sheets.
7. Bake for 15 to 20 minutes until golden.

Enjoy!

MBK'S TIPS

Use one or any combination of herbs that sound good for your meal. Rosemary comes through as a strong flavor, so I tend to use that by itself. Thyme goes well with gumbo and sage is delicious with poultry.

For leftovers, cut and reheat in the toaster and serve with eggs the next morning.

CHAPTER 8
desserts

blueberry pie 208

chocolate chip pecan cookies with ground flaxseed 211

chocolate glaze for chocolate espresso cake 212

flourless chocolate espresso cake 215

chocolate macaroon cake 216

key lime pie 219

nut and seed brittle 220

oatmeal cookies 223

strawberry tarts with pecan crust 224

pecan pie 227

thanksgiving pumpkin roll 228

Christmas butterballs 231

peanut butter cookies 232

Palates famous chocolate-covered grahams 235

I DO BELIEVE THAT SUGAR NEEDS TO BE MODIFIED in our diet. Desserts should indeed be a once in a while treat and only eaten in small portions. I love to bake and I love to make a homemade treat to share. Most of these recipes have a season or a holiday that they are associated with and are only made for that occasion. Others are cookies and treats that I have made for years for family and friends. Christmas calls for butterballs, just like a summer night calls for key lime pie. These foods are associated with wonderful memories and gatherings.

Dessert was never an after-dinner staple or daily habit; it was an occasional afternoon snack. Like Oscar Wilde said, "everything in moderation, including moderation!"

blueberry pie

I MAKE BLUEBERRY PIE MORE THAN ANY OTHER DESERT. Am I making it clear how much I love blueberries? It's a Thanksgiving must, even though it is not seasonal like apples, and it is a summer Fourth of July staple. In addition to the holidays, I make this whenever there is a special request from one of my children. Making a pie is not as challenging as it sounds, and after you have made a few, you never shy from the task. My sister K.C. is a beautiful pie maker. Whenever we are sharing a holiday, I happily hand her the responsibility. Maybe it's the fact that she is an architect that her pie always wins the prize for the prettiest and tastiest!

MBK'S TIPS

If blueberries are not in season, use frozen. Frozen fruit is picked in season and flash frozen and tastes so much better than out of season fruit that is sold all year long. It's also easy to find organic frozen fruit at most of the big grocery stores.

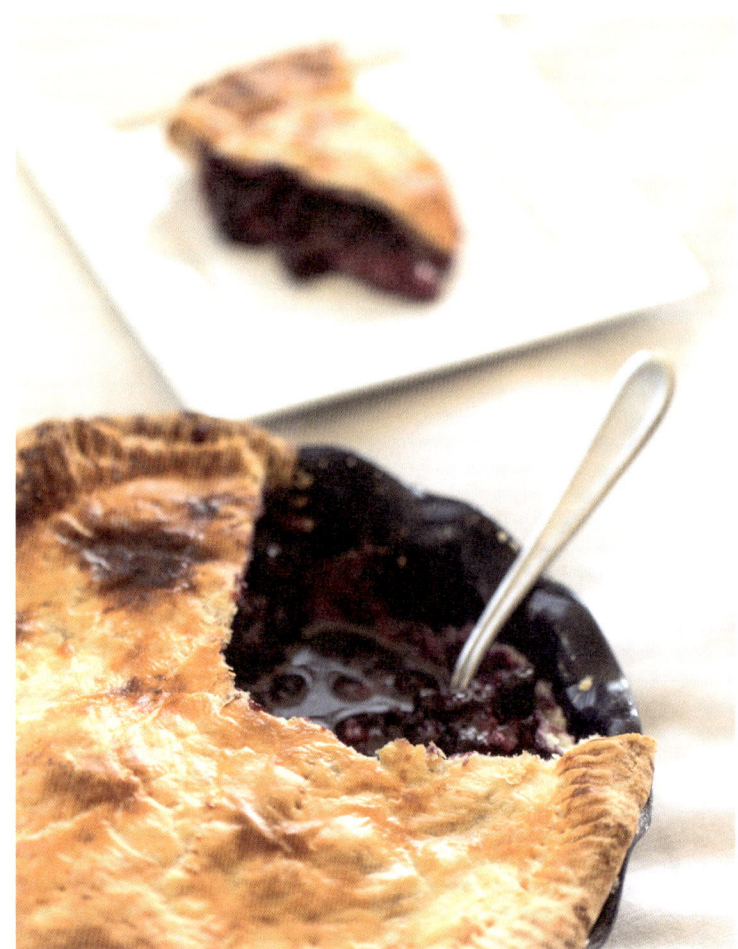

BASIC PIE DOUGH

2¼ cups all-purpose flour

2 teaspoons sugar

¾ teaspoon salt

2 sticks unsalted butter, cut into ½ inch cubes

½ cup and up to ⅔ cup ice-cold water

1. Mix flour, sugar and salt in a mixing bowl fitted with a pastry blade.

2. Slowly add butter, while incorporating into flour mixture on medium speed.

3. Drizzle ice water onto dough while dough is turning. Mix until pastry comes together and dough can be turned out onto a slightly floured surface.

4. Form 2 even balls of dough. Flatten, wrap in plastic and refrigerate for 1 hour or until ready to use.

PIE

7-8 cups fresh or frozen blueberries

1¼ cups of organic pure cane sugar *(can use light brown sugar or coconut sugar)*

3 tablespoons cornstarch

3 tablespoons tapioca

1 teaspoon lemon zest

¼ teaspoon salt

1 teaspoon cinnamon

1 scrambled egg + 1 tablespoon water, for egg wash

1. Preheat oven to 425°.

2. Place blueberries into a large bowl. Mix all other ingredients and gently toss with blueberries.

3. On a slightly flowered surface, roll out one disk of dough. Fit into a deep-dish 9-inch pie dish with extra dough hanging over the edge by 1/2 inch.

4. Load blueberry mixture into the dish. It will cook down, so pile it high, and fill the dish.

5. Roll out second disk and place evenly over pie with enough dough to crimp the edges and create a crust on the perimeter of the dish.

6. Poke holes in the top to vent the pie. Brush the top with egg wash. Place pie on a baking dish lined with aluminum foil.

7. Bake in a hot oven for 30 minutes. Reduce temperature to 375° and continue to bake until crust is golden and pie is bubbling hot, approximately 40 minutes longer.

8. Cool the pie completely *(3 hours)* before serving.

Enjoy!

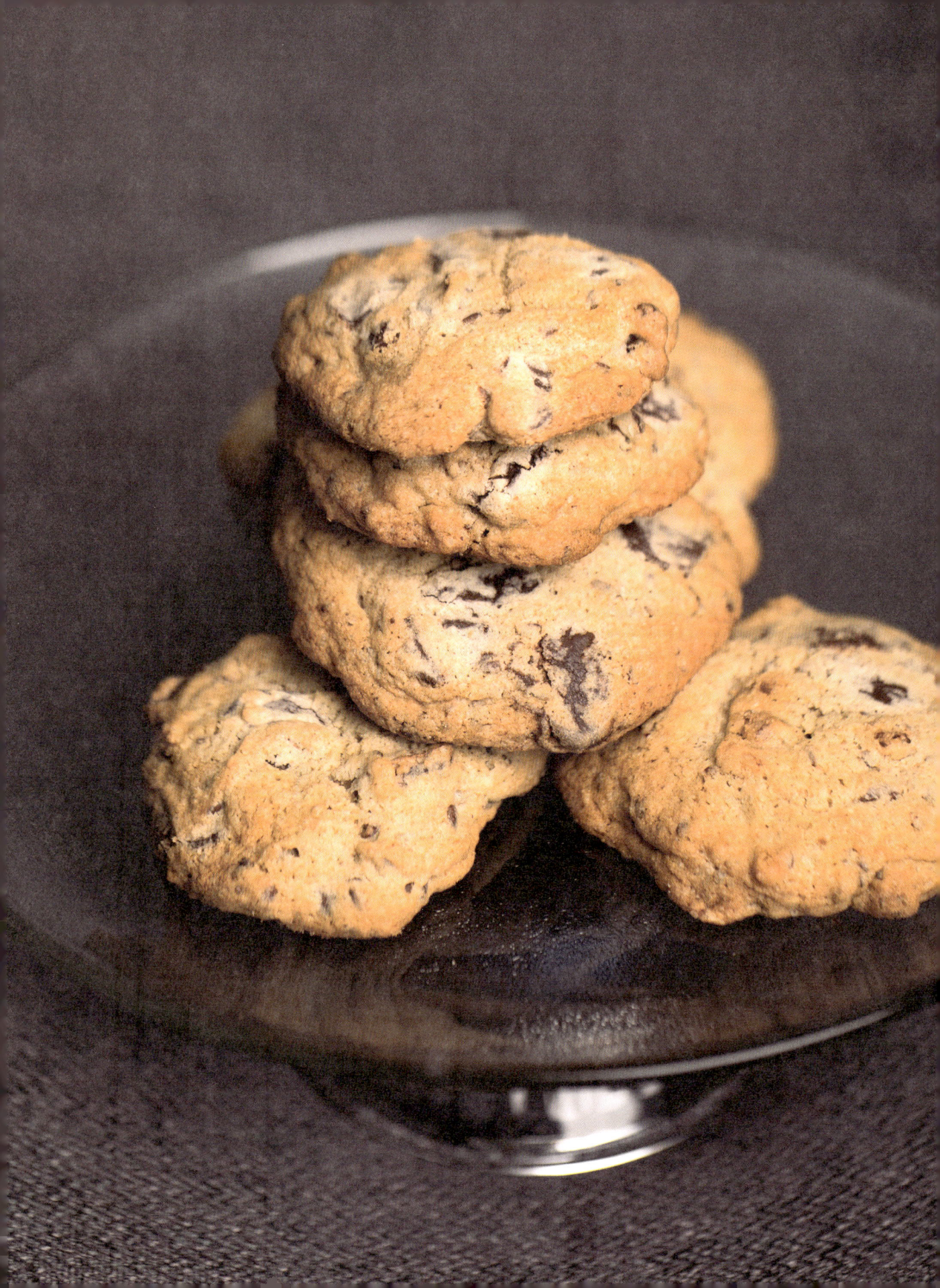

chocolate chip pecan cookies
with flax seed

THIS RECIPE IS MY BASIC CHOCOLATE CHIP COOKIE RECIPE that I just happened to have changed one day. I had leftover ground flaxseed that I needed to use, so I threw it in. I liked the added flavor so much that I now use it every time that I make a batch. I also use one half whole wheat flour to give it more depth and make it a bit healthier. Only homemade cookies go in the "healthy" category.

1 cup unbleached organic all-purpose flour

1 cup whole wheat organic flour

¼ cup ground flax seed

1 teaspoon baking soda

½ teaspoon salt

½ pound unsalted butter

¾ cup brown sugar

¾ cup fine white granulated sugar

2 eggs

1 teaspoon vanilla

16 ounces bittersweet chocolate chips

1 cup pecans, toasted and chopped

1. Preheat oven to 350° convection.
2. Mix dry ingredients and set aside.
3. Cream butter and sugars until smooth, approximately 2 minutes on medium-high speed.
4. Add eggs, incorporating one at a time, then vanilla.
5. Slowly incorporate dry ingredients, then chocolate and nuts. Do not overmix.
6. Drop cookies evenly, by the spoonful, on two cookie sheets. Bake in a convection oven for 10-12 minutes or until golden brown.

Enjoy!

MBK'S TIPS

Make sure to buy ground flaxseed instead of whole flaxseed. The intense flavor of whole flaxseed will overpower the taste of the cookie.

chocolate glaze
for chocolate espresso cake

THIS GLAZE IS NOT ONLY GOOD FOR THE CAKE ON the following page, but for any cake that calls for chocolate to glaze its top. The espresso adds an intense, smoky coffee flavor. If you love coffee and chocolate, this is a winner.

NUTRITION EXTRAS

Dark chocolate is rich in antioxidants called flavonoids, which provide several health benefits, including longevity. It is also rich in minerals such as iron, magnesium, and zinc.

Coffee is also rich in therapeutic antioxidants that have an anti-inflammatory and potential anti-cancer effect.

GF

---

3 ounces bittersweet chocolate, 70% cacao, chopped

1½ tablespoons unsalted butter

2 teaspoons vanilla extract

⅓ cup heavy cream

⅓ cup fine sugar

2 teaspoons instant espresso powder

¼ teaspoon salt

---

1. Combine chocolate, butter, and vanilla in a heat resistant bowl.
2. Bring cream, sugar, espresso powder and salt to a boil in a small sauce pan, stirring until sugar and espresso powder have dissolved.
3. Pour over chocolate mixture and whisk by hand until smooth.
4. Let cool, then pour on top of cooled cake. Spread evenly.

Enjoy!

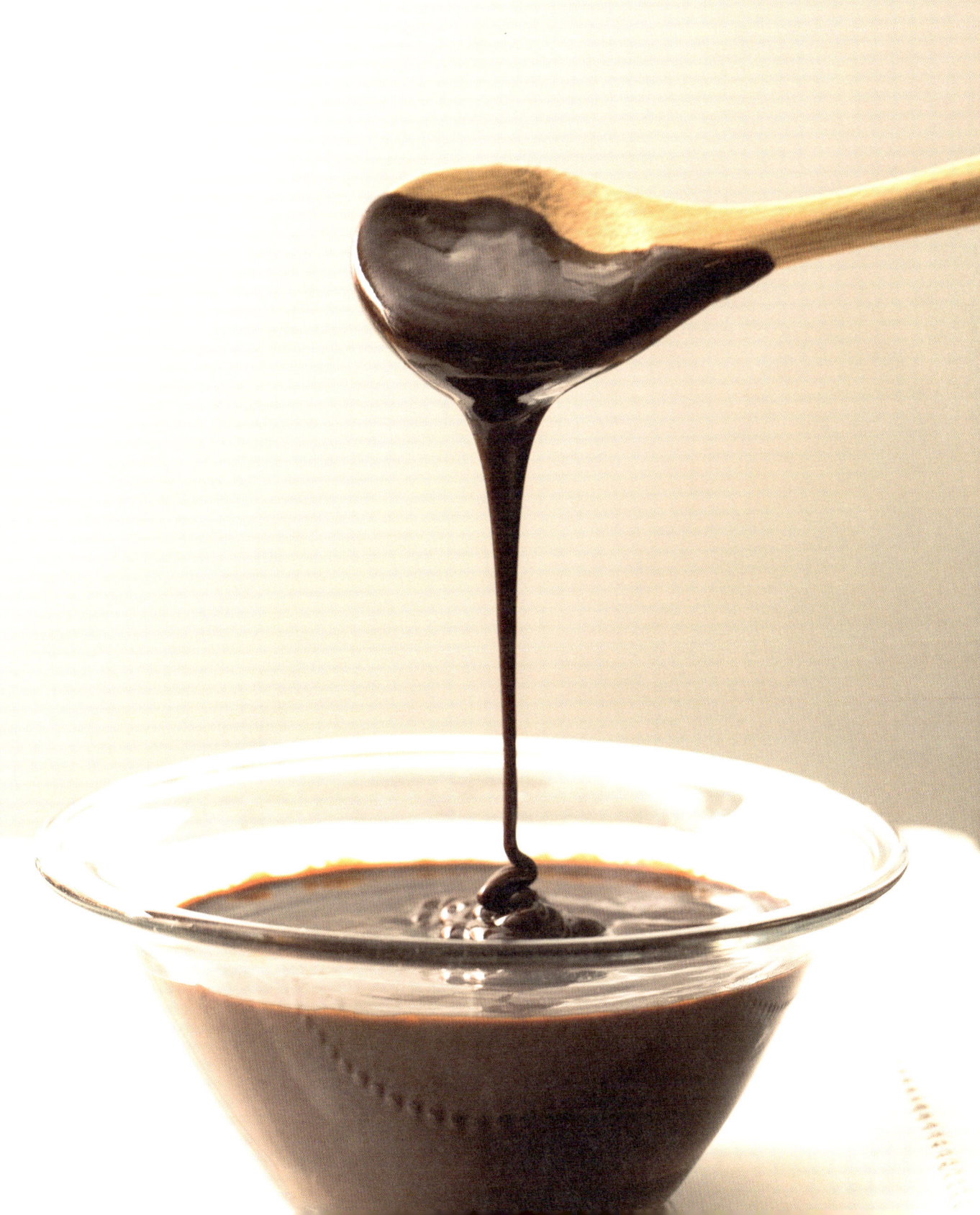

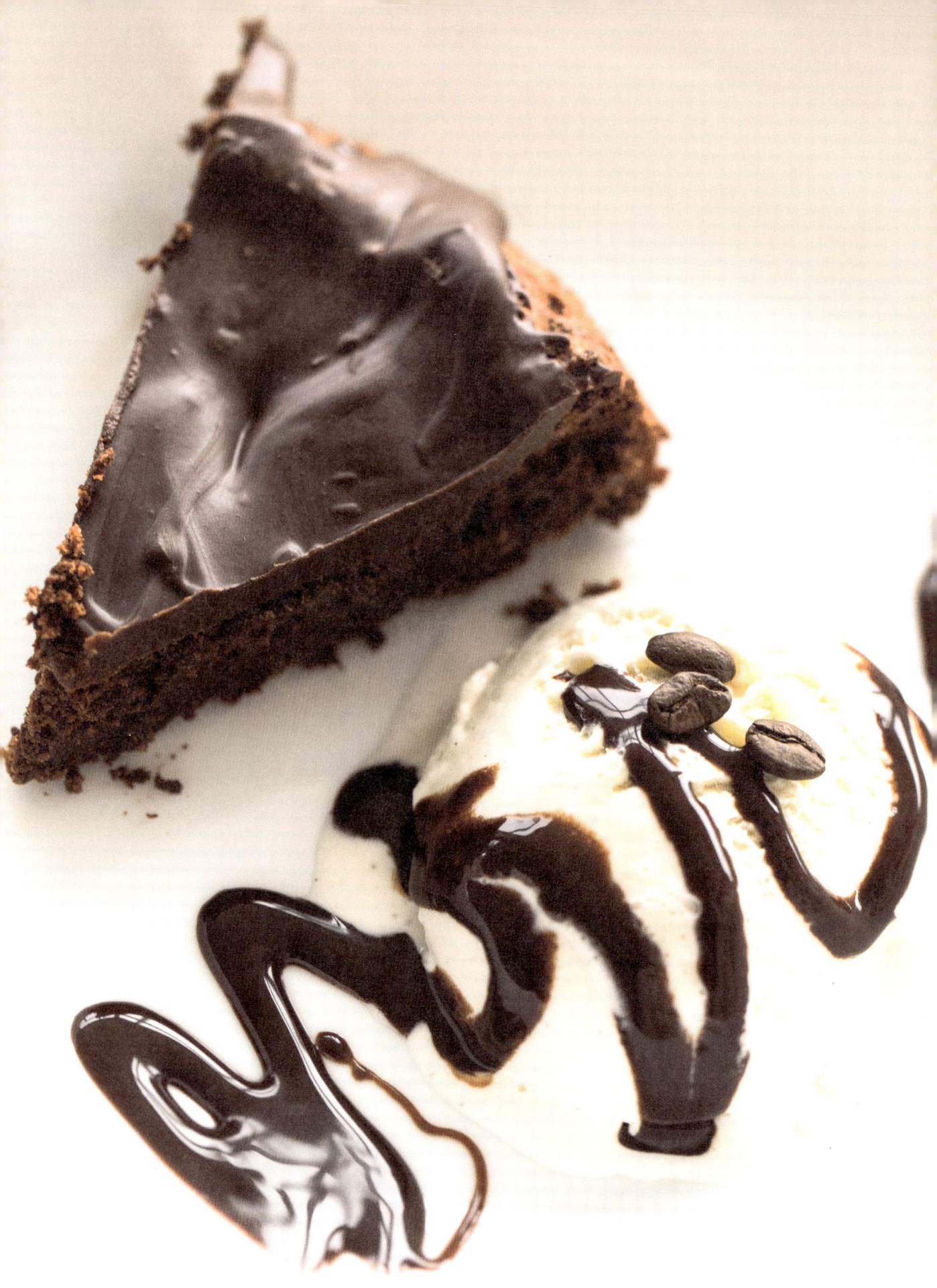

flourless chocolate espresso cake

IF YOU ARE LOOKING FOR A LITTLE DESSERT TO POWER you through a sleepy afternoon - this is the one! Between the dark chocolate and the espresso, you will feel a jolt from just a small portion of this desert. Everything in moderation, right? The icing for this cake also adds more chocolate and coffee, but you can always opt for whipped cream and fresh berries if you want to lighten the recipe.

- 3 tablespoons unsalted butter
- 6 ounces bittersweet chocolate, 70 percent cacao, chopped
- 6 large room temperature eggs, separated
- 1 cup sugar, divided
- 2 tablespoons instant espresso powder
- ¼ teaspoon salt
- 1 tablespoon vanilla

1. Pre-heat oven to 350°. Generously butter or spray a 9-inch springform pan with baking cooking spray until well coated.
2. Melt butter and chocolate in a small saucepan on low heat, stirring util smooth. Let cool.
3. Beat egg yolks and ½ cup sugar with a mixer on medium speed until thick and pale, about 3 minutes.
4. Add espresso and salt and continue to mix for one more minute.
5. Add chocolate and vanilla to egg yolks and beat for one additional minute.
6. In a separate bowl beat egg whites on medium-high speed, until foamy.
7. Increase speed to high and gradually add 1/2 cup of sugar, beating until stiff peaks form, about 5 minutes.
8. Fold egg whites into chocolate mixture in three batches, then transfer to cake pan to bake until set. The cake should be done in 35 - 45 minutes.
9. Let cool completely before removing from pan. Top with chocolate glaze if desired.

enjoy!

MBK'S TIPS

For successful egg white peaks:

First, make sure your eggs are room temperature. Secondly, make sure no yokes get into the egg white mix. If you still have trouble getting them to form peaks, you can add a teaspoon of cream of tartar or lemon juice.

GF

chocolate macaroon cake

THIS CAKE IS A LABOR OF LOVE that is worth every bit of time invested in making it. I discovered this in Bon Appetit years ago, and I shared it with my soon-to-be daughter in law Marissa, who like me, flipped for the taste. It has since been made several times, by both of us, for multiple family special occasions. If you loved an almond joy as a child, this is your cake. The ingredients are so healthy that you don' feel any guilt over eating dessert!

MBK'S TIPS

The ganache calls for coconut milk that is from a can. This is entirely different than the coconut milk sold in the dairy section *(mainly added water)*.

Give the milk a good shake before opening!

GF
DF
V

GANACHE

4-ounce semisweet or bittersweet chocolate, coarsely chopped

1 tablespoon agave or pure maple syrup

pinch of salt

½ cup canned unsweetened coconut milk

1. Combine chocolate, agave nectar and salt in a medium bowl.

2. In a small saucepan over low heat, bring coconut milk to a simmer and pour over chocolate. Let mixture stand for 5 minutes until chocolate is melted.

3. Beat the ganache on medium speed for approximately 6-8 minutes, until thick enough to hold soft peaks.

4. Spread quickly on top of cooled cake, spreading just to the edges with a small spatula.

5. Top cake with toasted coconut and almonds if desired.

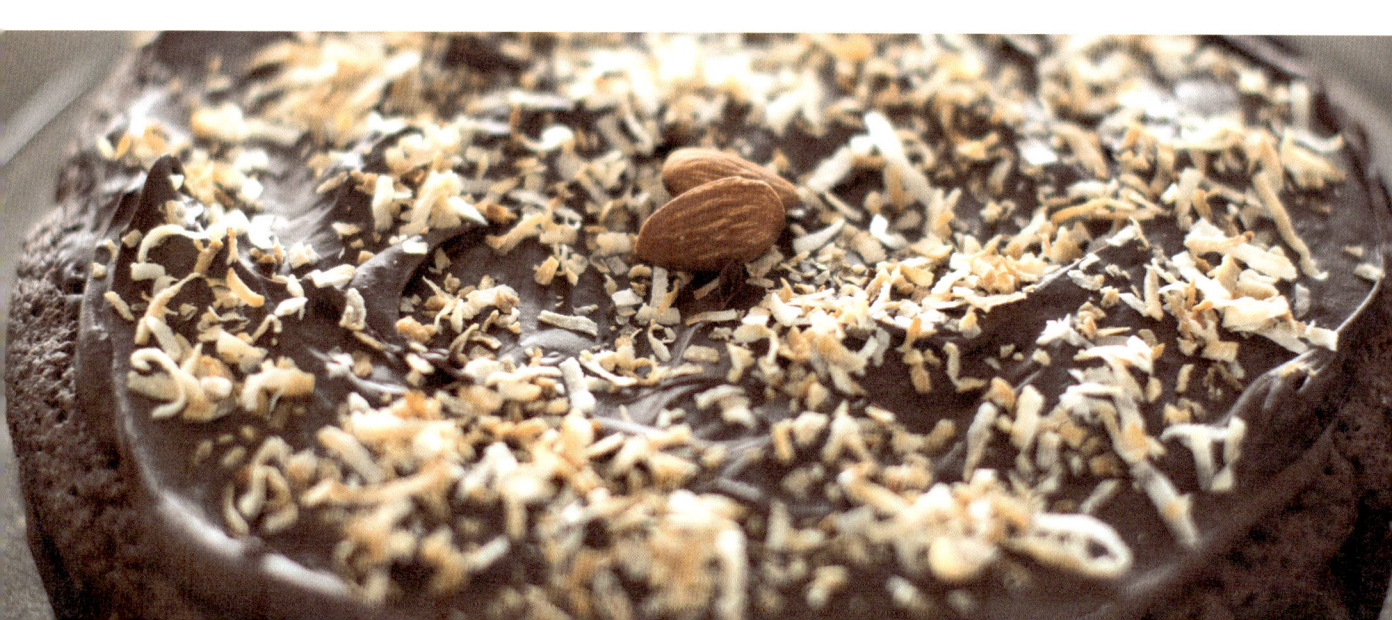

CAKE

1 cup raw almonds

1 cup virgin coconut oil *(plus more for pan)*, warmed to liquid

¼ cup unsweetened cocoa powder (additional for dusting pan)

8 ounces semisweet or bittersweet chocolate, coarsely chopped

1 teaspoon kosher salt

½ cup unsweetened shredded coconut

6 large eggs, room temperature

½ cup granulated sugar

½ cup packed light brown sugar

2 teaspoons vanilla extract

1. Preheat oven to 350°.

2. Toast almonds on a rimmed baking sheet *(during cooking, toss once until fragrant and slightly darkened)*, 8-10 minutes. Let cool completely.

3. Reduce oven to 325°.

4. Line bottom of springform pan with parchment paper. Oil sides and paper with coconut oil, dust with cocoa powder. Shake off excess.

5. In a medium heatproof bowl, set over saucepan of barely simmering water, heat bittersweet chocolate and oil. Stir often, until the mixture is smooth. Remove from heat.

6. Pulse almonds, salt and ¼ cup cocoa in a food processor, until nuts are finely ground. Add coconut and pulse a few times to combine.

7. Beat eggs on medium speed of stand up mixer with a whisk attachment, about 20 seconds. Add both sugars and vanilla, increase speed to high and beat until mixture is pale and thick, about 2 minutes.

8. Switch to the paddle attachment and with mixer on low speed gradualy add chocolate. Beat only to incorporate, then add almond mixture. Fold batter with a rubber spatula, then scrape into prepared pan.

9. Bake cake until a tester comes out clean and cake is firm to touch, approximately 35-45 minutes. Cool completely on wire rack.

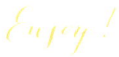

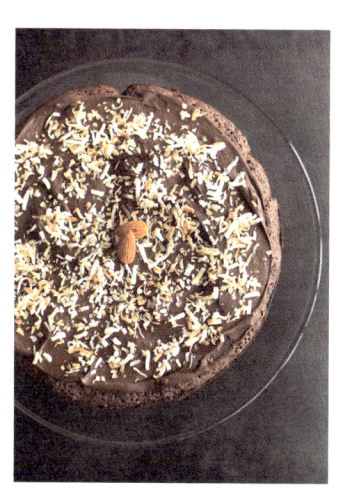

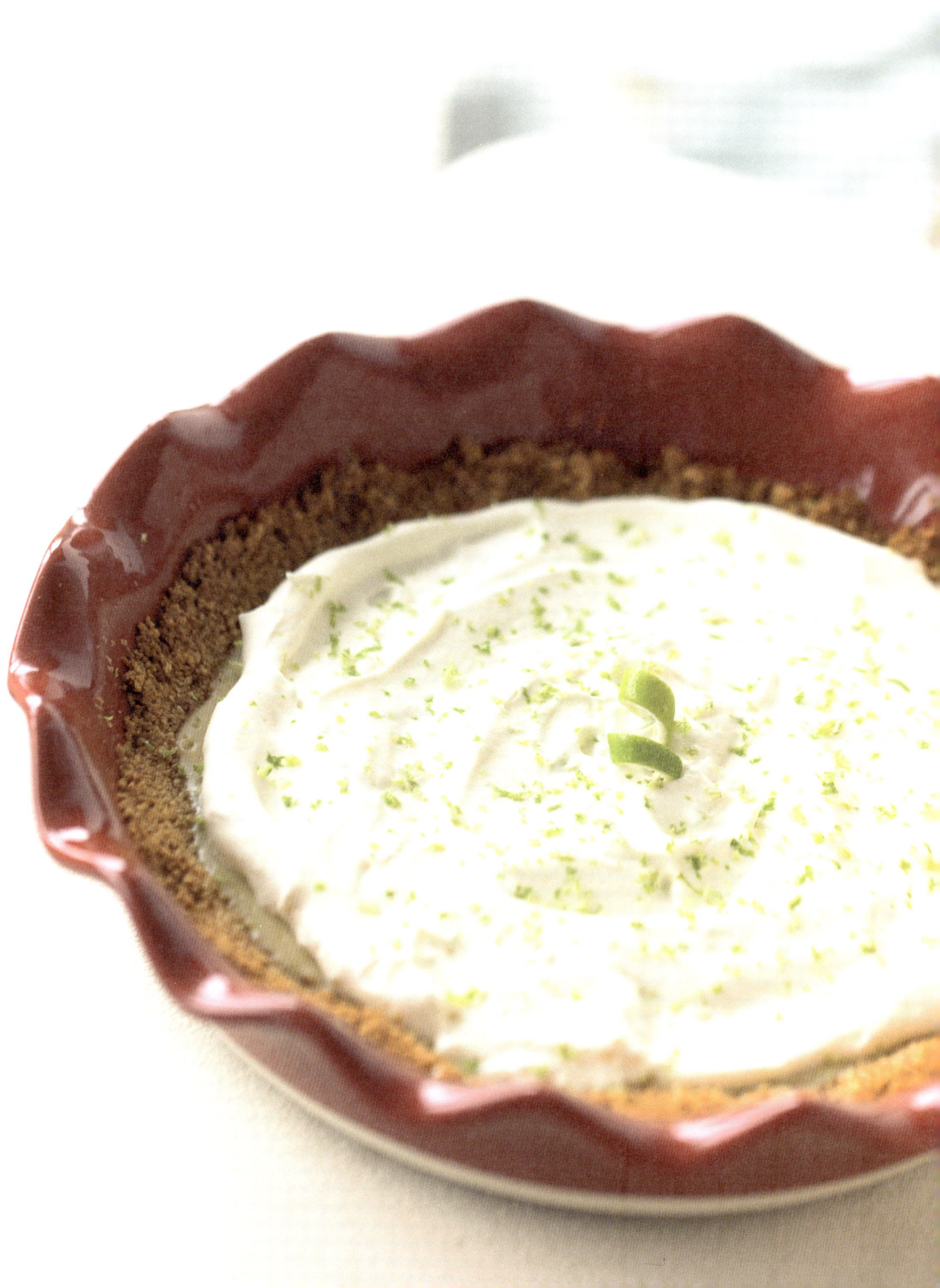

key lime pie

MY FAVORITE SUMMER DESSERT! During the months of relaxed entertaining, long days in the outdoors and lots of fresh seafood on the menu, this citrus delight is the perfect ending to dinner outdoors. I love key lime pie and love having this in the refrigerator during the summer months. This recipe is easy to pull off and always wows your guests. It's a light finish to a meal that is not too filling.

CRUST

coconut oil spray

1¼ cups organic graham cracker crumbs (⅓ of box)

2 tablespoons brown sugar (can use coconut sugar)

5 tablespoons unsalted butter, melted

FILLING

1 - 14-ounce can sweetened condensed milk

4 large egg yolks

½ cup organic key lime juice from concentrate

TOPPING

¾ cup heavy whipping cream

1 tablespoon confectioners' sugar

1 teaspoon vanilla

lime zest

1. Preheat oven to 350°. Set rack in the middle of the oven.

2. Spray a 9-inch pie plate with coconut oil.

3. Use a food processor to combine graham crackers, brown sugar and butter. Pulse until a course crumble occurs.

4. Press crust evenly onto the bottom and partially up the sides of the pie plate. Bake in the preheaded oven for 10 minutes. Leave oven on for later use.

5. Whisk together condensed milk and egg yolks until well combined. Add the lime juice and incorporate it thoroughly. Pour into prepared crust and return to oven for 15 minutes.

6. Remove from oven and cool the pie completely, then refrigerate for 6-8 hours.

7. In a mixer, beat cream with sugar and vanilla, until still peaks form. Spread on top of the cool pie and top with lime zest.

Enjoy!

MRK'S TIPS

I love key west organic lime juice, but it can be tricky to find. Look for ingredients long before you anticipate making this dish. It will keep in your pantry for months.

nut and seed brittle

BRITTLE IS A TASTY TREAT I LIKE TO MAKE FOR GIFTS around the Christmas holiday. I don't make this often, but when I produce a batch, it always reminds me how easy it is to pull together. Just a little bite of this is so delicious with my afternoon tea. As for the nuts, you can use any combination of nuts and seeds - they all work in brittle.

parchment paper

1 cup of sugar

½ cup of agave

1 cup raw pumpkin seeds, shelled

½ cup roasted salted nuts of choice (*peanuts or almonds*)

2 tablespoons unsalted butter

1 teaspoon fine salt

¾ teaspoon baking soda

⅛ teaspoon cinnamon

candy thermometer

MBK'S TIPS

Make sure you have a real candy thermometer. You want to be sure to get the sugar to the right temperature before adding the baking soda - kitchen chemistry at its best!

GF

1. Line a cookies sheet with parchment paper and set aside.

2. In a saucepan over medium heat add sugar, agave and 3 tablespoons of water. Bring to a boil, stirring to dissolve sugar. Fit saucepan with a thermometer and cook until thermometer registers 290°, 3-4 minutes.

3. Stir in pumpkin seeds, nuts, butter and salt. Continue cooking and stirring, until pale brown and thermometer registers 305°, 3-4 minutes.

4. Stir in baking soda and cinnamon (*mixture will bubble vigorously*), then immediately pour the caramel onto parchment paper. Using a heat resistant spatula quickly spread out brittle.

5. Let cool and break into pieces.

Enjoy!

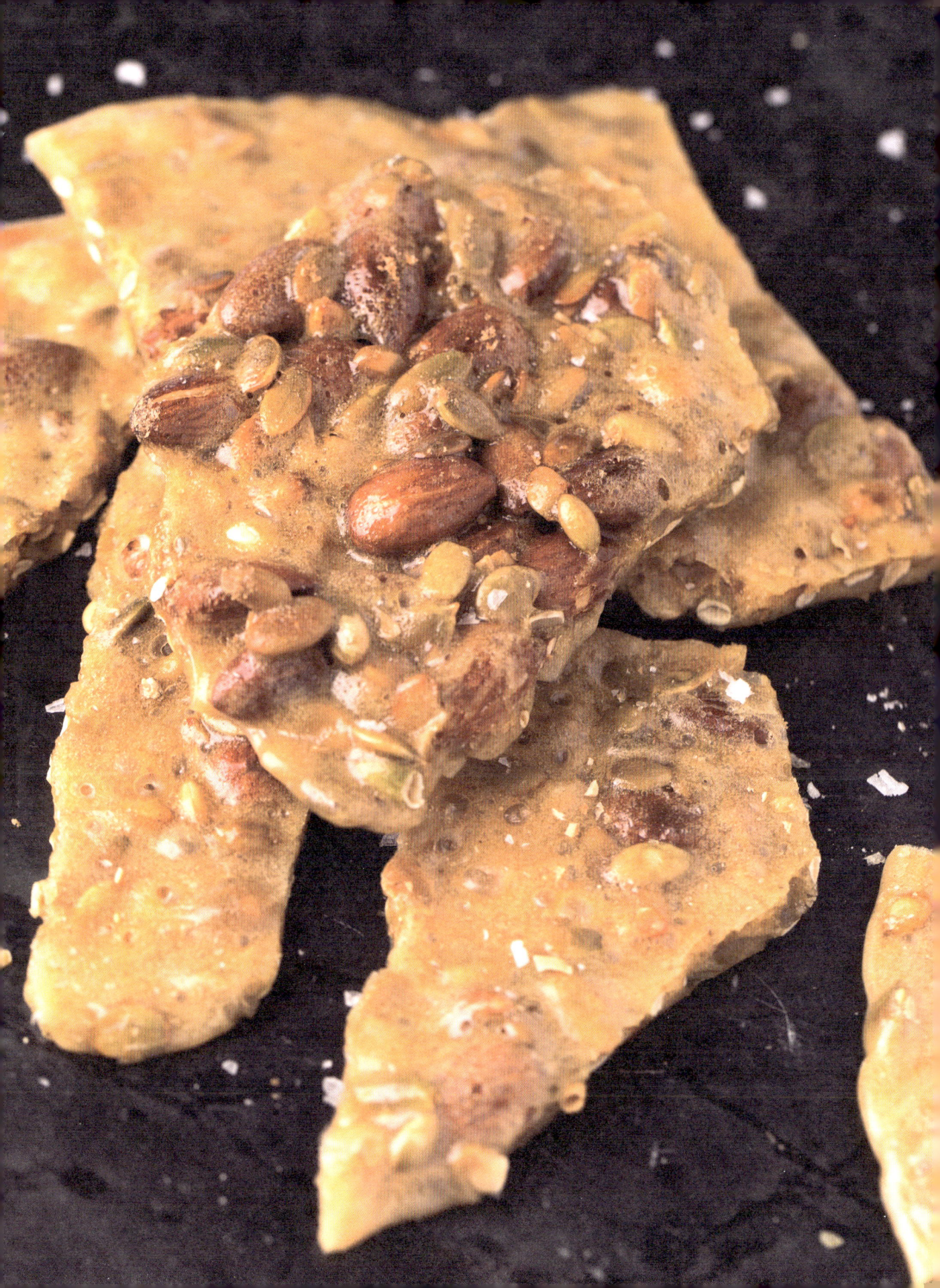

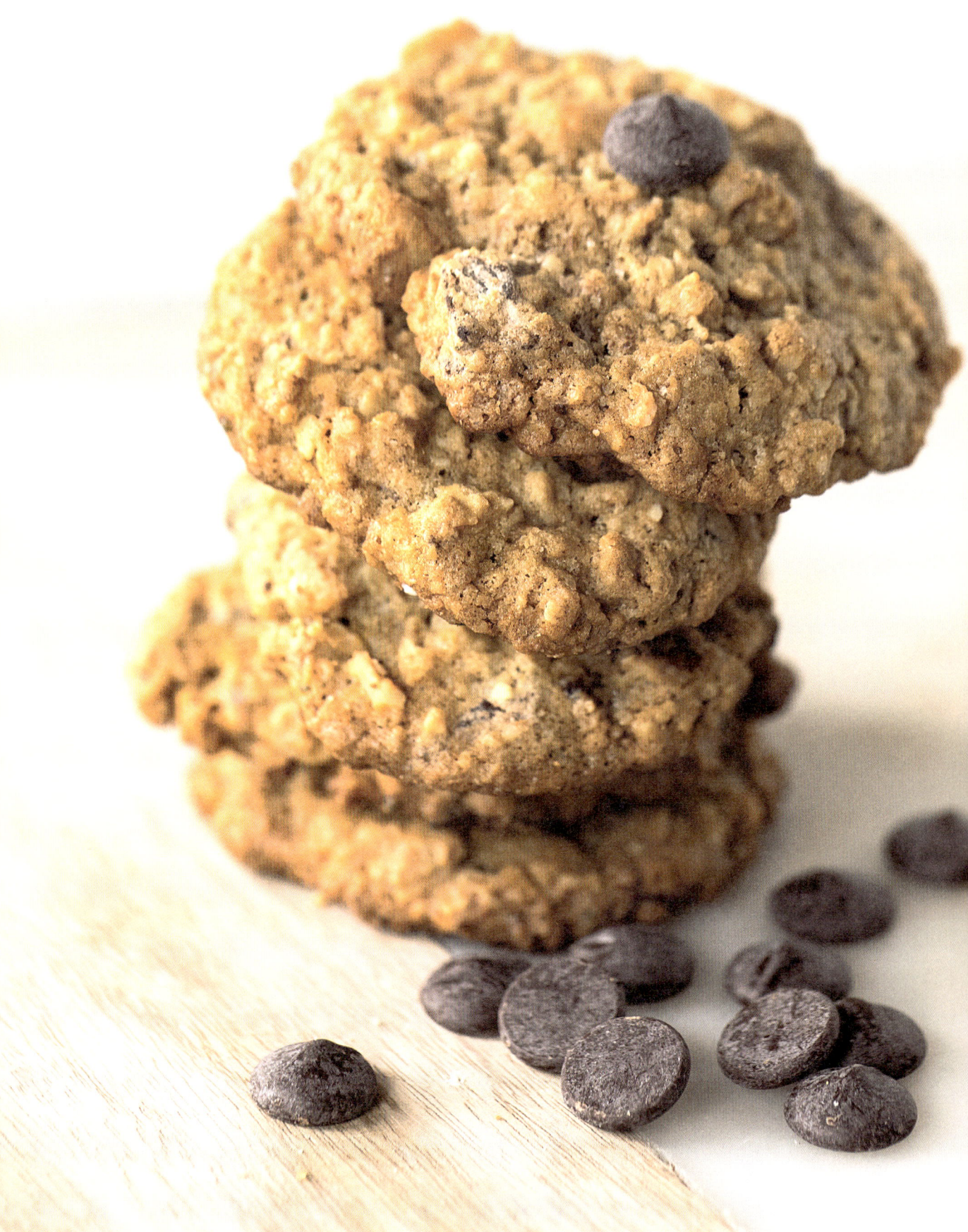

oatmeal chocolate walnut cookies

THE TEXTURE AND FLAVOR OF THESE COOKIES HITS your taste buds on all cylinders. You have the delicious dark chocolate, along with chewy oatmeal and the earthy walnuts. I love keeping a batch of these frozen in the house, for when the urge for a good cookie hits. These are crowd pleasers if you are in charge of bringing dessert. The recipe is sure to be requested!

3 cups old fashioned rolled oats

1¼ cups unbleached all-purpose flour

¼ cup ground flaxseed

1 teaspoon baking soda

1 teaspoon baking powder

½ teaspoon salt

1 teaspoon cinnamon

2 sticks unsalted butter, room temperature

1 cup dark brown sugar

1 cup fine sugar

2 eggs

1 teaspoon vanilla

2 cups semi-sweet chocolate baking chips

1½ cups walnuts, chopped

1. Preheat oven to 350°.
2. Mix the first seven dry ingredients in a medium-size bowl. Set aside.
3. Combine butter and sugars in mixing bowl and beat on medium speed until pale and fluffy, approximately 4 minutes.
4. Add eggs and vanilla to sugars and mix until well combined.
5. On low speed slowly add dry ingredients to wet ingredients and mix thoroughly.
6. Stir in chocolate and walnuts by hand.
7. With a large spoon or ice-cream scooper drop cookies 2-inches apart on a baking sheet. Bake for approximately 14 minutes, until golden brown and just set.
8. Once cool, cookies can be stored in air tight container at room temperature for several days.

Enjoy!

MBK'S TIPS

I make a full batch of dough and only make a dozen cookies at a time and freeze the rest of the dough for later use. Cookies are always best right out of the oven.

Be sure your ingredients are fresh and remember, freeze your flour if not using frequently.

strawberry tarts
with pecan crust

12 tarts

THESE GLUTEN-FREE TARTS ARE THE PERFECT LITTLE healthy sweet for the finishing touch on a summer meal. I love making these for all the patriotic holidays, like Memorial Day, Fourth of July and Labor Day. Strawberries are particularly delicious and best at the beginning of summer.

NUTRITION EXTRAS

Not too high in sugar and gluten-free makes this a winner for most people. Pecans, being a good source of healthy fat and protein, is an excellent alternative to a wheat crust.

GF
DF*
V*
* *(option)*

- coconut oil spray for muffin pan
- 2 cups unsalted pecans, toasted
- 5 tablespoons maple syrup
- 2 tablespoons almond flour
- 1 teaspoon ground ginger
- ½ teaspoon salt
- 2 tablespoons avocado or coconut oil *(warmed to liquid)*
- 1 pound fresh strawberries, hulled and thinly sliced
- 1 teaspoon lemon juice
- 1 vanilla bean, split lengthwise
- whipped cream, if desired

1. Lightly spray a 12 cup muffin pan with coconut oil.

2. Pulse pecans in a food processor until coarsely ground. Add 3 tablespoons of maple syrup, flour, ginger, salt and oil. Process until coarse dough forms.

3. Remove the ball from the food processor, divide the dough into one heaping tablespoon of mixture per muffin cup and press onto bottom and up the sides to form the tart base. Chill for 1 hour.

4. Preheat oven to 350°.

5. Bake crust for 8-10 minutes until golden around edges. Let cool entirely *(on the stovetop or a wire rack)* before removing.

6. Mix strawberries, lemon juice, remaining 2 tablespoons maple syrup and seeds from vanilla bean until well combined.

7. Fill shells and serve immediately. Top with fresh whipped cream, if desired.

Enjoy!

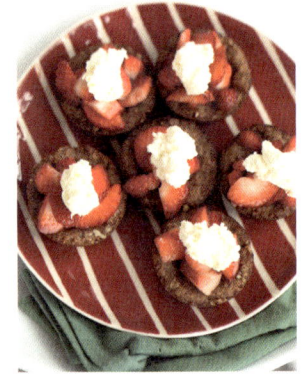

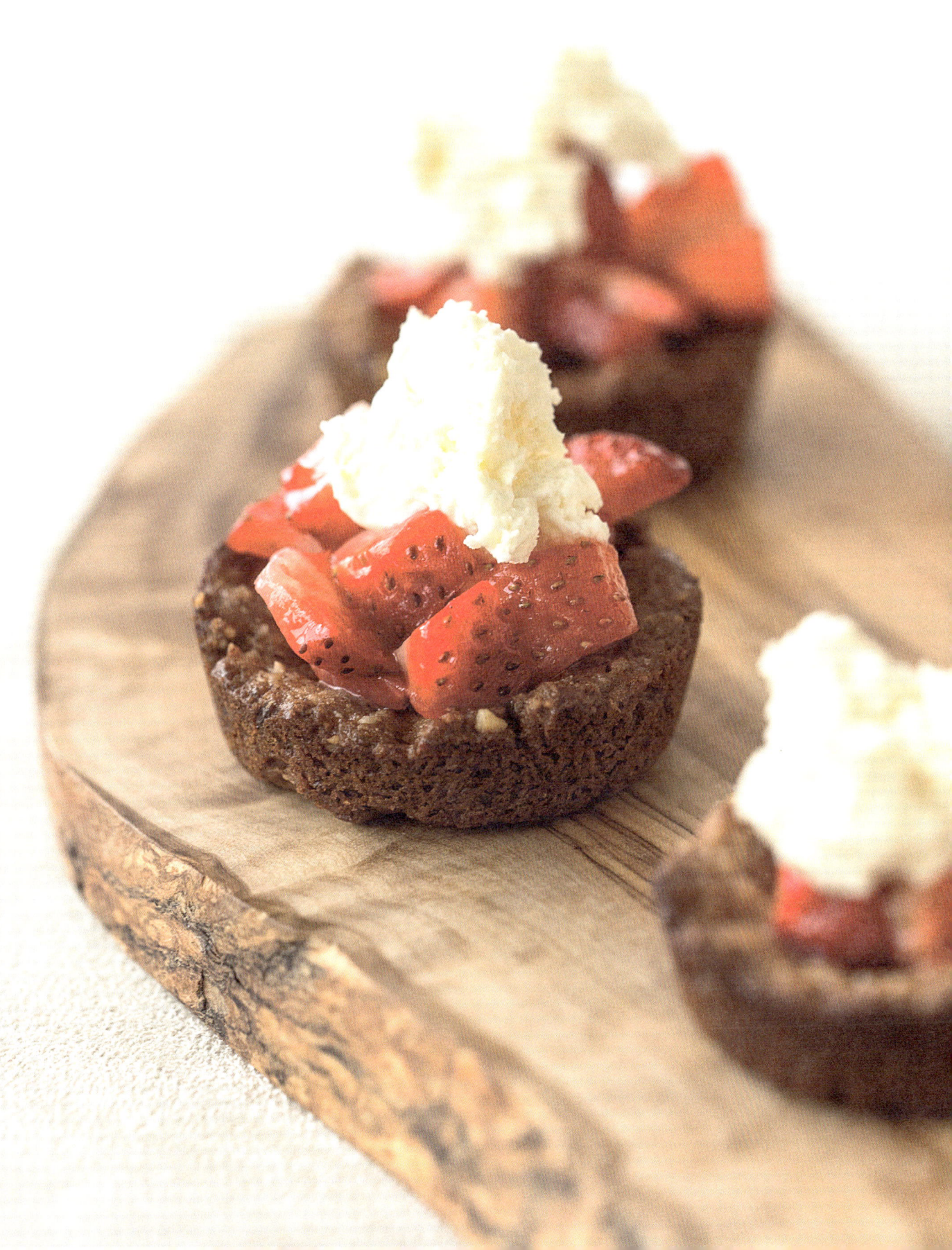

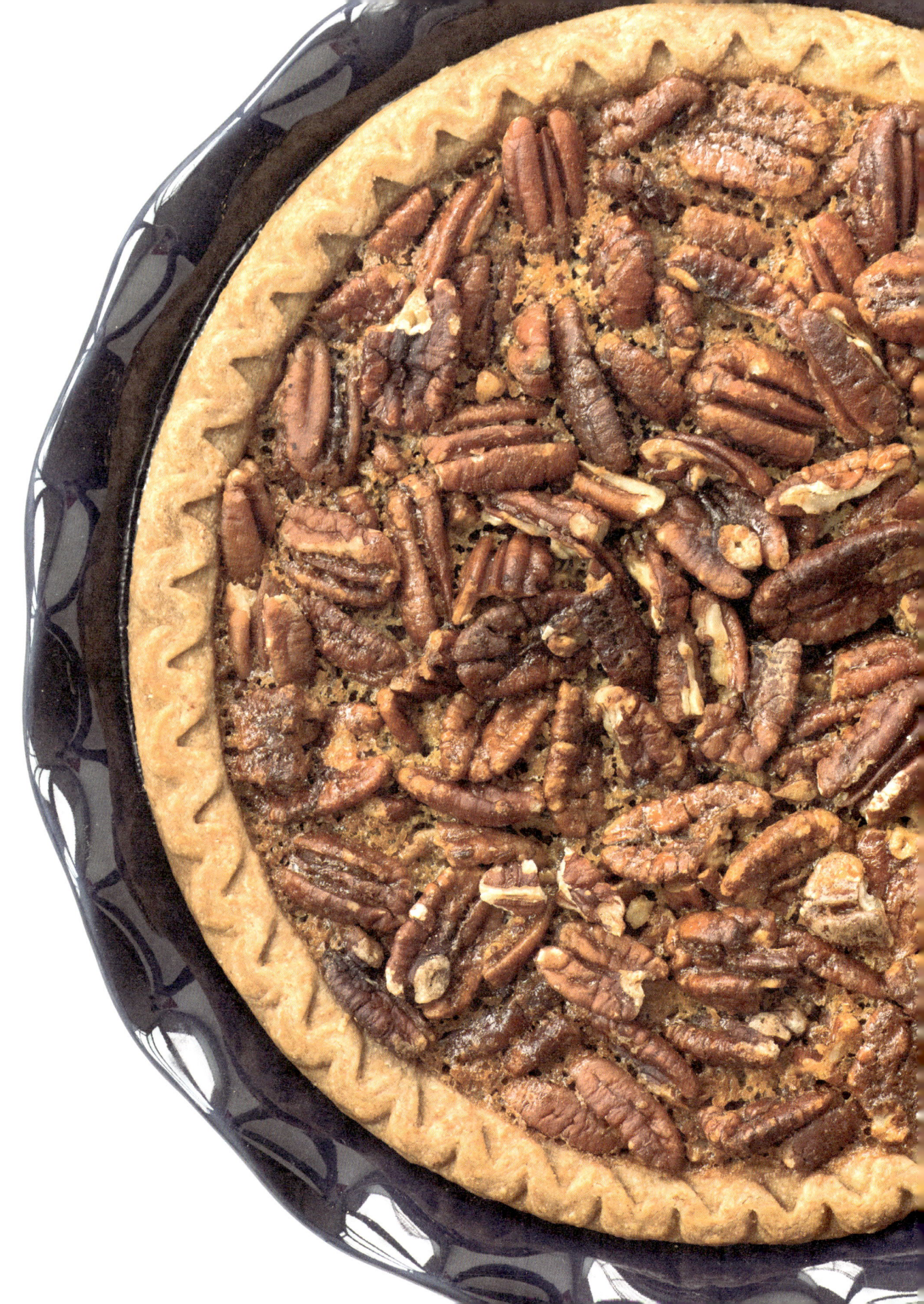

pecan pie

I ONLY MAKE THIS PIE ONCE A YEAR at Thanksgiving, and I have had my fill for the year. It's a very rich but delicious dessert that you can only eat on occasion. I happen to love sweet and salty together, so anything with a nut involved has my attention. This is the ultimate combination of those two palates.

9-inch pie crust

4 eggs

1 cup dark brown sugar

⅔ cup maple syrup

½ teaspoon salt

¼ cup melted unsalted butter, cooled

1 teaspoon vanilla

2 cups + toasted pecan halves

whipped cream or vanilla ice cream, if desired

1. Preheat oven to 400°. Bake an empty pie shell for 10 minutes before assembly until light golden brown. Cool entirely while leaving the oven on.

2. Beat eggs well with electric mixture. Add brown sugar, maple syrup, salt, butter and vanilla to the egg mixture.

3. Load the pecans evenly into the prepared pie crust. Pour egg mixture over the pecans, completely covering all of the exposed nuts. Set in the middle of the rack in a preheated oven and bake for 10 minutes.

4. Reduce heat to 325° and bake for an additional 30 minutes or until set. Remove from the oven and let cool completely. Serve with fresh whipped cream or vanilla ice cream.

Enjoy!

MBK'S TIPS

This is the one time I buy a ready-made *(organic)* crust to save on time. The crust is essential, but being that it's only on the bottom of the pie, you can cheat with a frozen premade variety. Be sure to toast your nuts to intensify the flavor. Do this in a 350° oven for approximately 10 minute, occasionally shaking to ensure even browning.

thanksgiving pumpkin roll

THIS IS ANOTHER ONE OF THOSE DESSERT RECIPE treasures that I only make on Thanksgiving and everyone is happy to see this after 12 months of absence! The smell of the spices throughout the house while this cake cooks will make you excited for the feast to come. This pumpkin roll tradition started when I was in my twenties and it has graced the table every year since.

3 eggs

1 cup sugar

⅔ cup canned pumpkin

1 teaspoon lemon juice

1 teaspoon baking powder

1 teaspoon dried ginger

2 teaspoons cinnamon

½ teaspoon salt

½ teaspoon nutmeg

¾ cup flour

2 cups of confectioners' sugar

1 - 8-ounce package cream cheese

½ cup unsalted butter, softened

½ teaspoon vanilla

1 cup walnuts, finely chopped

MBK'S TIPS

You can make this days ahead of the holiday. It tastes best when cold and keeps in the refrigerator without losing any of its flavors.

Wait until you serve the roll before you sprinkle the powdered sugar on top.

1. Preheat oven to 375°. Grease and flour a 15x10x1 inch jelly roll pan lined with parchment paper.

2. Beat eggs on high speed for 5 minutes. Gradually add sugar, mixing into the egg mixture. Stir in pumpkin and lemon.

3. Sift together dry ingredients and gently fold into pumpkin mixture. Spread mixture onto prepared pan and bake for 15 minutes.

4. Remove cake from the pan while still warm. Roll cake using the parchment and set aside until cool.

5. Combine powdered sugar, cream cheese, butter and vanilla. Beat until smooth. Spread over cooled and unrolled cake.

6. Spread nuts evenly onto the frosting, then roll back up.

7. Refrigerate for several hours and up to 2 days.

8. Sprinkle powdered sugar on top.

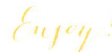

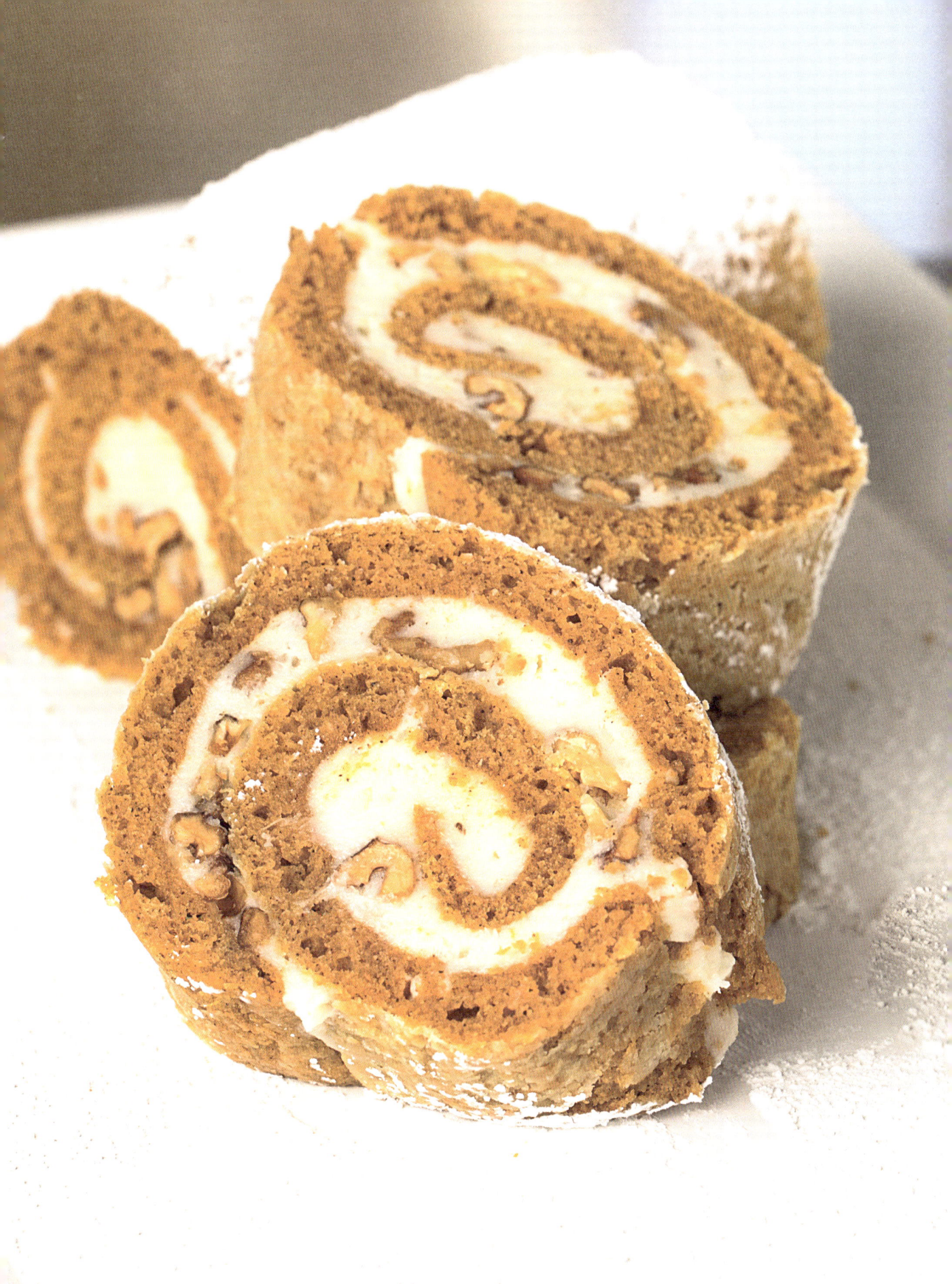

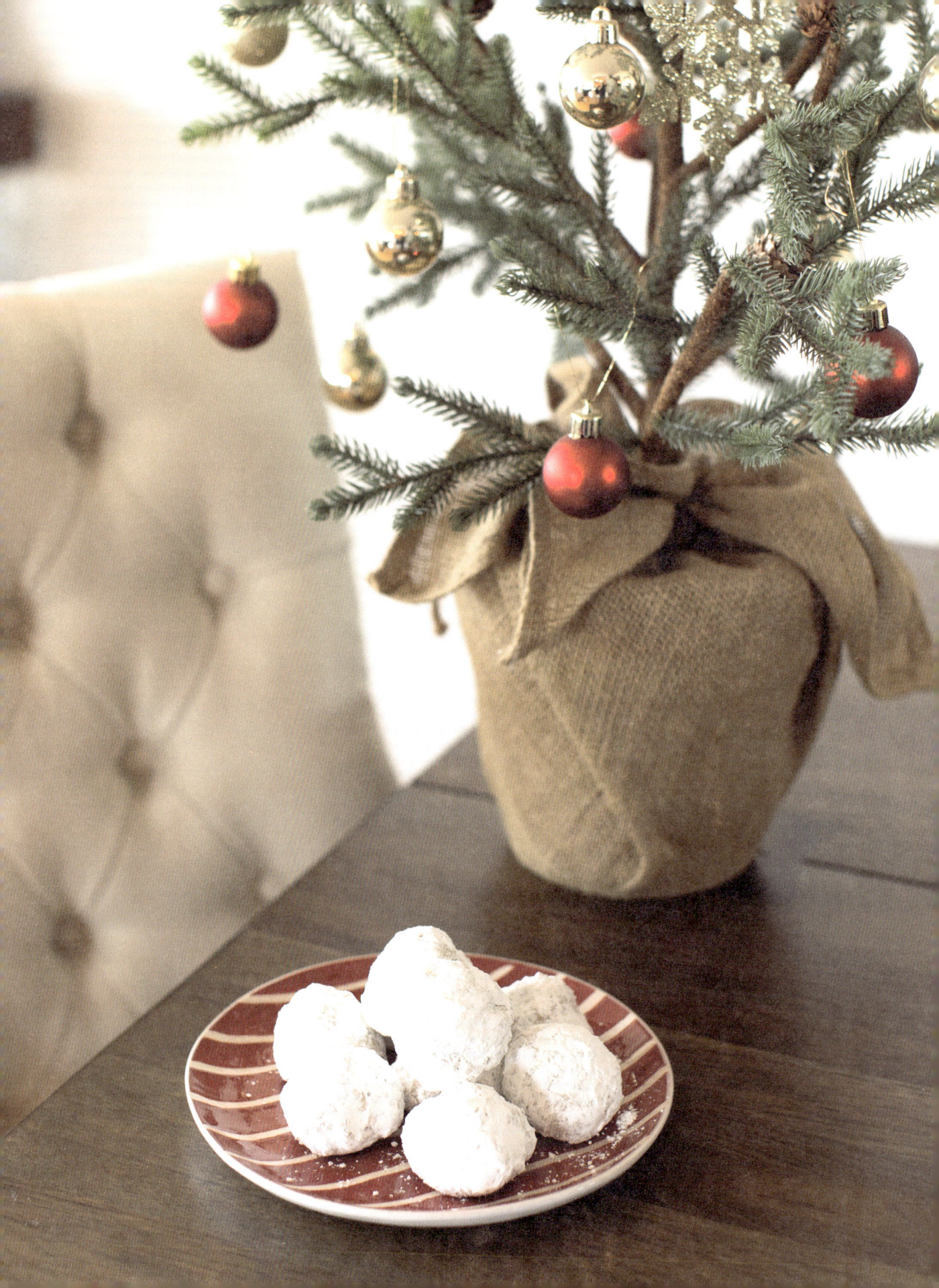

christmas butterballs

THERE ARE LOTS OF TRADITIONS AT CHRISTMAS TIME in our family, such as Grandma Rose's cutout sugar cookies with frosting and toppings, which I made often when the children were young. This particular cookie is one that our family can't go without during the Christmas season, even to this day. Years ago, I switched from using powdered sugar to sweeten the cookie, to honey, and never went back. These cookies melt in your mouth. It takes willpower to wait until December to pull this recipe out!

½ pound room temperature, unsalted sweet cream butter

6 tablespoons clover honey

1 tablespoon + 1 teaspoon vanilla extract

2 cups unbleached all-purpose flour

¾ teaspoon salt

2 cups roasted pecans, finely chopped

1½ cups confectioners' sugar

1. Cream butter and honey in the mixer on medium speed until smooth. Add vanilla and mix well. Gradually mix in flour, salt and pecans.

2. Wrap dough in foil and chill for 1 hour.

3. Preheat oven to 300°.

4. When the dough is ready, form into balls the size of quarters and space evenly on the baking sheet.

5. Bake in preheated oven for 20 minutes, until just starting to brown on the bottom. Remove from oven, let cool to touch and roll in confectioners sugar.

Enjoy!

MBK'S TIPS

Pull dough from refrigerator and rest for 15 minutes while the oven warms.

You can roll these in powdered sugar twice, if you like them extra sweet!

peanut butter cookies

THESE COOKIES FIRST STARTED CIRCULATING on the sidelines of my daughter Brittany's high school lacrosse games and quickly became requested anytime I was asked to bring snacks. I was never fond of the store-bought cookies that came out at tailgates and told the girls that if they were going to eat cookies, to make sure they are worth eating. That same group is still close friends to this day, and on occasion, my cookies are still requested.

MBK'S TIPS

The consistency of natural peanut butter varies from jar to jar, which is why a little added water is sometimes necessary to soften the dough. I have made this with almond flour and they turn out beautifully if you prefer to make these gluten-free.

NUTRITION EXTRAS

Peanut butter is a good source of protein, so this is a nice afternoon snack that is not too sweet when you need a little lift.

GF*

* (option)

Ingredients

- ½ cup unsalted butter room temperature
- 1½ cups natural organic creamy peanut butter
- 1 cup packed brown sugar
- 1 egg
- 1 cup unbleached white flour
- ¾ cup whole wheat flour
- ½ teaspoon baking powder
- ½ teaspoon salt
- ¼ cup water

Instructions

1. Preheat oven to 350°.
2. Cream butter, peanut butter and brown sugar together for 3 minutes, until pale and fluffy. Add egg and mix well.
3. Mix dry ingredients separately and slowly add to egg mixture until thooughly incorporated. Add ¼ cup water if dough appears dry.
4. Form dough into symmetrical balls *(about the size of a quarter)* and flatten with the back of a fork.
5. Bake for 16-20 minutes or until just starting to brown on edges.

Enjoy!

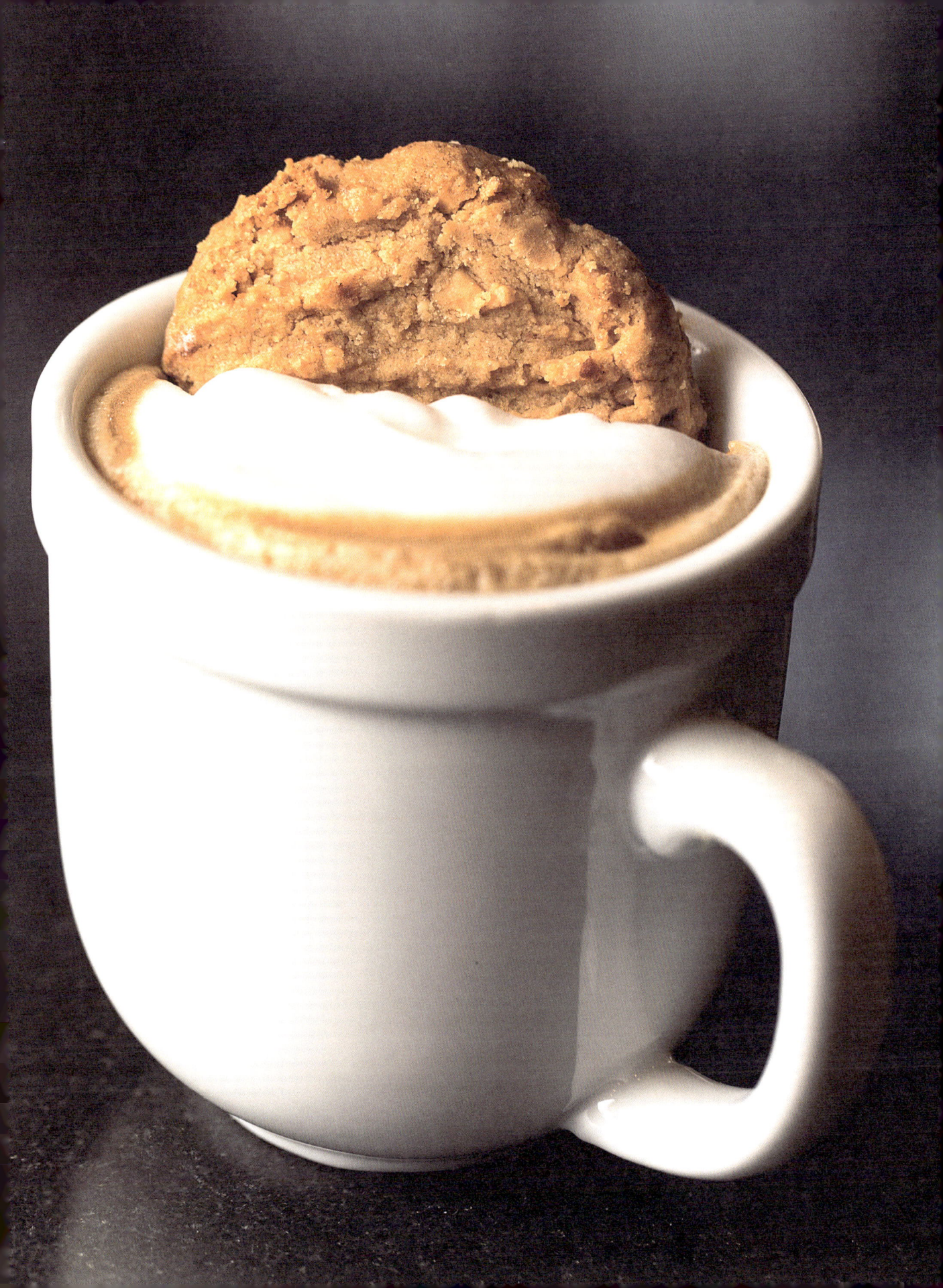

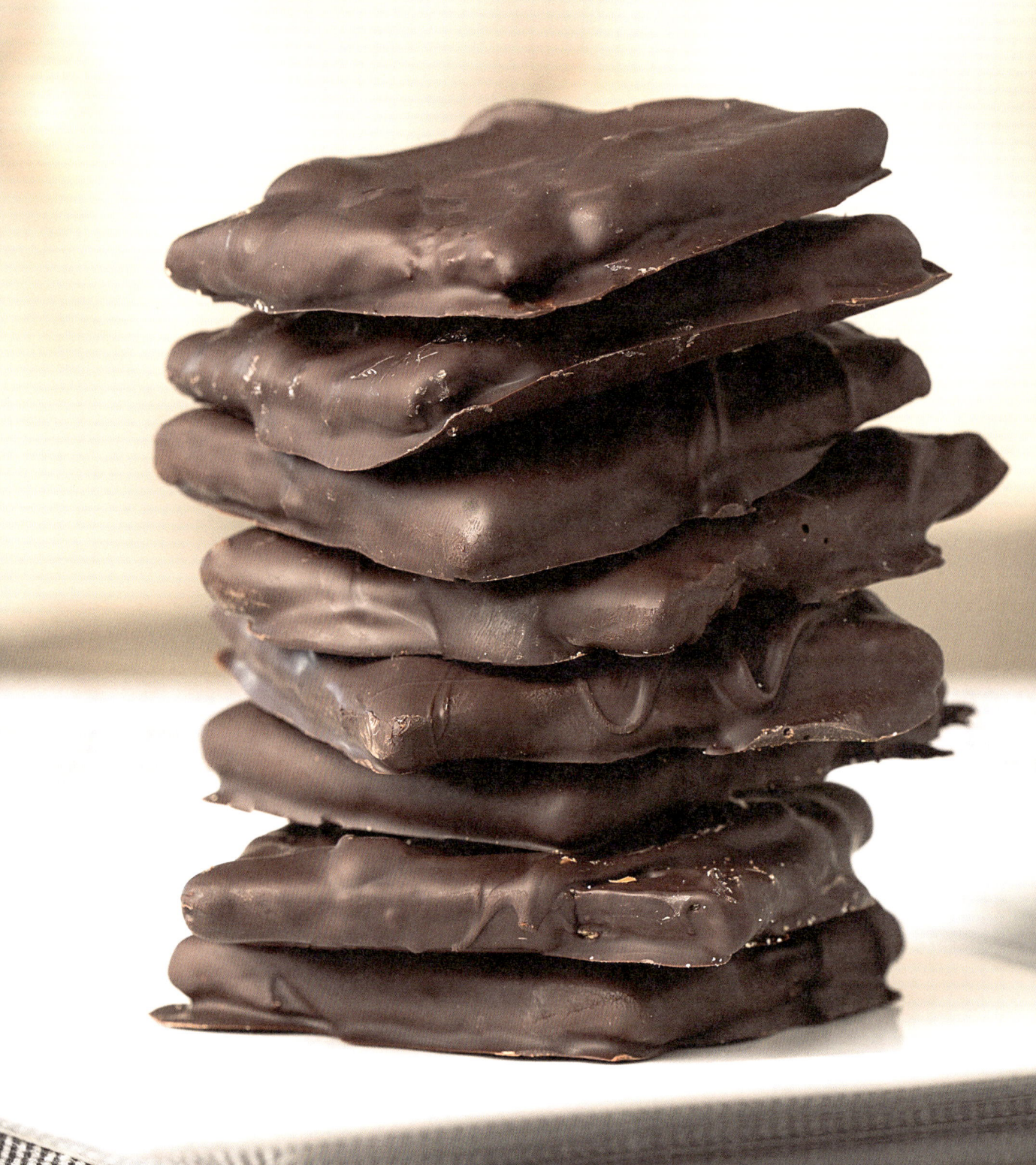

Palates famous
chocolate covered grahams

THESE COOKIES LAUNCHED A SMALL BUSINESS FOR ME in the 90's called Palates, where I made and sold these weekly for our local Nordstrom department store cafe. My husband called it my, "not for profit chocolate business." Truthfully, he was not far-off the mark on that term. It was a lot of work, not a lot of money, but lots of glory. I even got a shout out in our local newspaper. The chocolate is so good, because of the quality of the chocolate I use and because it's not tempered. It's that simple! This is a graham that puts all other graham's that you have eaten to shame.

1 pound bittersweet Callebaut chocolate

good quality store-bought graham crackers, such as Trader Joe's or Whole Foods, cut into 2x2 inch squares

1. Line a baking sheet with parchment paper.
2. In a double boiler slowly warm chocolate until melted and smooth.
3. Dip grahams in chocolate, one at a time, shaking off any excess before laying flat on wax paper. Repeat until all chocolate is used.
4. Take the back of a knife and create a design on the cookie's face, while chocolate is still warm.
5. Place a tray in the refrigerator until chocolate is completely cooled and hardened.
6. Peel off wax paper and store in an airtight container in the fridge. Cookies stay fresh for several weeks.

Enjoy!

MBK'S TIPS

I reference the type of chocolate I buy, but you may prefer local artisanal chocolate, which is fine. High-quality dark chocolate is all you need.

DF
V

giving thanks

I want to thank my husband and four children and their spouses, who have encouraged me to write this book for a long time. Their nurturing efforts were continually pushing me to finish this project. My husband has always been supportive of my dreams, my career and my personal goals. He has always appreciated that he eats really well and happily remains my sole tester in the kitchen on an average day.

I want to thank my parents who were incredible mentors to me and my nine siblings. They taught us all manners, respect and the love of dining *(which started as two picnic tables in their first kitchen)*. My parents' traditions have carried on for two generations, as the love of gathering around the table with good food and laughter permeates our homes.

I want to thank my siblings who continue to inspire me with new ideas from their own kitchens. Whether eating in our homes or traveling together, we love to explore local epicurean delights as our top priority. We all cherish the joy of a shared meal.

Thanks to all the friends and clients who have persuaded me for years to put my recipes in a hardbound book. I have appreciated every one of your kind encouraging words.

This book could not have happened without the help of Tara Hope Thompson. She is the photographer behind these beautiful photographs and the talent behind the design layout. My dear friend Susan Jones, who always supported my vision of creating this book, introduced me to her accomplished cousin, Tara. We immediately connected and have worked side by side for over a year, developing a deep respect and friendship for one another. Her creative ability behind the camera and design concepts have pulled this ambitious venture together, just as I had imagined.

Thank - you, thank - you, thank - you!

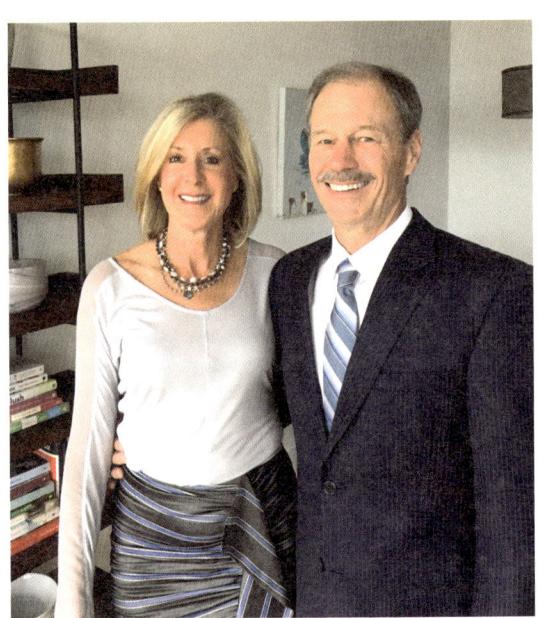

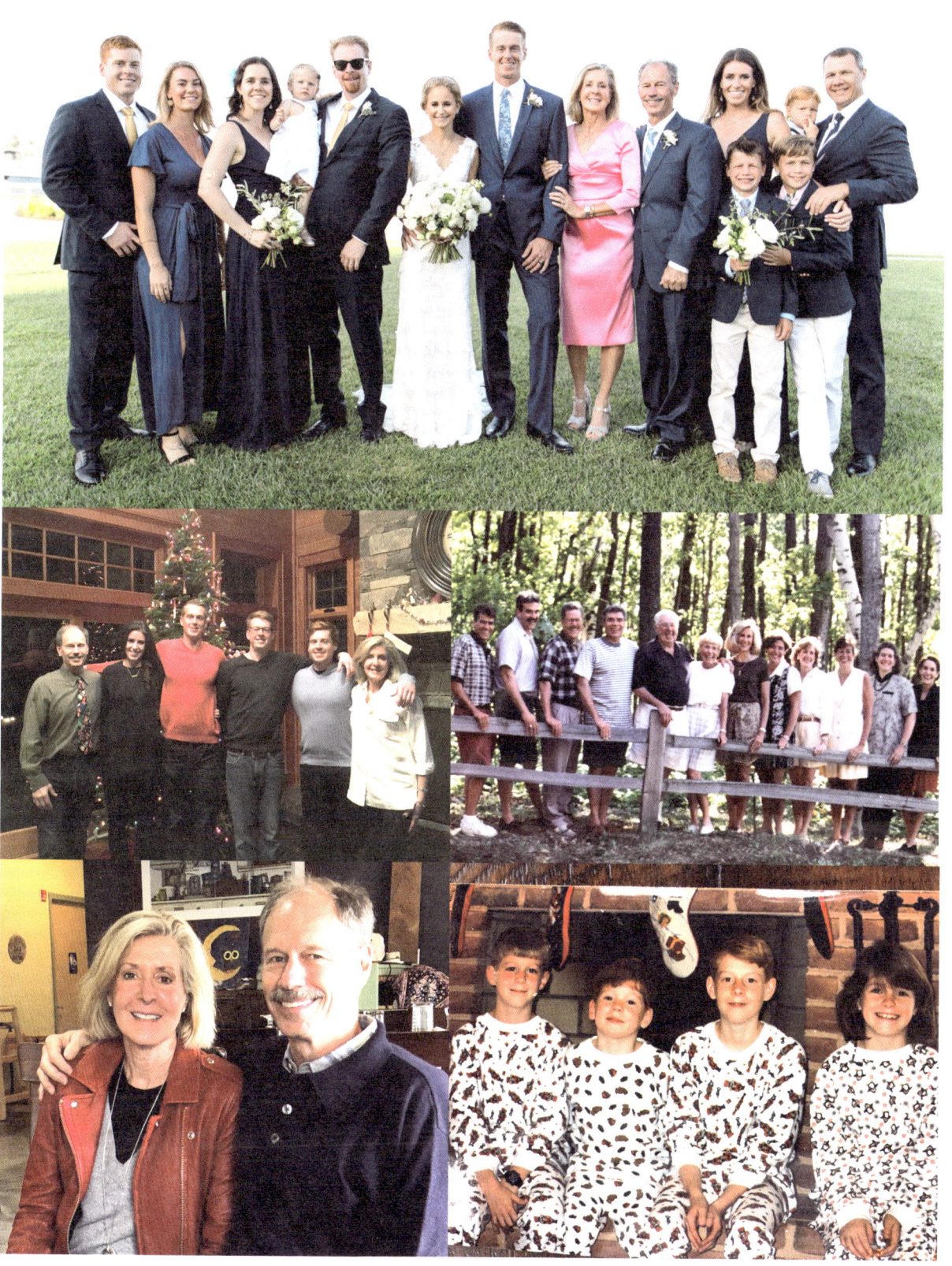

children's letters

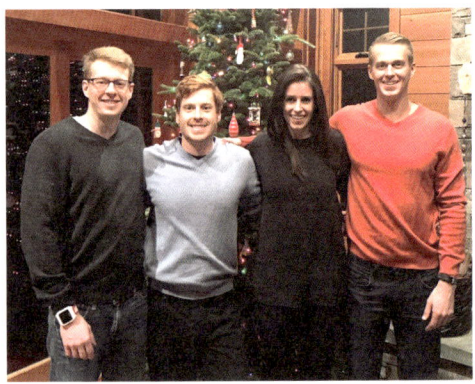

BLAKE

My mother has a rule: the first one to pull their phone out at the table does the dishes. In a world of constant pulls and pushes, people and things vying for your attention, the table is a sacred place. The table has become a place of gratitude, a place of sharing each other's lives, of being a family again. In our case, it didn't hurt that there was great food in front of us. Making great tasting food is easy - my mother will show you how in this book. Creating a tradition takes time. Over and over again as a child and now as an adult, when my mother says, "Come To The Table," we all scamper. We put our phones away, we shut off work, we share our gratitude and we eat great tasting and great for you food. When my wife and I moved into our first house, my parents gifted me a kitchen table, so we can pass on the tradition of, "Come to the Table" to the next generation. And I look forward to you joining in that tradition.

RUSSELL

As a kid, I used to get upset at my mom for not having junk food and soda in the house. All of the other kids on the block got to have them, why couldn't we? At the time, I didn't realize she was trying to raise four healthy children by feeding them good meals and real food!

Today, I am eternally grateful to have such an upbringing. As a result, I eat a healthy balanced diet. I don't crave junk food. I want to put healthy food into my body when hungry. I drink water when I am thirsty.

Organizing the chaos and hectic schedules of our family was a full-time job - four children, all a year and a half apart. Three of them were three-sport athletes and the fourth was involved in many other extracurricular activities. But somehow, we all managed to convene at dinner time for a delicious home-cooked meal and everyone stayed at the table until everyone had finished. It gave us a chance to catch up with each other on how our days went and check-in as a family. I genuinely believe her cooking was integral in creating the tight-knit family we have today! I hope to instill the same tradition of family mealtime on my children one day. Thanks, Mom!

BRITTANY

When my mom announced the title of her cookbook, "Come to the Table", memories from my childhood through my adulthood, flooded my mind: the dinner bell, the six of us seated around our wood table, saying grace and sharing stories of our day. It did not matter what activity or sporting event or how much homework you had – when that dinner bell rang, you better come running. Looking back, I am in awe of how my mother managed to put together a deliciously balanced meal while wrangling four very active kids and one extremely hard-working husband/father. Every. Single. Night. I am so grateful. It was the only time of the day that all six of us were together. And to this day, I cherish and look forward to those moments with my family.

I don't think I could ever fully appreciate what a task that was until I had my own children and family. Dinner is an ORDEAL. But my mom always looked so "at home" in the kitchen. She has passed on her love of cooking and food to each of us. I am so glad and proud that she is sharing her passion in this book. My personal favorite *(and always requested birthday dish)* is her chicken parmesan with homemade sauce – Enjoy!!

WARREN

"Warren Michael...come to the table!" I would push the time limit when it came to returning home while enjoying every minute of being outside, but I learned to respect that call when I heard my middle name. My mother always held to her firm belief that it was paramount for our development to bring our busy family together for a wholesome cooked meal every single night. She created an atmosphere of love and friendship by making family dinner a weeknight habit, hardening our families bond every time we sat together, that still holds steady to this day.

My brothers and sister are now spread out between the west and east coast, but her love and dedication still brings us back regularly to spend quality time around the kitchen table. My brother Russ and I have a tradition to weigh ourselves before and after holiday meals to see who can eat the most. And while it may not be the healthiest "game," my Mom's cooking is THAT good!

Mom - I love you, and I am so grateful that you have managed to bring the art of your craft to paper and picture. You have had an impact on all of our lives. It matriculates to our families, patients and loved ones - and to the readers that see the true importance of this book. Quality family time, healthy food, grace and gratitude - these are the qualities you brought to our lives. We are eternally thankful.

index

A

Agave
  Homemade Granola, 24
  Chocolate Macaroon Cake, 216
  Nut & Seed Brittle, 220
Allium Fmaily of Vegetables, 110
Almonds
  Kale & Shaved Brussels Sprouts Salad with Cranberry Vinaigrette, 104
  Chocolate Macaroon Cake, 216
Almond Flour
  Strawberry Tarts with Pecan Crust, 224
Almond Milk
  All Day Energy Smoothie, 29
  Blueberry Kale Smoothie, 30
  Berry Chocolate Protein Powerhouse Smoothie, 30
Appetizers, 34
  Bacon-Wrapped Dates with Goat Cheese, 36
  Guacamole, 38
  Hot & Spicy Mexican Dip, 39
  Summer Salsa, 43
  Roasted Carrot Hummus, 44
  Lime & Avocado Sea Scallops, 47
  Spicy Shrimp, 48
  Sweet Potato Chips, 51
  Baked Tequila Lime Chicken Drumsticks, 52
Artichoke Hearts
  Creamy Artichoke Soup, 62
Arugula
  White Bean & Farro Salad, 91
Asparagus
  Asparagus Frittata, 22-23
  Asparagus Soup, 76
  Pasta with Shrimp & Mixed Vegetables, 124
  Fresh Roasted Asparagus, 184

Avocado
  All Day Energy Smoothie, 29
  Guacamole, 39
  Summer Salsa, 43
  Lime & Avocado Sea Scallops, 47
  Quinoa with Kale, Mixed Vegetables & Garbanzo Beans, 92
  Southwest Quinoa Salad, 96
  Crab Cakes, 144
  Strawberry Tarts with Pecan Crust, 224
  Oven-Roasted Fresh Corn with Summer Squash and Avocado, 183
Avocado Oil
  Healthy Chicken Stir-Fry, 131
  Coconut Chicken, 139

B

Baby Back Ribs, 127
Bacon
  Asparagus Frittata, 22-23
  Bacon-Wrapped Dates With Goat Cheese, 36
  Pumpkin Soup, 75
  Summer Farmer's Market Corn Chowder, 80
  Tagliatelle with Bacon & Leeks, 119
  Twice Baked Potatoes with a Sweet Twist, 166
Baked Potatoes, 166
Baking Powder
  Corn Muffins, 198
  Blueberry Muffins, 202
  Herb Biscuits, 205
  Oatmeal Cookies, 223
  Thanksgiving Pumpkin Roll, 228
  Peanut Butter Cookies, 232
Baking Soda
  Christmas Pecan Sour Cream Coffee Cake, 20-21
  Oatmeal Muffins, 26
  Whole Wheat Banana Muffins, 197
  Herb Biscuits, 205
  Chocolate Chip Pecan Cookies with Ground Flax, 211
  Nut and Seed Brittle, 220
  Oatmeal Cookies, 223
Balsamic Vinegar
  Summer Caprese Salad, 87
  Basic Balsamic Vinaigrette, 107
  Grilled Rosemary Lamb Chops, 136
  Fresh Roasted Asparagus, 184
Banana
  Morning Power Smoothie, 29
  Blueberry Kale Smoothie, 30
  Berry Chocolate Protein Powerhouse Smoothie, 30
  Carrot Cake Banana Muffins, 194
  Whole Wheat Banana Muffins, 197
Barbecue Sauce
  Slow-Cooked Ribs, 116
  Baby Back Ribs for the Barbecue, 127
Basil
  Megan's Minestrone, 69
  Summer Caprese Salad, 87
  Chicken Cacciatore, 123
  Fresh Tomato Sauce, 140
  Fresh Pizza with the Works, 156
Basmati Rice
  Healthy Chicken Stir-Fry, 131
Bay Leaf
  Easy Chicken Noodle, 65
  French Onion Soup, 66
  New Orleans Gumbo with the Works, 72-73
  Summer Farmer's Market Corn Chowder, 80
Beans (*black*)
  Summer Salsa, 43
  Mexican Tortilla Soup, 70
  Quinoa with Black Beans & Nectarine, 88
  Southwest Quinoa Salad, 96
Beans (*cannellini*))
  Megan's Minestrone, 69

White Bean & Farro Salad, 91
White Bean & Tuna Salad, 95
Beans *(garbanzo)*
    Roasted Carrot Hummus, 44
    Quinoa with Kale, Mixed Vegetables & Garbanzo Beans, 92
Beans *(kidney)*
    Turkey Chili, 79
Beans *(refried)*
    Hot & Spicy Mexican Dip, 40
Beef
    Beer-Braised Brisket, 115
    Slow-Cooked Ribs, 116
    Taco Meat, 120
    Baby Back Ribs for the Barbecue, 127
    Meatballs, 143
Beer
    Beer-Braised Brisket, 115
Beets
    Roasted Beets, 179
Berries *(frozen)*
    Morning Power Smoothie, 29
Blueberries
    Blueberry Kale Smoothie, 30
    Berry Chocolate Protein Powerhouse Smoothie, 30
    Blueberry Scones, 201
    Blueberry Muffins, 202
    Blueberry Pie, 208
Blue Cheese
    Kale & Shaved Brussels Sprouts Salad with Cranberry Vinaigrette, 104
Bones *(beef, ham or lamb)*
    Megan's Minestrone, 69
Bran
    Oatmeal Muffins, 26
Breadcrumbs
    Meatballs, 143
    Eggplant Parmesan, 152
    Chicken Parmesan, 163
    Roasted Brussels Sprouts with Lemon, 176
Breakfast & Smoothies, 16
Brisket, 115

Broccoli
    Broccoli Soup, 58
    Turkey Chili, 79
    Broccoli & Mushroom Salad, 100
    Broccoli Cheddar Quinoa Muffins, 191
Brown Sugar
    Cristmas Pecan Sour Cream Coffee Cake, 20-21
    Oatmeal Muffins, 26
    Fajita Marinade, 108
    Beer-Braised Brisket, 115
    Fresh Tomato Sauce, 140
    Whole Wheat Banana Muffins, 197
    Chocolate Chip Pecan Cookies with Ground Flax, 211
    Key Lime Pie, 219
    Oatmeal Cookies, 223
    Pecan Pie, 227
    Peanut Butter Cookies, 232
Brussel Sprouts, 176
    Kale & Shaved Brussels Sprouts Salad with Cranberry Vinaigrette, 104
    Roasted Vegetables, 175
    Roasted Brussels Sprouts with Lemon, 176
Buttermilk
    Oatmeal Muffins, 26
    Whole Wheat Banana Muffins, 197
    Corn Muffins, 198
    Herb Biscuits, 205
Butternut Squash
    Butternut Squash Soup, 61
    Coconut Chicken, 139

C

Cabbage *(purple)*
    Potato Salad with Shrimp, 103
Canola Oil
    New Orleans Gumbo with the Works, 72-73
Caprese Salad, 87

Carrot
    Roasted Carrot Hummus, 44
    Butternut Squash Soup, 61
    Easy Chicken Noodle Soup, 62
    Megan's Minestrone, 69
    Pumpkin Soup, 75
    Turkey Chili, 79
    Turkey Orzo Soup, 83
    Pasta & Spinach Sauce, 128
    Healthy Chicken Stir-Fry, 131
    Post-Thanksgiving Shepard's Pie, 149
    Roasted Chicken with Vegetables, 151
    Carrot Yam Puree, 188
    Carrot Cake Banana Muffins, 194
Cashew Hemp Milk
    All Day Energy Smoothie, 29
Cayenne Pepper
    Hot and Spicy Mexican Dip, 40
    Roasted Carrot Hummus, 44
    New Orleans Gumbo with the Works, 72-73
    Turkey Chili, 79
    Beer-Braised Brisket, 115
    Crab Cakes, 144
    Southwest Sweet Corn Succotash, 169
    Oven-Roasted Fresh Corn with Summer Squash & Avocado, 183
Celery
    Easy Chicken Noodle Soup, 65
    Megan's Minestrone, 69
    New Orleans Gumbo with the Works, 72-73
    Pumpkin Soup, 75
    Turkey Chili, 79
    Turkey Orzo Soup, 83
    Quinoa with Kale, Mixed Vegetables & Garbanzo Beans, 92
    White Bean & Tuna Salad, 95

Celery *(continued)*
    Celery and Fennel Salad, 99
    Healthy Chicken Stir-Fry, 131
    Post-Thanksgiving Shepard's Pie, 149

Cheese *(blue)*
    Kale & Shaved Brussels Sprouts Salad with Cranberry Vinaigrette, 104

Cheese *(cheddar)*
    Twice Baked Potatoes with a Sweet Twist, 166
    Broccoli Cheddar Quinoa Muffins, 191

Cheese *(feta)*
    White Bean & Farro Salad, 91

Cheese *(goat)*
    Scalloped Potatoes with Goat Cheese and Herbs De Provence, 172

Cheese *(gruyere)*
    French Onion Soup, 66
    Mexican Tortilla Soup, 70
    Summer Farmer's Market Corn Chowder, 80

Cheese *(mascarpone)*
    Creamy Artichoke Soup, 62

Cheese *(mozzarella)*
    Eggplant Parmesan, 152
    Fresh Pizza with the Works, 156
    Chicken Parmesan, 163

Cheese *(parmesan)*
    Spicy Shrimp, 48
    Celery and Fennel Salad, 99
    Tagliatelle with Bacon & Leeks, 119
    Chicken Cacciatore, 123
    Pasta with Shrimp & Mixed Vegetables, 124
    Pasta and Spinach Sauce, 128
    Meatballs, 143
    Eggplant Parmesan, 152
    Fresh Pizza with the Works, 156
    Pasta with Kale & Tuna, 159
    Chicken Parmesan, 163
    Parmesan Potatoes, 180
    Fresh Roasted Asparagus, 184

Cheese *(sharp cheddar)*
    Hot and Spicy Mexican Dip, 40

Chia Seed
    Morning Power Smoothie, 29

Chicken
    Baked Tequila Lime Chicken Drumsticks, 52
    Easy Chicken Noodle Soup, 65
    Mexican Tortilla Soup, 70
    New Orleans Gumbo with the Works, 72-73
    Chicken Cacciatore, 123
    Healthy Chicken Stir-Fry, 131
    Coconut Chicken, 139
    Roasted Chicken with Vegetables, 151
    Chicken Picatta, 160
    Chicken Parmesan, 163

Chicken Stock
    Broccoli Soup, 58
    Butternut Squash Soup, 61
    Creamy Artichoke Soup, 62
    Easy Chicken Noodle Soup, 65
    French Onion Soup, 66
    Pumpkin Soup, 75
    Asparagus Soup, 76
    Chicken Cacciatore, 123
    Pasta with Shrimp & Mixed Vegetables, 124
    Healthy Chicken Stir-Fry, 131
    Spring Green Risotto, 135
    Shrimp & Grits with Chorizo & Kale, 147
    Post-Thanksgiving Shepard's Pie, 149
    Roasted Chicken with Vegetables, 151
    Chicken Picatta, 160
    Scalloped Potatoes with Goat Cheese and Herbs De Provence, 172
    Carrot Yam Puree, 188

Chili, 79

Chili Paste
    Spicy Shrimp, 48

Chili Powder
    Hot and Spicy Mexican Dip, 40
    Baked Tequila Lime Chicken Drumsticks, 52
    Mexican Tortilla Soup, 70
    Turkey Chili, 79
    Fajita Marinade, 108
    Slow-Cooked Ribs, 116
    Taco Meat, 120

Chips, 51

Chives
    Twice Baked Potatoes with a Sweet Twist, 166

Chocolate
    Chocolate Glaze for Chocolate Espresso Cake, 212
    Flourless Chocolate Espresso Cake, 215
    Chocolate Macaroon Cake, 216
    Chocolate Macaroon Cake, 216
    Palates Famous Chocolate-Covered Grahams, 235

Chocolate Chips
    Chocolate Chip Pecan Cookies with Ground Flax, 211
    Oatmeal Cookies, 223

Chorizo Sausage
    Shrimp & Grits with Chorizo & Kale, 147

Cilantro
    Guacamole, 39
    Summer Salsa, 43
    Lime & Avocado Sea Scallops, 47
    Baked Tequila Lime Chicken Drumsticks, 52
    Mexican Tortilla Soup, 70
    Quinoa with Black Beans & Nectarine, 88
    Southwest Quinoa Salad, 96
    Southwest Sweet Corn Succotash, 169
    Oven-Roasted Fresh Corn with Summer Squash and Avocado, 183

Cinnamon
    Christmas Pecan Sour Cream Coffee Cake, 20-21

Homemade Granola, 24
Carrot Cake Banana Muffins, 194
Blueberry Scones, 201
Blueberry Muffins, 202
Blueberry Pie, 208
Nut and Seed Brittle, 220
Oatmeal Cookies, 223
Thanksgiving Pumpkin Roll, 228

Cloves
Lime & Avocado Sea Scallops, 47
Butternut Squash Soup, 61
Fajita Marinade, 108

Cocoa Powder
Berry Chocolate Protein Powerhouse Smoothie, 30
Chocolate Macaroon Cake, 216

Coconut
Sesame-Nut Bars, 19
Homemade Granola, 24
Chocolate Macaroon Cake, 216

Coconut Chicken, 139

Coconut Oil
Oatmeal Muffins, 26
Carrot Cake Banana Muffins, 194
Strawberry Tarts with Pecan Crust, 224

Coconut Sugar
Homemade Granola, 24
Oatmeal Muffins, 26
Hot and Spicy Mexican Dip, 40
Roasted Carrot Hummus, 44
Carrot Cake Banana Muffins, 194

Coconut Water
Morning Power Smoothie, 29
Berry Chocolate Protein Powerhouse Smoothie, 30

Coffee Cake, 20

Condensed Milk
Summer Farmer's Market Corn Chowder, 80
Coconut Chicken, 139
Chocolate Macaroon Cake, 216
Key Lime Pie, 219

Confectioners' Sugar
Key Lime Pie, 219
Thanksgiving Pumpkin Roll, 228
Christmas Butterballs, 231

Corn
Summer Salsa, 43
Easy Chicken Noodle Soup, 65
Megan's Minestrone, 69
Mexican Tortilla Soup, 70
Turkey Chili, 79
Summer Farmer's Market Corn Chowder, 80
Turkey Orzo Soup, 83
Southwest Sweet Corn Succotash, 169
Oven-Roasted Fresh Corn with Summer Squash and Avocado, 183

Cornmeal
Fresh Pizza Dough, 155
Fresh Pizza with the Works, 156
Corn Muffins, 198

Corn Starch
Healthy Chicken Stir-Fry, 131
Post-Thanksgiving Shepard's Pie, 149
Blueberry Pie, 208

Crab Cakes, 144

Cranberries (dried)
Kale & Shaved Brussels Sprouts Salad with Cranberry Vinaigrette, 104

Cream (heavy)
Tagliatelle with Bacon & Leeks, 119
Blueberry Scones, 201
Pasta with Shrimp & Mixed Vegetables, 124
Pasta and Spinach Sauce, 128
Shrimp & Grits with Chorizo & Kale, 147

Creamed Cheese
Thanksgiving Pumpkin Roll, 228

Cucumber (English)
Quinoa with Kale, Mixed Vegetables & Garbanzo Beans, 92

Cumin
Guacamole, 39
Turkey Chili, 79
Beer-Braised Brisket, 115
Slow-Cooked Ribs, 116
Taco Meat, 120

Fajita Marinade, 108
Beer-Braised Brisket, 115
Southwest Sweet Corn Succotash, 169

D

Dates (Medjool)
All Day Energy Smoothie, 29
Bacon-Wrapped Dates With Goat Cheese, 36

Desserts
Blueberry Pie, 208
Chocolate Chip Pecan Cookies with Ground Flax, 211
Chocolate Glaze for Chocolate Espresso Cake, 212
Flourless Chocolate Espresso Cake, 215
Chocolate Macaroon Cake, 216
Key Lime Pie, 219
Nut and Seed Brittle, 220
Oatmeal Cookies, 223
Strawberry Tarts with Pecan Crust, 224
Pecan Pie, 227
Thanksgiving Pumpkin Roll, 228
Christmas Butterballs, 231
Peanut Butter Cookies, 232
Palates Famous Chocolate-Covered Grahams, 235

Dijon Mustard
Lemon Vinaigrette Dressing, 107
Basic Balsamic Vinaigrette, 107
Beer-Braised Brisket, 115

Dill
Turkey Chili, 79
White Bean & Farro Salad, 91

Dressings, 84

Dried Fruit
Homemade Granola, 24
Oatmeal Muffins, 26

Dry Mustard
Crab Cakes, 144

Dry Yeast
Fresh Pizza Dough, 155

E

Eggplant Parmesan, 152

Eggs
- Asparagus Frittata, 23
- Meatballs, 143
- Crab Cakes, 144
- Eggplant Parmesan, 152
- Broccoli Cheddar Quinoa Muffins, 191
- Carrot Cake Banana Muffins, 194
- Whole Wheat Banana Muffins, 197
- Corn Muffins, 198
- Blueberry Muffins, 202
- Blueberry Pie, 208
- Flourless Chocolate Espresso Cake, 215
- Chocolate Macaroon Cake, 216
- Key Lime Pie, 219
- Oatmeal Cookies, 223
- Pecan Pie, 227
- Thanksgiving Pumpkin Roll, 228
- Peanut Butter Cookies, 232

Espresso Powder
- Chocolate Glaze for Chocolate Espresso Cake, 212
- Flourless Chocolate Espresso Cake, 215

F

Farro
- White Bean & Farro Salad, 91

Fennel Bulb
- Celery and Fennel Salad, 99
- Spring Green Risotto, 135

Feta Cheese
- White Bean & Farro Salad, 91

File Powder
- New Orleans Gumbo with the Works, 72-73

Flax Seed
- Morning Power Smoothie, 29
- Blueberry Kale Smoothie, 30
- Oatmeal Cookies, 223

Flour
- New Orleans Gumbo with the Works, 72-73
- Carrot Cake Banana Muffins, 194
- Whole Wheat Banana Muffins, 197
- Corn Muffins, 198
- Blueberry Scones, 201
- Blueberry Muffins, 202
- Herb Biscuits, 205
- Blueberry Pie, 208
- Chocolate Chip Pecan Cookies with Ground Flax, 211
- Thanksgiving Pumpkin Roll, 228
- Christmas Butterballs, 231

French Onion Soup, 66

Frittata, 23

G

Garlic
- Guacamole, 39
- Roasted Carrot Hummus, 44
- Creamy Artichoke Soup, 62
- French Onion Soup, 66
- Mexican Tortilla Soup, 70
- New Orleans Gumbo with the Works, 72-73
- Asparagus Soup, 76
- Summer Farmer's Market Corn Chowder, 80
- White Bean & Tuna Salad, 95
- Lemon Vinaigrette Dressing, 107
- Beer-Braised Brisket, 115
- Kale & Shaved Brussels Sprouts Salad with Cranberry Vinaigrette, 104
- Chicken Cacciatore, 123
- Pasta and Spinach Sauce, 128
- Grilled Rosemary Lamb Chops, 136
- Coconut Chicken, 139
- Fresh Tomato Sauce, 140
- Roasted Chicken with Vegetables, 151
- Pasta with Kale & Tuna, 159
- Chicken Picatta, 160
- Scalloped Potatoes with Goat Cheese and Herbs De Provence, 172
- Roasted Brussels Sprouts with Lemon, 176
- Carrot Yam Puree, 188

Ginger
- Strawberry Tarts with Pecan Crust, 224
- Thanksgiving Pumpkin Roll, 228

Goat Cheese
- Bacon-Wrapped Dates With Goat Cheese, 36
- Scalloped Potatoes with Goat Cheese and Herbs De Provence, 172
- Broccoli Cheddar Quinoa Muffins, 191

Graham Crackers
- Key Lime Pie, 219
- Palates Famous Chocolate Covered Grahams, 235

Granola, 24

Grated Parmesan Cheese
- Meatballs, 143

Grits
- Shrimp & Grits with Chorizo & Kale, 147

Gumbo, 72

Gruyere Cheese
- Asparagus Frittata, 22-23
- Christmas Butterballs, 231

Guacamole, 39

H

Half & Half
- Pumpkin Soup, 75

Heavy Cream
- Broccoli Soup, 58
- Pasta with Shrimp & Mixed Vegetables, 124
- Pasta and Spinach Sauce, 128
- Shrimp & Grits with Chorizo & Kale, 147
- Tagliatelle with Bacon & Leeks, 119
- Scalloped Potatoes with Goat Cheese and Herbs De Provence, 172
- Blueberry Scones, 201
- Chocolate Glaze for Chocolate Espresso Cake, 212

Key Lime Pie, 219
Hemp Seeds
    Berry Chocolate Protein Powerhouse Smoothie, 30
Herbs and Spices, 32
Herbs de Provence
    Scalloped Potatoes with Goat Cheese and Herbs De Provence, 172
Honey
    Sesame-Nut Bars, 19
    Baked Tequila Lime Chicken Drumsticks, 52
    Kale & Shaved Brussels Sprouts Salad with Cranberry Vinaigrette, 104
    Basic Balsamic Vinaigrette, 107
    Fresh Pizza Dough, 155
    Christmas Butterballs, 231
Hot & Spicy Mexican Dip, 40
Hummus, 44

K

Kale
    Asparagus Frittata, 22-23
    Blueberry Kale Smoothie, 30
    Berry Chocolate Protein Powerhouse Smoothie, 30
    Broccoli Soup, 58
    Quinoa with Kale, Mixed Vegetables & Garbanzo Beans, 92
    Kale & Shaved Brussels Sprouts Salad with Cranberry Vina grette, 104
    Pasta with Kale & Tuna, 159

L

Lamb
    Roast Leg of Lamb with Crispy Tomatoes, 132
    Grilled Rosemary Lamb Chops, 136
Leek
    Creamy Artichoke Soup, 62
    French Onion Soup, 66
    Asparagus Soup, 76
    Tagliatelle with Bacon & Leeks, 119

Leek (continued)
    Spring Green Risotto, 135
    Charred Onions and Sauteed Greens, 187
Lemon
    Roasted Carrot Hummus, 44
    Spicy Shrimp, 48
    Quinoa with Kale, Mixed Vegetables & Garbanzo Beans, 92
    White Bean & Tuna Salad, 95
    Lemon Vinaigrette Dressing, 107
    Celery and Fennel Salad, 99
    Kale & Shaved Brussels Sprouts Salad with Cranberry Vinaigrette, 104
    Roast Leg of Lamb with Crispy Tomatoes, 132
    Spring Green Risotto, 135
    Grilled Rosemary Lamb Chops, 136
    Crab Cakes, 144
    Pasta with Kale & Tuna, 159
    Chicken Picatta, 160
    Roasted Brussels Sprouts with Lemon, 176
    Charred Onions and Sauteed Greens, 187
    Blueberry Pie, 208
    Strawberry Tarts with Pecan Crust, 224
    Thanksgiving Pumpkin Roll, 228
Lettuce (Boston)
    White Bean & Tuna Salad, 95
Lime
    Guacamole, 39
    Baked Tequila Lime Chicken Drumsticks, 52
    Quinoa with Black Beans & Nectarine, 88
    Southwest Quinoa Salad, 96
    Fajita Marinade, 108
    Oven-Roasted Fresh Corn with Summer Squash and Avocado, 183
    Key Lime Pie, 219

M

Main Courses
    Beer-Braised Brisket, 115
    Slow-Cooked Ribs, 116
    Tagliatelle with Bacon & Leeks, 119
    Taco Meat, 120
    Chicken Cacciatore, 123
    Pasta with Shrimp & Mixed Vegetables, 124
    Baby Back Ribs for the BBQ, 127
    Pasta and Spinach Sauce, 128
    Healthy Chicken Stir-Fry, 131
    Roast Leg of Lamb with Crispy Tomatoes, 132
    Spring Green Risotto, 135
    Grilled Rosemary Lamb Chops, 136
    Coconut Chicken, 139
    Fresh Tomato Sauce, 140
    Meatballs, 143
    Crab Cakes, 144
    Shrimp & Grits with Chorizo & Kale, 147
    Post-Thanksgiving Shepard's Pie, 149
    Roasted Chicken with Vegetables, 151
    Eggplant Parmesan, 152
    Fresh Pizza Dough, 155
    Fresh Pizza with the Works, 156
    Pasta with Kale & Tuna, 159
    Chicken Picatta, 160
    Chicken Parmesan, 163
Maple Syrup
    Homemade Granola, 24
    Chocolate Macaroon Cake, 216
    Strawberry Tarts with Pecan Crust, 224
    Pecan Pie, 227
Marinade
    Fajita Marinade, 108
Mashed Potatoes, 170
    Post-Thanksgiving Shepard's Pie, 149
Matcha Green Tea Powder
    All Day Energy Smoothie, 29

M (continued)

Mayonnaise
    Crab Cakes, 144
Meatballs, 143
Mexican Dip, 40
Mexican Tortilla Soup, 70
Milk
    Summer Farmer's Market Corn Chowder, 80
    Corn Muffins, 198
    Blueberry Muffins, 202
Minestrone Soup, 69
Mozzarella Cheese
    Summer Caprese Salad, 87
    Fresh Pizza with the Works, 156
    Chicken Parmesan, 163
Muffins & Biscuits
    Carrot Cake Banana Muffins, 194
    Whole Wheat Banana Muffins, 197
    Corn Muffins, 198
    Blueberry Scones, 201
    Blueberry Muffins, 202
    Herb Biscuits, 205
Mushrooms
    Asparagus Frittata, 22
    Broccoli Soup, 58
    Asparagus Soup, 76
    Broccoli & Mushroom Salad, 100
    Chicken Cacciatore, 123
    Healthy Chicken Stir-Fry, 131
    Fresh Pizza with the Works, 156
    Chicken Picatta, 160
Mustard (dry)
    Baby Back Ribs for the Barbecue, 127
    Crab Cakes, 144

N

Nectarine
    Quinoa with Black Beans & Nectarine, 88
New Orleans Gumbo, 72
Nutmeg
    Pumpkin Soup, 75
    Thanksgiving Pumpkin Roll, 228

Nuts
    Homemade Granola, 24
    Sesame-Nut Bars, 19
    Nut and Seed Brittle, 220
Nuts (pecans)
    Chocolate Chip Pecan Cookies with Ground Flax, 211
    Strawberry Tarts with Pecan Crust, 224
    Pecan Pie, 227
    Christmas Butterballs, 231
Nuts (pine)
    Celery and Fennel Salad, 99
Nuts (walnut)
    Carrot Cake Banana Muffins, 194
    Whole Wheat Banana Muffins, 197
    Thanksgiving Pumpkin Roll, 228

O

Oats
    Homemade Granola, 24
    Oatmeal Muffins, 26
    Oatmeal Cookies, 223
Oat Bran
    Oatmeal Muffins, 26
Okra
    New Orleans Gumbo with the Works, 72-73
Old Bay
    Crab Cakes, 144
Onion
    Hot & Spicy Mexican Dip, 40
    Summer Salsa, 43
    Broccoli Soup, 58
    Butternut Squash Soup, 61
    Easy Chicken Noodle Soup, 65
    French Onion Soup, 66
    Megan's Minestrone, 69
    Mexican Tortilla Soup, 70
    New Orleans Gumbo with the Works, 72-73
    Pumpkin Soup, 75
    Asparagus Soup, 76
    Turkey Chili, 79
    Summer Farmer's Market Corn Chowder, 80

Onion (continued)
    Turkey Orzo Soup, 83
    Broccoli & Mushroom Salad, 100
        Potato Salad with Shrimp, 103
    Beer-Braised Brisket, 115
    Chicken Cacciatore, 123
    Pasta and Spinach Sauce, 128
    Healthy Chicken Stir-Fry, 131
    Fresh Tomato Sauce, 140
    Post-Thanksgiving Shepard's Pie, 149
    Roasted Chicken with Vegetables, 151
    Fresh Pizza with the Works, 156
    Southwest Sweet Corn Succotash, 169
    Roasted Vegetables, 175
    Oven-Roasted Fresh Corn with Summer Squash and Avocado, 183
    Charred Onions and Sauteed Greens, 187
    Carrot Yam Puree, 188
    Broccoli Cheddar Quinoa Muffins, 191
Oregano
    Spicy Shrimp, 48
    Baked Tequila Lime Chicken Drumsticks, 52
    Megan's Minestrone, 69
    New Orleans Gumbo with the Works, 72-73
    Turkey Chili, 79
    Chicken Cacciatore, 123
    Pasta and Spinach Sauce, 128
    Fresh Tomato Sauce, 140
    Meatballs, 143
    Fresh Pizza with the Works, 156
Orzo
    Turkey Orzo Soup, 83
Oysters
    New Orleans Gumbo with the Works, 72-73

P

Panko
    Crab Cakes, 144

Paprika
- Beer-Braised Brisket, 115
- Baby Back Ribs for the Barbecue, 127
- Broccoli Cheddar Quinoa Muffins, 191

Parmesan
- Spicy Shrimp, 48
- Celery and Fennel Salad, 99
- Tagliatelle with Bacon & Leeks, 119
- Chicken Cacciatore, 123
- Pasta with Shrimp & Mixed Vegetables, 124
- Pasta and Spinach Sauce, 128
- Eggplant Parmesan, 152
- Fresh Pizza with the Works, 156
- Pasta with Kale & Tuna, 159
- Chicken Parmesan, 163
- Fresh Roasted Asparagus, 184

Parmesan Potatoes, 180

Parsley
- Crab Cakes, 144
- Shrimp & Grits with Chorizo & Kale, 147
- Pasta with Kale & Tuna, 159
- Chicken Picatta, 160

Pasta
- Easy Chicken Noodle, 65
- Megan's Minestrone, 69
- Tagliatelle with Bacon & Leeks, 119
- Pasta with Shrimp & Mixed Vegetables, 124
- Pasta & Spinach Sauce, 128
- Pasta with Kale & Tuna, 159

Peanut Butter
- Peanut Butter Cookies, 232

Peas
- Pasta with Shrimp & Mixed Vegetables, 124
- Spring Green Risotto, 135

Peanuts/Peanut Butter
- Sesame-Nut Bars, 19
- Nut & Seed Brittle, 220
- Peanut Butter Cookies, 232

Pecans
- Pecan Pie, 227
- Chocolate Chip Pecan Cookies with Ground Flax, 211
- Strawberry Tarts with Pecan Crust, 224
- Christmas Butterballs, 231

Pepper (*green bell*)
- New Orleans Gumbo with the Works, 72-73
- Fresh Pizza with the Works, 156

Pepper (*jalapeno*)
- Hot & Spicy Mexican Dip, 40
- Baked Tequila Lime Chicken Drumsticks, 52
- Mexican Tortilla Soup, 70
- Southwest Quinoa Salad, 96
- Southwest Sweet Corn Succotash, 169

Pepper (*poblano*)
- Hot & Spicy Mexican Dip, 40
- Summer Salsa, 43
- Summer Farmer's Market Corn Chowder, 80

Pepper (*red bell*)
- Quinoa with Black Beans & Nectarine, 88
- Chicken Cacciatore, 123
- Pasta with Shrimp & Mixed Vegetables, 124
- Healthy Chicken Stir-Fry, 131
- Shrimp & Grits with Chorizo & Kale, 147
- Southwest Sweet Corn Succotash, 169

Pepper (*serrano*)
- Guacamole, 39
- Hot and Spicy Mexican Dip, 40
- Summer Salsa, 43

Pepper (*yellow bell*)
- Healthy Chicken Stir-Fry, 131

Pepperoni
- Fresh Pizza with the Works, 156

Pizza
- Fresh Pizza with the Works, 156

Pizza Dough, 155

Pork (*ground*)
- Meatballs, 143

Potato (*yellow skin*)
- Parmesan Potatoes, 180

Potato (*russet*)
- Megan's Minestrone, 69
- Twice Baked Potatoes with a Sweet Twist, 166
- Scalloped Potatoes with Goat Cheese & Herbs De Provence, 172

Potato (*sweet*)
- Sweet Potato Chips, 51
- Roasted Vegetables, 175
- Carrot Yam Puree, 188

Potato (*Yukon gold*)
- Sour Cream Mashed Potatoes, 170

Protein Powder
- Blueberry Kale Smoothie, 30

Protein Powder (*pea*)
- Morning Power Smoothie, 29
- Berry Chocolate Protein Powerhouse Smoothie, 30

Potato
- Creamy Artichoke Soup, 62
- Summer Farmer's Market Corn Chowder, 80
- Potato Salad with Shrimp, 103
- Roast Leg of Lamb with Crispy Tomatoes, 132
- Roasted Chicken with Vegetables, 151

Pumpkin Puree
- Pumpkin Soup, 75
- Thanksgiving Pumpkin Roll, 228

Pumpkin Seeds
- Nut and Seed Brittle, 220

Pumpkin Soup, 75

Q

Quinoa
- Quinoa with Black Beans & Nectarine, 88
- Quinoa with Kale, Mixed Vegetables & Garbanzo Beans, 92
- Southwest Quinoa Salad, 96
- Broccoli Cheddar Quinoa Muffins, 191

R

Radishes
    Quinoa with Black Beans & Nectarine, 88

Raisins
    Carrot Cake Banana Muffins, 194

Red Pepper
    Lime & Avocado Sea Scallops, 47
    Megan's Minestrone, 69
    Fresh Tomato Sauce, 140

Red Wine
    Chicken Cacciatore, 123
    Healthy Chicken Stir-Fry, 131
    Fresh Tomato Sauce, 140

Ribs, 116, 127

Rice (*basmati*)
    Healthy Chicken Stir-Fry, 131
    Spring Green Risotto, 135

Risotto, 135

Roasted Carrot Hummus, 44

Roasted Chicken with Vegetables, 151

Roasted Vegetables, 175

Rolled Oats
    Oatmeal Cookies, 223

Rosemary
    Roast Leg of Lamb with Crispy Tomatoes, 132
    Grilled Rosemary Lamb Chops, 136
    Roasted Chicken with Vegetables, 151

S

Sage
    Butternut Squash Soup, 61

Salads, 84
    Summer Caprese Salad, 87
    White Bean & Tuna Salad, 95
    White Bean & Farro Salad, 91
    Quinoa with Kale, Mixed Vegetables & Garbanzo Beans, 92
    Quinoa with Black Beans & Nectarine, 88
    Southwest Quinoa Salad, 96
    Celery and Fennel Salad, 99
    Broccoli & Mushroom Salad, 100

Salads (*continued*)
    Kale & Shaved Brussels Sprouts Salad with Cranberry Vinaigrette, 104
    Potato Salad with Shrimp, 103

Salt
    A Touch of Salt, 54

Sausage (*andouille*)
    New Orleans Gumbo with the Works, 72-73

Sausage (*chorizo*)
    Shrimp & Grits with Chorizo & Kale, 147

Sausage (*turkey*)
    Turkey Chili, 79

Scalloped Potatoes, 173

Scallops
    Lime & Avocado Sea Scallops, 47

Seeds (*sesame, pumpkin, flax*)
    Homemade Granola, 24
    Nut and Seed Brittle, 220

Sesame-Nut Bars, 19

Shallot
    Guacamole, 39
    White Bean & Farro Salad, 91
    Kale & Shaved Brussels Sprouts Salad with Cranberry Vinaigrette, 104
    Pasta with Shrimp & Mixed Vegetables, 124
    Shrimp & Grits with Chorizo & Kale, 147
    Scalloped Potatoes with Goat Cheese and Herbs De Provence, 172

Shepherd's Pie, 149

Shrimp
    Spicy Shrimp, 48
    New Orleans Gumbo with the Works, 72-73
    Potato Salad with Shrimp, 103
    Pasta with Shrimp & Mixed Vegetables, 124
    Shrimp & Grits with Chorizo & Kale, 147

Sides, 164
    Twice Baked Potatoes with a Sweet Twist, 166
    Southwest Sweet Corn Succotash, 169
    Sour Cream Mashed Potatoes, 170
    Scalloped Potatoes with Goat Cheese and Herbs De Provence, 172
    Roasted Vegetables, 175
    Roasted Brussels Sprouts with Lemon, 176
    Roasted Beets, 179
    Parmesan Potatoes, 180
    Oven-Roasted Fresh Corn with Summer Squash and Avocado, 183
    Fresh Roasted Asparagus, 184
    Charred Onions and Sauteed Greens, 187
    Carrot Yam Puree, 188
    Broccoli Cheddar Quinoa Muffins, 191

Slow Cooked Ribs, 116

Smoothies, 16
    All Day Energy, 29
    Morning Power, 29
    Blueberry Kale, 30
    Berry Chocolate Protein Powerhouse, 30

Soups
    Broccoli Soup, 58
    Butternut Squash Soup, 61
    Creamy Artichoke Soup, 62
    Easy Chicken Noodle, 65
    French Onion Soup, 66
    Megan's Minestrone, 69
    Mexican Tortilla Soup, 70
    New Orleans Gumbo with the Works, 72-73
    Pumpkin Soup, 75
    Asparagus Soup, 76
    Turkey Chili, 79
    Summer Market Chowder, 80
    Turkey Orzo Soup, 83

Sour Cream
　Hot & Spicy Mexican Dip, 40
　Twice Baked Potatoes with a
　　Sweet Twist, 166
　Sour Cream Mashed Potatoes, 170
Sour Cream Coffee Cake, 20
Soy Sauce
　Lime & Avocado Sea Scallops, 47
　Fajita Marinade, 108
　Healthy Chicken Stir-Fry, 131
Spicy Shrimp, 48
Spinach
　Morning Power Smoothie, 29
　Broccoli Soup, 58
　Easy Chicken Noodle Soup, 65
　Megan's Minestrone, 69
　Turkey Chili, 79
　Turkey Orzo Soup, 83
　Pasta and Spinach Sauce, 128
Squash
　Oven-Roasted Fresh Corn with
　　Summer Squash and Avocado, 183
　Butternut Squash Soup, 61
Strawberries
　Strawberry Tarts with Pecan
　　Crust, 224
Stir-Fry, 131
Succotash, 169
Sugar
　Fajita Marinade, 108
　Beer-Braised Brisket, 115
　Fresh Tomato Sauce, 140
　Whole Wheat Banana Muffins, 197
　Corn Muffins, 198
　Blueberry Scones, 201
　Blueberry Muffins, 202
　Blueberry Pie, 208
　Chocolate Chip Pecan Cookies
　　with Ground Flax, 211
　Chocolate Glaze for Chocolate
　　Espresso Cake, 212
　Flourless Chocolate Espresso
　　Cake, 215
　Chocolate Macaroon Cake, 216
　Key Lime Pie, 219
　Nut and Seed Brittle, 220

　Oatmeal Cookies, 223
　Thanksgiving Pumpkin Roll, 228
　Peanut Butter Cookies, 232
　Homemade Granola, 24
　Hot and Spicy Mexican Dip, 40
　Roasted Carrot Hummus, 44
　Carrot Cake Banana Muffins, 194
　Pecan Pie, 227
Summer Salsa, 43
Sweetened Condensed Milk
　Summer Farmer's Market Corn
　　Chowder, 80
　Coconut Chicken, 139
　Chocolate Macaroon Cake, 216
　Key Lime Pie, 219
Sweet Potato
　Sweet Potato Chips, 51
　Roasted Vegetables, 175
　Carrot Yam Puree, 188

T

Tapioca
　Blueberry Pie, 208
Taco Meat, 120
Tequila
　Baked Tequila Lime Chicken
　　Drumsticks, 52
Thyme
　French Onion Soup, 66
　Megan's Minestrone, 69
　New Orleans Gumbo with the
　　Works, 72-73
　Pumpkin Soup, 75
　Summer Farmer's Market Corn
　　Chowder, 80
　Turkey Orzo Soup, 83
　Slow-Cooked Ribs, 116
　Tagliatelle with Bacon & Leeks, 119
　Post-Thanksgiving Shepard's Pie, 149
Tomato
　Hot & Spicy Mexican Dip, 40
　Summer Salsa, 43
　Summer Caprese Salad, 87
　Quinoa with Kale, Mixed Vege-
　　tables & Garbanzo Beans, 92
　Southwest Quinoa Salad, 96
　Fresh Pizza with the Works, 156
　Pasta with Kale & Tuna, 159

Tomato (canned)
　Mexican Tortilla Soup, 70
　New Orleans Gumbo with the
　　Works, 72-73
　Turkey Chili, 79
　Chicken Cacciatore, 123
　Pasta and Spinach Sauce, 128
　Fresh Tomato Sauce, 140
Tomato (paste)
　Megan's Minestrone, 69
　Taco Meat, 120
　Chicken Cacciatore, 123
Tomato (sauce)
　Eggplant Parmesan, 152
　Fresh Pizza with the Works, 156
　Chicken Parmesan, 163
Tomato Sauce, 140
Tortillas (corn)
　Mexican Tortilla Soup, 70
Tumeric
　Turkey Chili, 79
　Slow-Cooked Ribs, 116
　Southwest Sweet Corn Succotash, 169
Tuna
　White Bean & Tuna Salad, 95
　Pasta with Kale & Tuna, 159
Turkey
　Turkey Chili, 79
　Turkey Orzo Soup, 83
　Post-Thanksgiving Shepard's
　　Pie, 149

V

Vanilla
　Blueberry Scones, 201
　Chocolate Chip Pecan Cookies
　　with Ground Flax, 211
　Chocolate Glaze for Chocolate
　　Espresso Cake, 212
　Flourless Chocolate Espresso
　　Cake, 215
　Chocolate Macaroon Cake, 216
　Key Lime Pie, 219
　Oatmeal Cookies, 223
　Strawberry Tarts with Pecan
　　Crust, 224

Vanilla *(continued)*
    Pecan Pie, 227
    Thanksgiving Pumpkin Roll, 228
    Christmas Butterballs, 231
Vegetable Stock
    Summer Farmer's Market Corn Chowder, 80
Vinegar *(apple cider)*
    Broccoli & Mushroom Salad, 100
Vinegar *(balsamic)*
    Summer Caprese Salad, 87
    Basic Balsamic Vinaigrette, 107
    Grilled Rosemary Lamb Chops, 136
    Fresh Roasted Asparagus, 184
Vinegar *(red wine/champagne)*
    Quinoa with Black Beans & Nectarine, 88
    White Bean & Tuna Salad, 95
    Lemon Vinaigrette Dressing, 107
    Potato Salad with Shrimp, 103
Vinegar *(sherry)*
    White Bean & Farro Salad, 91
Vinaigrettes
    Basic Balsamic Vinaigrette, 107
    Basil Lemon Vinaigrette, 107

W

Walnuts
    Carrot Cake Banana Muffins, 194
    Whole Wheat Banana Muffins, 197
    Oatmeal Cookies, 223
    Thanksgiving Pumpkin Roll, 228
White Pepper
    Crab Cakes, 144
White Wine
    French Onion Soup, 66
    Chicken Cacciatore, 123
    Healthy Chicken Stir-Fry, 131
    Spring Green Risotto, 135
    Chicken Picatta, 160
    Scalloped Potatoes with Goat Cheese and Herbs De Provence, 172

Whole Wheat Flour
    Oatmeal Muffins, 26
    Carrot Cake Banana Muffins, 194
    Whole Wheat Banana Muffins, 197
    Chocolate Chip Pecan Cookies with Ground Flax, 211
    Peanut Butter Cookies, 232